MANAGEMENT OF INFLAMMATORY BOWEL DISEASE

Management of Inflammatory Bowel Disease

Burton I. Korelitz, M.D.
Chief, Section of Gastroenterology
Lenox Hill Hospital
Cornell University Medical College
New York, New York

Norman Sohn, M.D.
Associate Physician
Lenox Hill Hospital
Department of Surgery
Clinical Assistant Professor of Surgery
Cornell University Medical College
New York, New York

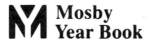

Mosby Year Book

St. Louis   Baltimore   Boston   Chicago   London   Philadelphia   Sydney   Toronto

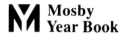
Mosby
Year Book
Dedicated to Publishing Excellence

Sponsoring Editor: Stephanie Manning
Editorial Assistant: Colleen Boyd
Assistant Managing Editor, Text and Reference: George Mary Gardner
Production Supervisor: Carol A. Reynolds

1   2   3   4   5   6   7   8   9   0   CL   MB   96   95   94   93   92

Library of Congress Cataloging-in-Publication Data
Korelitz, Burton I., 1926-
    Management of inflammatory bowel disease / Burton I. Korelitz,
Norman Sohn.
        p.   cm.
    Includes bibliographical references and index.
    ISBN 0-8016-6493-4
    1. Inflammatory bowel diseases.   I. Sohn, Norman.   II. Title.
    [DNLM: 1. Inflammatory Bowel Diseases—drug therapy.
2. Inflammatory Bowel Diseases—surgery.   WI 522 K84m]
RC862. I53K67   1991   91-32516
616.3'44—dc20   CIP
DNLM/DLC
for Library of Congress

CONTRIBUTORS

Daniel Adler, M.D.
Adjunct Physician
Section of Gastroenterology
Lenox Hill Hospital
New York, New York

Theodore Bayless, M.D.
Professor of Medicine
The Johns Hopkins University
  Clinical Director
The Meyerhoff Digestive
  Diseases – Inflammatory Bowel
  Disease Center
The Johns Hopkins Hospital
Baltimore, Maryland

Zane Cohen, M.D.
Professor, University of Toronto
Head, Department of Colorectal
  Surgery
Toronto General Hospital
Toronto, Canada

Steven M. Faber, M.D.
Past Fellow in Gastroenterology
Lenox Hill Hospital
New York, New York

Joseph B. Felder, M.D.
Fellow in Gastroenterology
Lenox Hill Hospital
New York, New York

Michael S. Frank, M.D.
Adjunct Physician
Section of Gastroenterology
Lenox Hill Hospital
New York, New York

Myron D. Goldberg, M.D.
Associate Physician
Section of Gastroenterology
Assistant Chief
Gastrointestinal Endoscopy Unit
Lenox Hill Hospital
New York, New York

Bette Harig, M.D.
Attending Physician
Department of Radiology
Lenox Hill Hospital
New York, New York

Arthur D. Heller, M.D.
Adjunct Physician
Section of Gastroenterology
Lenox Hill Hospital
New York, New York

Henry Janowitz, M.D.
Chief Emeritus
Division of Gastroenterology
Department of Medicine
Mount Sinai Medical Center
New York, New York

Marvin A. Kaplan, M.D.
Adjunct Physician
Section of Psychiatry
Lenox Hill Hospital
New York, New York

Albert B. Knapp, M.D.
Adjunct Physician
Section of Gastroenterology
Lenox Hill Hospital
New York, New York

Burton I. Korelitz, M.D.
Chief
Section of Gastroenterology
Lenox Hill Hospital
Cornell University Medical College
New York, New York

Michael P. Krumholz, M.D.
Adjunct Physician
Section of Gastroenterology
Lenox Hill Hospital
New York, New York

Gregory V. Lauwers, M.D.
Fellow
Department of Pathology
Memorial Hospital
New York, New York

Raul N. Lugo, M.D.
Adjunct Surgeon
Lenox Hill Hospital
New York, New York

Robert A. Mendelsohn, M.D.
Fellow in Gastroenterology
Lenox Hill Hospital
New York, New York

Mark A. Peppercorn, M.D.
Associate Professor of Medicine
Harvard Medical School
Physician, Beth Israel Hospital
Section of Gastroenterology
Department of Medicine
Boston, Massachusetts

Daniel H. Present, M.D.
Clinical Professor of Medicine
Mount Sinai School of Medicine
Attending Physician
Section of Gastroenterology
Department of Medicine
Mount Sinai Medical Center
New York, New York

David B. Sachar, M.D.
Professor of Medicine
Mount Sinai School of Medicine
Director, Division of Gastroenterology
Department of Medicine
New York, New York

Norman Sohn, M.D.
Associate Physician
Lenox Hill Hospital
Department of Surgery
Clinical Assistant Professor of Surgery
Cornell University Medical College
New York, New York

Stephan R. Targan, M.D.
Professor of Medicine
University of California at Los Angeles
Director, UCLA Center for Health
  Sciences
Inflammatory Bowel Disease Research
  and Clinical Center
Los Angeles, California

Jerome D. Waye, M.D.
Clinical Professor of Medicine
Mount Sinai School of Medicine
Chief, Gastrointestinal Endoscopy Unit
Lenox Hill Hospital
New York, New York

Michael A. Weinstein, M.D.
Associate Physician
Department of Surgery
Lenox Hill Hospital
New York, New York

Audrey Woolrich, M.D.
Assistant Adjunct Physician
Section of Gastroenterology
Lenox Hill Hospital
New York, New York

PREFACE

The rationale for grouping ulcerative colitis with Crohn's disease (inflammatory bowel disease) has historical support. The medical literature included descriptions of both diseases in the latter half of the 19th century, both cause inflammation of the colon, they share many symptoms, in some instances the differential diagnosis may be very difficult, and the cause of each remains unknown. Furthermore, one member of a family may have Crohn's disease, and another have ulcerative colitis. Both processes are prone to the late complication of carcinoma at a site of previous involvement. Finally, the investigators and students of one disease usually have contributed to understanding of the other disease as well.

The prevalence of Crohn's disease is remarkable when we consider that 60 years ago, as the classic description from Mt. Sinai Hospital was being prepared, the disease was rare. Although the cause remains elusive, we must acknowledge the natural course, complications, choices of drug therapy and both their positive and negative effects, and the risks of surgical intervention, including the likelihood of recurrence and its own subsequent complications. Therapy must try to combat this disease as skillfully as possible, with consideration of indications and timing of drug and surgical intervention. In this regard, the choice forms of management have been controversial even among the most experienced.

The incidence of ulcerative colitis seems to be stable. Nonsurgical management has improved, however, and urgent surgery is much less often required. This has provided many patients the opportunity to have pouches shaped by the surgeon on an elective basis. Successful nonsurgical management also has created the opportunity for greater likelihood of development of carcinoma of the rectum or colon. These considerations also introduce controversy.

Burton I. Korelitz, M.D.
Norman Sohn, M.D.

CONTENTS

PART 1

Overview and Etiology

Chapter 1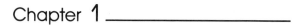

Recent Developments in Inflammatory Bowel Disease

Burton I. Korelitz

There have been many developments in *inflammatory bowel disease* (IBD) during the past 4 years. First, however, what has not changed?

1. The causes of both Crohn's disease and ulcerative colitis remain unknown.
2. Evidence for an infectious cause, which dominated the scene a few years ago, has really not been sustained.
3. Crohn's disease is not cured by any form of surgery; that remains a fact.
4. Many resections continue to be performed for perirectal abscesses and fistulas, small bowel obstruction, and toxic megacolon despite the efficacy of minor operative procedures and nonoperative techniques.
5. The role of antibiotics in the treatment of Crohn's disease has not yet been submitted to any trials.

What is it that has changed?

1. New epidemiologic factors have been identified that influence cause and course, and these are challenging.
2. Provocation of IBD by nonsteroidal anti-inflammatory drugs has become recognized.
3. New types of colitis, such as collagenous and microscopic colitis, have been defined.
4. The mechanism of diversion colitis is now being explained, and it is of particular pertinence in Crohn's disease.

5. The need for surgery in ulcerative colitis has been decreased.
6. As a corollary to the preceding, more patients retain the colon and are at risk of development of carcinoma.
7. The need for surgery in Crohn's disease has been at least postponed if not reduced; therefore we see less malabsorption and less short bowel syndrome.
8. The risk of cancer complicating long-standing Crohn's disease, particularly when it involves the colon, is increasing and is approaching that of ulcerative colitis.
9. The role of both oral and rectal 5-aminosalicylic acid (5-ASA) preparations is becoming better established, the first not only for ulcerative colitis but also for Crohn's disease.
10. New steroids that are absorbed but have no glucocorticoid effect, and others not absorbed at all, are now available for trial.
11. Utilization of immunosuppressive drugs has increased as experience with efficacy and toxicity has accumulated. The role of 6-mercaptopurine (6-MP) in treatment of Crohn's disease has been established, and its use in treatment of resistant cases has now been acknowledged by gastroenterologists all over the country. Cyclosporine has arrived, as have methotrexate and hydroxychloroquine sulfate (Plaquenil).
12. The role of surveillance for dysplasia in carcinoma has become better established, and the clinical recommendations based on these findings are being clarified.
13. The early enthusiasm resulting from the introduction of the ileo-pouch-anal anastomosis for ulcerative colitis has now been tempered to some extent. There is renewed enthusiasm for some of the older procedures. The best choice of operation for the individual patient is being sought.
14. Experience has led us not only to new approaches in therapy but also to recognition of errors that have occurred in the past.

Chapter 2 _____

Progress in Understanding the Pathogenesis of Inflammatory Bowel Disease: Infectious and Immunologic Factors

Stephan Targan

_____

Advances in understanding the cause, genetic factors, and infectious process of inflammatory bowel disease (IBD) have been made recently. These advances have identified new directions for study of the cause of, and new treatments for, IBD.[13a] Potential contributors to the pathogenesis of IBD include elements that might predispose to, trigger, and perpetuate the disease. Tissue damage might be due to a direct attack by the mucosal immune system on a specific target, such as the surface, or glandular, epithelial cell. A nonspecific outcome of disordered mucosal immune regulation, with uncontrolled overreactivity to environmental antigens based on a defective down-regulation of this response, may perpetuate the damage. Genetic predisposing factors might operate at the level of the "target" cell or at the level of the mucosal immune system.

Evidence to suggest genetic predisposing factors in these diseases is based on the percentage of concordance in monozygotic twins and dizygotic twins. In Crohn's disease, 67% of monozygotic twins are concordant, vs. only 3% of dizygotic twins. Among twins with ulcerative colitis, 27% of monozygotic twins are concordant, and no dizygotic twins are concordant.[18] The concordance among monozygotic twins, then, is greater than among dizygotic twins. There was no concordance among mixed pairs. Given the evidence of genetic predisposition, studies have begun in an attempt to demonstrate linkage. Linkage refers to the existence of two loci located so close together on chromosomes that they are inherited as a unit.[18]

Demonstrating HLA linkage in IBD is particularly complicated. In work performed previously, linkage analyses of IBD and HLA were limited to samples of affected sib-pairs. Furthermore, the various forms of these diseases could reflect a genetic heterogeneity that greatly limits the power of the sib-pair method. Geneticists have recently developed a new linkage method for extended pedigrees, which employs the study of affected relative pairs.[18] This method searches for shared alleles among affected relatives. Since the chance of concordance decreases the more distantly related pairs of patients with disease may be, fewer patients or pairs are required to establish significance. A significant association could be made within as few as one family if concordance among third cousins can be determined.

This method has been applied to families of patients with IBD. Recent genetic investigations have determined an HLA linkage to the presence of IBD in families with multiple affected members. The fact that 20 years of prior research have not yielded consistent findings regarding linkage is due to the likelihood that these diseases are genetically heterogeneous. The evidence points to forms of IBD that can be demonstrated to be linked to HLA, and forms of IBD in which no linkage can be determined (Rotter et al, unpublished data).

The HLA region has been identified in IBD. Candidate genes for IBD have been advanced. Genetic studies have defined an HLA (HLA-DR, DQ haplotype) and C3 (C3F related) abnormality to be associated with Crohn's disease (H. Toyoda, unpublished data). An HLA (HLA-DR2 haplotype) may be associated with ulcerative colitis. Using subclinical markers, family studies of patients with Crohn's disease have defined C3 dysfunctional and intestinal permeability to be increased in family members of patients with Crohn's disease. Antibodies to epithelial antigens are increased in a very large number of family members of patients with IBD; suggesting this represents a common infectious exposure and not an underlying genetic susceptibility. Family studies will soon be performed to investigate the relationship of colonic mucins and antineutrophil cytoplasmic antibodies in ulcerative colitis.

The implication of the inconsistency of genetic data among various groups is that genetically distinct forms of the disease exist. This signals the need to begin considering subgroups of IBD in future investigations. The development of "reagent grade" patients is required to perform such studies adequately. Such reagent grade patients can be determined by analysis of all available clinical and subclinical markers, and then groups of individuals with like profiles considered individually in both clinical and basic investigations. The ultimate goal would be to tailor investigations to groups of patients based on clinical and subclinical profiles.

Increasing amounts of data are illustrating the connections between genetics and immune-mediated processes. What makes IBD unique among other immune-mediated conditions such as arthritis, thyroiditis, and diabetes is the organ. The intestine is the largest immunologic organ in the body with its own intrinsic immune system. As stated earlier, the immune system of the gut plays a role in gut inflammation, either through some direct autoimmune injury or a nonspecific innocent bystander injury.

Immunologic studies to date point to the innocent bystander attack as the most likely mechanism of epithelial cell injury in IBD. This hypothesis implies the existence of some defect in the regulation of mucosal immunity leading to a poorly regulated response to a variety of exogenous antigens (virus, bacteria, or protein). Such an event would lead to the generation of highly activated T cells that generate cytokines capable of direct epithelial damage and others that recruit effector cells (i.e., neutrophils, eosinophils, mast cells, and macrophages). The arrival of these auxiliary effectors is associated with release of various mediators such as arachidonate metabolites and oxygen radicals, which are locally injurious in a nonspecific fashion. The inability to limit this injury to acute inflammation with healing in IBD, yielding chronic epithelial damage, could be related either to the release of greater levels or different repertoires of T cell–associated cytokines, a defective ability to down-regulate cytokine production or release (or both), or an enhanced susceptibility of target tissue to these cytokines combined with other inflammatory mediators. Interactions between the immune system and the other components of the mucosal microenvironment, such as the neuroendocrine system and the nature of the mucosal barrier, are also important in modulating the inflammatory response.

To date no specific antigen has been defined to be responsible for initiating the onset of IBD. It has been reported recently that viral and bacterial infections are capable of triggering the immune system, inducing an uncontrolled release of cytokines that may destroy the epithelial cells, as previously outlined. The goal of investigations of IBD would be to develop a way to inhibit and halt the uncontrolled release of cytokines and to down-regulate the immune system once it has been turned on.

At present, no good disease markers of Crohn's disease or ulcerative colitis have been established. Results do suggest a shift in immunoglobulin isotype to IgG1 in ulcerative colitis and to IgG2 in the mucosa of patients with Crohn's disease, however. These findings have stimulated a long search for antibodies as disease markers for IBD. A variety of autoantibodies have been reported previously in ulcerative colitis.[6] Most notable among these have been lymphocytotoxic antibodies[13] and colonic epithelial antibodies.[6, 19, 20] Although these may have genetic and pathophysiologic implications, they have not been useful diagnostically, either because of low frequency of occurrence or lack of specificity.

Recently studies to determine the presence of antineutrophil cytoplasmic autoantibodies (ANCA) in the sera of patients with IBD were performed. Previous studies of ANCA were completed on patients with Wegener's granulomatosis. A granular cytoplasmic pattern was observed on immunofluorescence, and data have shown that ANCA are a good disease marker for Wegener's granulomatosis.[7] Subsequently the antigen in Wegener's granulomatosis has been identified to be a 29 kd elastinolytic protease. ANCA are also found in patients with crescentic glomerulonephritis.[11] The immunofluorescence pattern is perinuclear, although additional studies have determined the antigen to be myeloperoxidase. Therefore ANCA in crescentic glomerulonephritis are not diagnostic.

Sera from patients with ulcerative colitis and Crohn's disease were tested for ANCA. The pattern produced upon immunofluorescence was very distinct from Wegener's granulomatosis in that it was cytoplasmic with perinuclear highlighting. The frequency of this occurrence was determined with use of enzyme-linked immunosorbent assay (ELISA). Results showed that the majority of patients with ulcerative colitis tested positive for ANCA. Ultimately more than 300 sera samples collected from around the country were tested. Eight percent were shown to be positive for ANCA. By comparison, only 10% of patients with Crohn's disease were positive for ANCA with use of ELISA, and only 5% produced the characteristic perinuclear pattern with use of immunofluorescence assay. Even comparison between patients with Crohn's disease of the colon with ulcerative colitis showed that the majority of those with ulcerative colitis tested positive for ANCA, while test results in the great majority of those with Crohn's colitis were negative for ANCA.[4]

The presence of ANCA in collagenous colitis was compared with that in ulcerative colitis. Approximately 10% of sera from patient with collagenous colitis are positive for ANCA. Further investigations are required to determine the relationship of collagenous colitis to ANCA. On the other hand, a negative relationship between ANCA in ulcerative colitis and that in radiation colitis, irritable bowel syndrome, diarrhea, and rectal bleeding was found. Therefore the presence of positive ELISA findings and an immunofluorescence pattern of perinuclear highlighting shows a high degree of specificity (94% for ulcerative colitis).[5]

Sera from patients with primary sclerosing cholangitis, which is clinically similar to ulcerative colitis, were investigated for the presence of ANCA in an attempt to define an immune link between the two diseases.[10] The great majority of patients with primary sclerosing cholangitis tested positive for ANCA with use of ELISA and displayed the characteristic perinuclear pattern on immunofluorescence staining. Patients with primary sclerosing cholangitis with no evidence of colitis proved by endoscopy also tested positive for ANCA. In contrast, primary biliary cirrhosis, chronic hepatitis, and non-A and non-B hepatitis tested positive for ANCA with use of ELISA, but had varying immunofluorescence patterns. The combination of positive findings with use of ELISA and a perinuclear immunofluorescence pattern gave a specificity of 100% for primary sclerosing cholangitis. Characterization of the antigen to which these antibodies react will allow characterization of distinct subsets of patients with ulcerative colitis.

If one considers that the normal mucosa is a model of controlled inflammation, the hypothesis of ulcerative colitis as unregulated immune activity provides the basic model for immune studies of the mechanism of IBDs. The normal intestinal immune response is regulated and includes selected trafficking of antigen-primed cells. Antigens that are exposed to the mucosa induce an immune response, which proliferated, enters the mesenteric lymph nodes back through the thoracic duct and repopulates the mucosa. Immunosuppressive interventions are one possible route of investigation, if they can be designed to modulate specific immune components within the mucosa.

A series of recent observations provides support for the central role of T cells and associated cytokines in the nonspecific indirect injury to epithelial cells as a mechanism of tissue injury in IBD, particularly Crohn's disease. Organ culture studies of human fetal jejunum have elegantly shown that T cell activation can lead to local tissue injury. Mitogen stimulation of direct T cell activation with use of monoclonal antibodies to the CD3 component of the T cell receptor led to a marked enteropathy consisting of villous atrophy (epithelial injury) and crypt cell hyperplasia. Histologic studies of early focal lesions in patients with Crohn's disease have provided indirect evidence for the role of activated T cells in the pathogenesis of tissue injury. T cells may mediate tissue and epithelial injury indirectly, by the release of cytokines. The demonstration of increased major histocompatibility complex (MHC) class II expression on epithelial cells overlying inflamed areas in IBD tissues and the ability of recombinant cytokines interferon gamma (INF-γ) or tumor necrosis factor (TNF-α) (or both) to induce such expression in vitro suggest that cytokine release plays a critical role in epithelial function and viability in IBD.

IFN-γ and TNF-α are likely candidates as T cell–associated cytokines that are responsible for epithelial injury in IBD. TNF-α and INF-γ have been shown to be capable effector molecules in immune destruction of self tissues.[8–10] Individually, or in combination, INF-γ or TNF-α is capable of destroying target tissues of known autoimmune responses. This has been demonstrated recently in an animal model of diabetes in which isolated CTL-22 or a combination of IFN-γ and TNF-α destroyed isolated pancreatic islet cells in vitro.[1] In addition, mTNF-α has been identified in lesions from brain tissues of patients who have multiple sclerosis.[12] Both TNF-α and IFN-γ have been implicated in the enteropathy associated with graft-vs.-host reaction (GVHR). Treatment of GVHR mice with anti–IFN-γ prevents crypt cell proliferation and villous atrophy.[14, 15] TFN-α has been identified in the serum of GVHR mice, and addition of exogenous TNF-α to normal mice mimics the villous atrophy seen in GVHR mice.[14, 15] Analysis of the specificity of these cytotoxic/cytostatic lymphokines has demonstrated that not all cells are equally sensitive to their effects. The ability of IFN-γ to up-regulate a variety of cellular receptors, including those for TNF-α, suggests that cytokine abnormalities in IBD may not be limited to alterations in levels, but probably include alterations in tissue sensitivity.[17] Sensitivity of targets to TNF-α and IFN-γ may be related to expression of certain antigens or receptors on their cell surface or to effects of viral products on cellular metabolism. This has been demonstrated most recently in the destruction of virally infected human targets by cytotoxic thymus (-dependent) lymphocyte–released lymphokines[16] and the enhanced lysis of fibroblasts infected with adenovirus by TNF-α.[3]

Results demonstrate that colonic mucosal T cells, triggered through the T cell receptor, produce TNF-α and IFN-γ in vitro.[2] A combination of both of these cytokines is required for killing the human colonic epithelial target cell line, HT-29. This study suggests that human mucosal T cells may be involved in indirect, cytokine-mediated damage to colonic mucosa during immune reactions. This finding is an important step in determining the mechanism of action of mucosal inflammation in IBDs.

In conclusion, significant progress has been made in understanding the pathogenesis of IBD genetic, infectious, and immunologic factors. Evidence of a genetic predisposition has been uncovered based on the presence of concordance in monozygotic and dizygotic twins. The observation has been made that family members of patients with IBD have subclinical markers suggestive of a possible common infectious exposure. The high specificity of the combination of sera positive for ANCA with use of ELISA with a perinuclear pattern on immunofluorescence is indicative of an excellent disease marker for ulcerative colitis.

REFERENCES

1. Campbell IL, Iscaro A, Harrison LC: IFN-gamma and tumor necrosis factor-alpha cytotoxicity to murine islets of Langerhans. *J Immunol* 1988; 141:2325–2329.|
2. Deem RL, Shanahan F, Targan SR: Triggered human mucosal T-cells release tumour necrosis factor-alpha and interferon-gamma which kill human colonic epithelial cells. *Clin Exp Immunol* 1991; 83:79–84.
3. Duerksen-Hughes P, Wold WSM, Gooding LR: Adenovirus ElA renders infected cells sensitive to cytolysis by tumor necrosis factor. *J Immunol* 1989; 143:4193–4200.
4. Duerr R, Targan S, Landers C, et al: Neutrophil autoantibodies in ulcerative colitis: Comparison with other colitides/diarrheal illnesses. *Gastroenterology* 1991; 100:1590–1596.
5. Duerr RH, Targan SR, Landers CJ, et al: Neutrophil autoantibodies: A link between primary sclerosing cholangitis and ulcerative colitis. *Gastroenterology* 1990; 98:(part 2):A584.
6. Elson CO: The immunology of IBD, in Kirsner J, Shorter R (eds): *Inflammatory Bowel Disease.* Philadelphia, Lea & Febiger, 1988, pp 97–174.
7. Falk RJ, Jennette JC: Anti-neutrophil cytoplasmic autoantibodies with specificity for myeloperoxidase in patients with systemic vasculitis and idiopathic necrotizing and crescentric glomerulonephritis. *N Engl J Med* 1988; 3118:1651–1657.
8. Granger GA, Hiserodt JC, Ware CF: In Cohen S, Pick E, Oppenheim J, (eds): *Biology of Lymphokines.* New York, Academic Press, 1979.
9. Green LM, Stern ML, Haviland DL, et al: Cytotoxic lymphokines produced by cloned human cytotoxic T-lymphocytes. I. *J Immunol* 1985; 135:4034–4043.
10. Green LM, Reade JL, Ware CF, et al: Cytotoxic lymphokines produced by cloned human cytotoxic T-lymphocytes. II. *J Immunol* 1986; 137:3488–3493.
11. Gross WL, Ludemann G, Kiefer G, et al: Anticytoplasmic antibodies in Wegener's granulomatosis. *Lancet* 1985; 1:425–429.
12. Hofman FM, Hinton DR, Johnson K, et al: Tumor necrosis factor identified in multiple sclerosis brains. *J Exp Med* 1989; 170:607–612.
13. Korsmeyer SJ, Williams RC Jr, Wilson ID, et al: Lymphocytotoxic antibody in IBD. A family study. *N Engl J Med* 1975; 293:1117.
13a. MacDermott RP, Stenson WF: The immunology of idiopathic IBD. *Adv Immunol* 1988; 42:285–328.
14. Mowat AM, Felstein MV: Experimental studies of immunologically mediated enteropathy. Development of cell mediated immunity and intestinal

pathology during a graft-vs-host reaction in irradiated mice. *Gut* 1988; 29:949–956.

15. Mowat AM, Felstein MV: Experimental studies of immunologically mediated enteropathy: Correlation between immune effector mechanisms and type of enteropathy during a GvHR in neonatal mice of different ages. *Clin Exp Immunol* 1988; 79:279–284.

16. Paya CV, Kenmotsu N, Schoon RA, et al: Tumor necrosis factor and lymphotoxin secretion by human natural killer cells leads to antiviral cytotoxicity. *J Immunol* 1988; 141:1989–1995.

17. Rosenblum MG, Donato NJ: Tumor necrosis factor alpha: A multifaceted peptide hormone. *Crit Rev Immunol* 1989; 9:21–44.

18. Shohat T, Vadheim C, Rotter GI: The genetics of inflammatory bowel diseases, in Gitnick G (ed): *Inflammatory Bowel Disease: A physician's guide.* New York, Igaku-Shoin, in press.

19. Shanahan F: Inflammatory bowel disease, in Targan SR, moderator: Immunologic mechanisms in intestinal diseases. *Ann Intern Med* 1987; 106:853.

20. Strober W, James SP: The immunologic basis of intestinal diseases. *J Clin Immunol* 1986; 91:746.

Progress in Understanding the Pathogenesis of Inflammatory Bowel Disease: Historic and Epidemiologic Factors

Theodore Bayless

The prevalence of ulcerative colitis remains relatively stable at perhaps 5 per 100,000 people.[19] In Olmstead County, Minnesota, in a very good study, there are about 10 per 100,000, however.[7] There are presumably 400,000 to 500,000 patients with ulcerative colitis in the United States. At least half have inflammation only in the distal area of the colon. Studies indicate that disease in the distal area is becoming more common. Physicians in medical centers are seeing more people with resistant proctocolitis, but perhaps this is also because we now have 5-aminosalicylic acid agents to treat these particular patients.

Another important point about ulcerative colitis is that, in contrast to Crohn's disease, smoking clearly is protective. Nonsmokers or recent withdrawal subjects are at greater risk of developing ulcerative colitis.[17]

As another feature, multiple problems may exist in the same patient. Since irritable bowel syndrome (IBS) affects 10% of the population, there are bound to be patients with both proctitis and IBS. It is important to try to distinguish these two illnesses when both affect the same individual.[4]

The prevalence of Crohn's disease has gradually increased during the past 30 years. Chapter 4 concerning older patients will make the point that we have been seeing more Crohn's disease in the distal area of the colon than in the past. Patients with Crohn's disease smoke more than is expected in the general population, and this may be an environmental factor in its pathogenesis.

Subsequently we will discuss scarring and obstruction in ileitis as well as the role of the lumenal constituents in the pathogenesis of ileocolitis and colitis. This dependence on the fecal stream to maintain Crohn's disease activity can be demonstrated by diverting the fecal stream, by using bowel rest and total parenteral nutrition (TPN) or by elemental diets such as Vivonex. These measures can temporarily decrease the inflammation in the ileum. Long-term medical therapy is usually needed to maintain a remission induced by bowel rest, however.[16]

Among the other epidemiologic factors, the tendency to family occurrences highlights the importance of genetic forces. This was discussed in Chapter 2. In terms of dietary factors, increased sugar intake in Crohn's disease has been cited as a factor. Stress and psychologic factors do not seem to be basic to the pathogenesis of these illnesses.

At another level of pathogenesis, lumenal short-chain fatty acids (SCFAs) seem to be important in maintaining the integrity of the colonic mucosa. Left-side colonic cells readily utilize lumenal short-chain fatty acids, especially butyric acid and acetic acid, for energy. They actually prefer these lumenal SCFAs to blood-borne glucose. The absence of this process may play a role in diversion colitis[9] and ulcerative colitis[4] (see Chapter 16). The lack of SCFAs in the lumen in diversion colitis and their therapeutic role led to the evaluation in ulcerative colitis.[4] There is a trial of SCFA in ulcerative colitis going on now.

With Crohn's disease, Dr. Targan (see Chapter 2) discusses increased permeability in patients and perhaps in relatives. Is this a mechanism by which a dietary antigen plays a role in pathogenesis? Is this why the elemental diets such as Vivonex help, or why bowel rest may play some role? The possibility that the relatives also may have altered gut permeability is interesting but awaits confirmation.

Mucopolysaccharide differences in ulcerative colitis, as described by Podolsky and Isselbacher,[14] may be primary or secondary. Since smoking apparently influences the mucus content in the colon, could this be the mechanism by which smoking is protective in the patient with ulcerative colitis?

Some of the demographic factors for inflammatory bowel disease (IBD) include a relatively equal sex ratio. There is a slight increase in female patients in some studies; in others, proctitis seems to be more common in men. IBD is more common in whites than in non-whites and is more common in Jews. Worldwide the highest prevalence is in the Northern Hemisphere. The illnesses involve predominantly teenagers and young adults. There are a number of older patients with IBD as well. The special problems of these elderly patients will be stressed in Chapter 4. Family history has been discussed in Chapter 2.

The average age of onset of IBD is 27, so one should have a high index of suspicion for Crohn's disease and ulcerative colitis in young people.* There have been changes in the prevalence of IBD. Ulcerative colitis has remained relatively stable, but perhaps shifting more toward disease of the distal area. Crohn's disease had increased in prevalence and also apparently shifting more toward colonic disease and disease of the distal area. The prevalence has perhaps stabilized now.[19]

Worldwide prevalence is also interesting. Rotter and his colleagues at University of California at Los Angeles have noted that of the many Ashkenazi Jews in Los Angeles with Crohn's disease, more came from Germany and Austria than would have been expected by emigration patterns. Most of the Jewish immigrants to California are thought to be from Russia and Poland. However, among the IBD patients, there were more from Germany and Austria than expected. What that means is not clear.[15]

Neuroticism does not seem to be the cause of ulcerative colitis. Certainly anxiety and depression are much more common in the irritable bowel than in the general population. If a person is upset, psychologic symptoms are more prevalent. When one looks at precipitating causes before relapses, however, IBS does stand out, while the occurrence of stressful factors, ulcerative colitis, and Crohn's disease probably is not different than in the general population. Psychosocial factors are important in IBD, as in any chronic illness, but they are probably not etiologic.

There is a subgroup of people who have both IBS and IBD. Because about 10% of the population have IBS, it is not unexpected that one will see both IBS and IBD in the same patient. There is probably a family tendency for IBS as well as for IBD. In history taking, ask about childhood and teenage bowel habits. It is important to think about IBS before onset of IBD, and to hear about the mother's colitis and constipation. Also, the muscle spasm due to rectal inflammation obviously can increase the symptoms of IBS. As another aspect of this issue, avoid using the ileum of a patient with coexistent IBS for an ileoanal pouch. These patients may become very unhappy if an ileoanal pouch is created for them. The irritable ileum, which shares the hyperactivity of the colon, does not enjoy accepting 300 mL of fluid regularly.[2, 3]

---

*Editor's Note: My own studies and those of some others suggest a still younger mean age of onset, particularly in Crohn's disease.

ENVIRONMENTAL FACTORS

Smoking seems to be a strong environmental factor in the pathogenesis of IBD. The data are quite impressive.[17] It seems clear that Crohn's disease risk correlates with increased smoking. Conversely, in ulcerative colitis the relative risk is raised for a nonsmoker. Recent withdrawal also seemed to increase the risk of ulcerative colitis. For a current smoker, the risk of Crohn's disease is 1.8 times greater than for the general population. For one who has smoked, the risk is higher than is expected for nonsmokers. If one is smoking at the time of onset of Crohn's disease, the risk obviously is even greater.

At present no one is urging people with ulcerative colitis to continue smoking or to start smoking. These are, however, some preliminary results of a favorable effect of nicotine gum in patients with ulcerative colitis. A recent letter to the editor in *Annals of Internal Medicine* suggests that marijuana also seemed to provide protection from ulcerative colitis.[1] Use of the information on nicotine gum and on marijuana is left at one's own discretion. Some British workers also believe that a heavy sugar intake adds to this risk from smoking.

It has been hypothesized by Targan et al.,[10] at the University of California at Los Angeles, that there is a genetic predisposition such as the HLA pattern. Add an environmental factor, perhaps smoking, and the decision is reached that Crohn's disease will develop or, in a nonsmoker, that ulcerative colitis will develop. Although I do not think these two diseases are commonly linked genetically, this is an interesting hypothesis.

There is a recent article on epidemiology from Japan with some interesting hypotheses. The prevalence of ulcerative colitis in Japan has been increasing with time. Subsequently Crohn's disease has begun to appear, and its frequency, although still low, is gradually increasing. The authors[20] found an association between ulcerative colitis and the increased use of dairy products as well as the increased use of meat products in Japan. Seafood intake remained constant during this same period. To date these ideas are still inferential.[20]

In the United States initial reports linked use of birth control pills with Crohn's disease, but recent studies have probably eliminated this as an important role.[12]

CHARACTERISTICS OF ANY PUTATIVE CAUSATIVE AGENT

We do not know the cause of Crohn's disease. If a virus causes it, what would its features be? It would have a long dormant period to go with the late recurrences of Crohn's disease. It would have a latency period also because of the late postoperative recrudescences as well as the subtle illness in adolescence, affecting growth for 2 or 3 years before any symptoms appear.

If a microorganism is involved, it incites inflammation that is suppressible. Importantly, in the small bowel the inflammation heals with dense scarring of the intestinal wall. This process seems predictable and almost programmed. The dense scarring of the ileum occurs regardless of therapy. Whether one treats patients continuously with alternate-day steroids and sulfasalazine or only with intermittent anti-inflammatory therapy, scarring will occur in an almost predictable fashion.[13] I do not know if 6-mercaptopurine or azathioprine therapy can prevent this dense scarring.

DIFFERENT FORMS OF CROHN'S DISEASE

Among the adolescents we have seen, there was a group who required "early" surgery in the first 3 years for perforation, fistulization, abscesses, or growth problems. We had a larger group who had "late" surgery. They were usually operated on for obstruction, and an almost programmed reappearance of obstruction occurred in about two thirds of the patients.[13]

In 1971 de Dombal et al.[5] described separate "early" and postoperative "late" recurrence as perhaps two distinguishable forms of Crohn's disease. Greenstein, and colleagues,[8] at Mount Sinai Hospital, have shown similar data. They have looked at the indications for a second resection among patients who had a perforating indication for resection. If a second operation was needed, most (73%) had it for a perforating indication. It was about 4 years between operations. When patients who had an obstructive or nonperforating indication for their first operation needed a repeat operation, two-thirds needed it for obstruction. The lag between these "late" operations was 8.8 years. This also supports the concept of both an aggressive and a less aggressive form of Crohn's disease, especially in the small bowel.[6]

ROLE OF LUMENAL CONTENTS IN CROHN'S DISEASE

Diversion of the fecal stream is believed to help about two thirds of acutely ill patients who have ileocolitis. If one constructs a double-barrelled ileostomy, it helps, at least temporarily. In about half of the patients who were operated on in Oxford, England, subsequent reanastomosis was possible.[11] This provides evidence that the fecal stream plays a role in maintaining the activity of Crohn's disease in the lower part of the ileum and colon.

Bowel rest via TPN or via elemental diets is another way of diverting the fecal stream. We have successfully utilized bowel rest in Crohn's colitis to bring the disease into remission in 16 of 17 severely ill patients referred to us for surgery. Azathioprine (Imuran) or 6-mercaptopurine, though, was sometimes started during that admission, in addition to the bowel rest. Hospital and then home hyperalimentation for 6 to 8 weeks provided time for the immunomodulators to begin to become active. Continued medical therapy after hyperalimentation was usually essential to maintain remissions.[16] Elemental diets seem less helpful in the colon than with small bowel disease. Teahon and Levi,[18] in England, noted improvement in about 70% of patients with small bowel disease who were treated with an elemental diet (Vivonex).

Our patients with ulcerative colitis treated with TPN did not fare as well as the patients with Crohn's disease. Only six of 21 did not require surgery.

SUMMARY

The epidemiologic studies show that while the frequency of ulcerative colitis has stabilized, more disease of the distal area of the colon is being encountered. Importantly, nonsmoking seems to increase the risk of ulcerative colitis. In Crohn's disease environmental factors, such as excessive smoking, are also probably important. Certainly lumenal nutrients or fecal materials are important in the pathogenesis of active Crohn's disease. In addition, there seems to be a fixed program of scarring in the small bowel of patients with Crohn's disease that may require another form of medication besides anti-inflammatory drugs. Perhaps in the future we will be giving patients antifibrotic as well as anti-inflammatory medications.

REFERENCES

1. Baron J, Folan A, Kelley ML Jr: Ulcerative colitis and marijuana. *Ann Intern Med* 1990; 112:471.
2. Bayless TM: Coexistent irritable bowel syndrome and inflammatory bowel disease, in Bayless TM (ed): *Current Management of Inflammatory Bowel Disease.* Toronto, BC Decker, 1989, pp 59–62.
3. Bayless TM, Harris ML: IBD and irritable bowel syndrome. Med Clin *North Am* 1990; 74:21–28.

4. Breuer RI, Buto SK, Christ ML, et al: Short chain fatty acids for distal ulcerative colitis. *Gastroenterology* 1990; 98:A161.
5. de Dombal FT, Burton I, Goligher JC: Recurrence of Crohn's disease after primary excisional surgery. *Gut* 1971; 12:517–527.
6. Farmer RG, Whelan G, Fazio WV: Long-term follow up of patients with Crohn's disease: Relationship between the clinical pattern and prognosis. *Gastroenterology* 1985; 88:1818–1825.
7. Gollop JH, Phillips SF, Melton LJ, et al: Epidemiologic aspects of Crohn's disease: A population based study in Olmstead County, Minnesota, 1943–1982. *Gut* 1988; 29:49–56.
8. Greenstein AJ, Lachman P, Sachar DB, et al: Perforating and nonperforating indications for repeated operations in Crohn's disease: Evidence for two clinical forms. *Gut* 1988; 29:588–592.
9. Harig JM, Soergel KH: Treatment of diversion colitis with short chain fatty acid (SCFA) irrigation. *Gastroenterology* 1987; 92:1425.
10. Hellers G, Bedrnell O: Genetic aspects of IBD. *Med Clin North Am* 1990; 74:13–19.
11. Jewell DP, Kettlewell MG: Split ileostomy for Crohn's colitis, in Bayless TM (ed): *Current Management of IBD.* Toronto, BC Decker, 1989, pp 294–296.
12. Lashner BA, Kane SV, Hanauer SB: Lack of association between oral contraceptive use and ulcerative colitis. *Gastroenterology* 1990; 98:A160.
13. Levine E, Schwartz J, Bayless T: Distal ileal Crohn's disease: The time course of fixed bowel obstruction. *Gastroenterology* 1987; 95:1504.
14. Podolsky DK, Isselbacher KJ: Glycoprotein composition of colonic mucosa. Specific alteration in ulcerative colitis. *Gastroenterology* 1984; 87:991–998.
15. Roth MP, Petersen GM, McElree C, et al: Geographic origins of Jewish patients with IBD. *Gastroenterology* 1989; 97:900–904.
16. Sitzman JV, Converse RL Jr, Bayless TM: Favorable response to parenteral nutrition and medical therapy in Crohn's colitis. *Gastroenterology* 1990; 99:1–6.
17. Sutherland LR, Ramcharan S, Bryant H, et al: Effect of cigarette smoking on recurrence of Crohn's disease. *Gastroenterology* 1990; 98:1123–1128.
18. Teahon K, Levi J: Dietary management, in Bayless TM (ed): *Current Management of IBD.* Toronto, BC Decker, 1989, pp 223–230.
19. Whelan G: Epidemiology of inflammatory bowel disease. *Med Clin North Am* 1990; 74:1–12.
20. Yoshida Y, Murata Y: IBD in Japan: Studies of epidemiology and etiopathogenesis. *Med Clin North Am* 1990; 74:67–90.

PART 2

Special Considerations in Diagnosis and Management

Chapter 4 _____

Inflammatory Bowel Disease in Older Age

Audrey Woolrich

_____

The natural history of inflammatory bowel disease (IBD) in the elderly has not yet been clarified by published reports.

DIFFERENTIAL DIAGNOSIS

Early studies have erroneously included patients who eventually were found to not have ulcerative colitis or Crohn's disease but rather another inflammatory process of the bowel.[4] Ischemic bowel disease may mimic IBD, but patients with ischemic colitis usually have a spontaneous resolution of their symptoms with only 5% having recurrent episodes.[1-3] An acute presentation of IBD can be similar to an attack of diverticulitis, but the subsequent clinical course and histologic findings should clarify the diagnosis. Nevertheless, the two processes can coexist. Most individuals older than 65 years of age have diverticulosis; therefore, when an elderly patient with ulcerative or Crohn's colitis has abdominal pain, fever, and rectal bleeding, with or without diarrhea, at initial presentation, that specific diagnosis may not be apparent. Other forms of colitis or enterocolitis that should be excluded when a patient has these presenting symptoms are those due to infectious agents such as *Salmonella, Shigella, Escherichia coli, Campylobacter*, and *Amoeba*, and antibiotic-associated colitis, radiation colitis, or even neoplasm.

DEFINITION OF AGE

Previous reports have contributed to misconceptions concerning the course of IBD in the elderly by lack of availability of a standard definition of age. Some authors have considered a person elderly after the age of 50, while most have used the term *elderly* to refer to those more than 60 years of age. Furthermore, when trying to sort the natural course of any disease in older age, one should look at two subgroups, those with onset of disease at a young age who have become "elderly" and those with actual onset of disease in older age. A few reports in the literature have studied the course of IBD in the elderly in this manner.[5, 6, 8, 9, 11, 15, 16]

Ulcerative colitis has been reported to develop in 7% to 10% of all elderly patients without any sexual predilection.[13, 17] The onset of Crohn's disease at an older age occurs similarly in 3% to 11% of all patients, but occurs more often in female patients.[7, 12–14]

Korelitz and I[15, 16] have attempted to clarify the course of both ulcerative colitis and Crohn's disease in elderly patients. We reviewed the clinical features of 40 patients with onset of ulcerative colitis after the age of 60 (mean 70 years, range 60–86) and those of 45 patients more than 60 years of age who were under the age of 60 at the time of their initial presentation (mean 42 years, range 18–58).[15] Both groups had a mean of 7 years of disease after the age of 60 during the period of observation. We also reviewed the features of 89 patients 60 years of age and older who had Crohn's disease, 37 with onset after the age of 60 (mean 69 years, range 60–83) and 52 with onset before the age of 60 (mean 41 years, range 16–59).[16] Both groups had a mean of 7 years of disease after the age of 60.

EXTENT OF INVOLVEMENT

In studies performed in the 1960s it was reported that the disease at the time of the presenting attack usually involved the entire colon in ulcerative colitis, but in Crohn's disease colonic involvement was infrequent.[13] More recent reports, however, have noted a predilection for distal involvement in ulcerative colitis and more colonic with less ileal involvement in Crohn's disease in patients of older age.[4, 7, 10, 17] We found that only 10% of our patients with late-onset ulcerative colitis had universal disease[15]; 47% had left-sided involvement and 43% had proctitis alone compared with those more than 60 years of age with earlier onset whose distribution of extent of disease was 31%, 47%, and

22%, respectively. The extent of Crohn's disease at the time of presentation at an older age in our study was 16% proctitis, 32% colitis alone, 32% ileitis alone, and 8% ileocolitis, in comparison with the distribution in those patients more than 60 years of age with earlier onset, which was 2%, 17%, 55% and 27%, respectively, reflecting more ileal involvement in the young and colonic involvement in the elderly.[16]

PRESENTING SYMPTOMS

The major presenting symptoms of IBD in older age appear to be quite similar to those seen in the younger patient.

Ulcerative Colitis

In our study we found that hematochezia and bloody diarrhea were the most common symptoms of late-onset ulcerative colitis.[15] Zimmerman et al.[17] in reviewing 47 patients with ulcerative colitis diagnosed between 21 and 30 years of age and 26 patients with "late-onset" ulcerative colitis (age 51 years or older), found that the latter had more bowel movements per day and had a more protracted presentation.

Crohn's Disease

Diarrhea, abdominal pain, and weight loss were the most common symptoms of late-onset Crohn's disease in our study.[16] Harper et al.[7] compared 41 variables in 24 patients with Crohn's disease between the ages of 64 and 85 matched for sex and disease duration with younger patients between the ages of 20 and 61. They found that there was a long delay to the time of diagnosis in the older group and that, at initial presentation, they had more hematochezia, less abdominal pain, and less frequent occurrence of an abdominal mass. Stalnikowicz et al.[14] also found a significant delay or failure to diagnose Crohn's disease in the elderly. They reported more diarrhea, hematochezia, and abscess formation and generally a higher complication rate in their elderly population.

COURSE

Studies of the natural course of IBD in the elderly from the 1960s differ from more recent reports. Earlier recognition and appropriate treatment with new modalities may have influenced the course, its complications, and incidence of surgical intervention favorably. Some studies report a more aggressive course in their "elderly" populations, but they have included patients with onset of IBD before age 60 years. Softley et al.[13], reported that 42% of their IBD patients more than 60 years of age were free of symptoms with conservative therapy after their presenting attack, with only 8% requiring surgery.

Ulcerative Colitis

In our experience and in that of most authors of recently reported studies, the course of ulcerative colitis in the elderly, whether diagnosed before or after the age of 60, appears to be similar to that of young patients. Zimmerman et al.[17] reported a more fulminant course in those with "late onset," but included patients whose disease was diagnosed before the age of 60 and who had a delay in making their diagnosis that led to a delay in therapy.[17]

Crohn's Disease

In any elderly population, in a patient whose presenting symptoms are abdominal pain, weight loss, diarrhea, hematochezia, or an abscess or fistula, Crohn's disease must be considered in the differential diagnosis. If it is not treated correctly at its presentation, a more difficult course may result.[14, 16]

COMPLICATIONS

The nature of the bowel complications occurring after the age of 60 generally is similar in patients with late-onset and early-onset IBD.[13, 15-17] However, their frequency differs in the two subgroups.

Ulcerative Colitis

In our patients with late-onset-ulcerative colitis, three (7.5%) developed toxic megacolon, but there were no instances after the age of 60 in those with earlier onset. This may indeed reflect a complication that occurs before recognition of the diagnosis and an adequate trial of medical therapy, and is not unique to late onset. Dysplasia was found after the age of 60 slightly more frequently in the late-onset population, but carcinoma after the age of 60 occurred in four (8.9%) of those patients with early-onset ulcerative colitis and in only one (2.5%) of the patients in the late-onset group, probably correlating more with duration of disease than with age at presentation (see Chapters 20 and 21).

Crohn's Disease

In Crohn's disease the bowel complications again are similar at all ages, but abscesses and fistulas appear to occur at a somewhat greater frequency at older age than in younger patients. This phenomenon may result from a selection bias, with most studies being performed at referral centers that generally see more ill patients. In our study of Crohn's disease after the age of 60, the patients with late onset of the disease had slightly more abscesses and fistulas than those with earlier onset.[16] The high prevalence of diverticulosis in those more than 60 years of age, frequently coinciding in location with Crohn's disease, may confuse the clinical picture in older age and contribute to the higher complication rate.

TREATMENT

The medical therapy for IBD in the elderly includes all the agents available to the young patient. Steroids and immunosuppressive agents are not contraindicated in the older patient. However, the possible side effects of drugs at older age and the worsening effect of drugs on other preexisting conditions require judicious use. Coincident diseases that often complicate management include diabetes, hypertension, congestive heart failure, osteopenia and susceptibility to infections, and these are more common in the elderly. Older patients are particularly vulnerable to personality changes and depression when sulfasalazine is used. The risk of fractures occurs sooner when elderly patients with IBD are treated with corticosteroids. We have seen 6-mercaptopurine work successfully in the elderly, making it another good drug that can be used in older patients with IBD as well as in the young.

Ulcerative Colitis

Recent reports suggest that systemic steroids are used more frequently in the elderly with ulcerative colitis than in the young. In our review of treatment after the age of 60, we found that 58% of the late-onset group had been treated with oral prednisone and 30% with intravenous steroids compared with 29% and 11%, respectively, of the early-onset group.[15] Zimmerman et al.[17] also found that most of the late-onset group required steroids.

Crohn's Disease

Harper and coworkers[7] reported that the elderly with Crohn's disease received less steroids in their management than young patients. Stalnikowicz et al.,[14] however, found that steroid therapy was the major treatment modality for approximately 90% of elderly patients with Crohn's disease as well as for the young. They made no distinction between those with onset at older age vs. those of older age with early onset. We, too, found that in our elderly population, in both the early-onset and late-onset groups, more than 50% required steroids, and 25% were started on 6-mercaptopurine because of chronicity and inability to stop steroids.[16]

SURGERY AND RECURRENCE

The reports on the need for surgical intervention in IBD in older age vary considerably.

Ulcerative Colitis

Contrary to the findings of most investigators, Brandt[1] noted that half of their elderly patients with ulcerative colitis failed medical therapy and required surgery. Numerous other reports describe a 7% to 16% incidence of surgical intervention in both their old and young patients.[12, 16, 17] Our study also noted low surgical rates in both the late-onset and early-onset groups (16% and 13%, respectively). The indication for surgery in those with early onset was more often carcinoma, and in those with late onset it was usually intractability or toxic megacolon.

Crohn's Disease

Reports in the literature concerning surgery in Crohn's disease and recurrence rates in the older age group are also unclear. The surgical incidence varies from most patients to less than half.[10-14, 16] Shapiro et al.[12] noted that 19 of 32 patients (58%) more than 60 years of age (with Crohn's disease diagnosed after the age of 60) required surgery. This included 10 of 11 (91%) with colitis, 2 of 4 (50%) with ileocolitis, and 7 of 8

(39%) with ileitis. Resection was the most common surgical procedure (17 of 19 patients) in their study. We found that the drainage of abscesses or fistulas was the most common surgical procedure in older age regardless of age at onset.[16]

There are no large reported series on recurrence in Crohn's disease after surgical resection in older age, and the several reports that have been published are contradictory.[11] Shapiro et al.[12] noted that in the patients with ileal disease the cumulative clinical recurrence rate at 9 years was 21% and at 15 years, 37%. Roberts et al.[10] reviewed the records of 50 patients with presenting symptoms of Crohn's disease after the age of 50 who had surgery. Eight of ten patients (80%) with ileocolitis had a recurrence, which the authors defined as recurrent symptoms with radiologic, endoscopic, or histologic confirmation; median time to the development of recurrence was 45.6 months (range 2.1 to 60.9 months). Thirty-eight percent of patients with ileal disease had a recurrence at a median time of 60.9 months (range 7.0 to 107.5 months) after initial resection. Of 26 patients with colitis only 17 had all obvious disease removed during resection. Of these, 6 had recurrent disease at a median time of 38.5 months (range 12.1 to 131.6 months). We have seen in the elderly, notably in those who had surgery after the age of 60, that recurrence defined by radiologic and histologic studies occurs both in those with early-onset and with late-onset Crohn's disease.

CONCLUSION

Reports from the 1960s indicated a poor prognosis for the elderly with IBD, but more recent studies suggest otherwise. Factors that are probably responsible for the improved statistics include, most importantly, a change in treatment modalities and emphasis on maintenance therapy.

In summary, the course of ulcerative colitis does not appear to differ in older age from younger age, nor does the age of onset significantly affect its course. Crohn's disease does not appear to "burn out" in older age, and may indeed have a more virulent course than in the young, especially in those with late onset of disease. Effort should be made to make an accurate diagnosis of IBD and its complications early, and aggressive treatment should follow; the most favorable outcome will result.

REFERENCES

1. Brandt LJ: Colitis in the elderly, in Bayless TM (ed): *Current Management of IBD*, Toronto, BC Decker, 1981.
2. Brandt LJ, et al: Colitis in the elderly, *Am J Gastroenterol* 1981; 76:239–245.
3. Brandt LJ, Boley SR, Mitsudo S: Clinical characteristics and natural history of colitis in the elderly. *Am J Gastroenterol* 1982; 77:382–386.
4. Brandt LJ, Dickstein G: Inflammatory bowel disease: Specific concerns in the elderly. *Geriatrics* 1989; 44:107–111.
5. Fabricus PJ, et al: Crohn's disease in the elderly. *Gut* 1985; 5:461–465.
6. Gupta S, et al: Is the pattern of IBD different in the elderly? *Age Aging* 1985; 6:366–370.
7. Harper PC, McAuliffe TL, Beeken WL: Crohn's disease in the elderly: A statistical comparison with younger patients matched for sex and duration of disease. *Arch Intern Med* 1986; 146:753–755.
8. Jones, HW, Hoare AM: Does ulcerative colitis behave differently in the elderly? *Age Aging* 1988; 6:410–414.
9. Mechjian HS, et al: Clinical features and natural history of Crohn's disease. *Gastroenterology* 1979; 77:898–906.
10. Roberts PL, et al: Clinical course of Crohn's disease in older patients. *Dis Colon Rectum* 1990; 33:458–462.
11. Rusch V, Simonowitz DA: Crohn's disease in the older patient. *Surg Gynecol Obstet* 1980; 150:184–186.
12. Shapiro PA, et al: IBD in the elderly. *Am J Gastroenterol* 1981; 76:132–137.
13. Softley A, et al: IBD in the elderly patient. *Scand J Gastroenterol* 1988; 144(suppl):27–30.
14. Stalnikowicz R, et al: Crohn's disease in the elderly. *J Clin Gastroenterol* 1989; 11:411–415.
15. Woolrich AJ, Korelitz BI: Ulcerative colitis in older age. *Am J Gastroenterol* 1988; 83:1060.
16. Woolrich AJ, Korelitz BI: Crohn's disease in older age. *Am J Gastroenterol* 1988; 83:1060.
17. Zimmerman J, Gavish D, Rachmilewitz D: Early and late onset ulcerative colitis: Distinct clinical features. *J Clin Gastroenterol* 1985; 7:492–498.

Chapter 5

Hepatic Complications of Inflammatory Bowel Disease

Albert B. Knapp

With regard to the liver and its association with inflammatory bowel disease (IBD), this chapter serves to dispel some myths, illustrate a few points, and then focus on two disease entities, namely, pericholangitis (PC) and primary sclerosing cholangitis (PSC).

Hepatic involvement in IBD is very common, with an incidence of approximately 10% of all affected patients in most large series. The rate of male to female patients is equal, and surprisingly the prevalence of hepatic involvement in Crohn's disease is equal to that of ulcerative colitis. IBD can affect the hepatic parenchyma, the hepatobiliary tree, or both. Pericholangitis, fatty liver, chronic hepatitis, primary biliary cirrhosis (PBC), cirrhosis, amyloidosis, and granulomatosis are the most common findings in parenchymal disease, while PSC, cholelithiasis, and cholangiocarcinoma are the major lesions of the hepatobiliary tree.

While not the most common pathologic entities associated with IBD, the two complications, one parenchymal (PC) and the other involving the hepatobiliary tree (PSC), are the most specifically identified. PC is defined pathologically as a chronic but limited portal tract inflammation usually relegated to the small bile ducts. There is an increased prevalence of PSC involved with PC, and this relationship will be explored later. The most important issue regarding PC is that it is a benign finding. It may "burn out," it may progress a bit, but only a minority of patients develop cirrhosis.

What causes PC? Possibilities include biliary infection, a change in bile acid composition with more lithocholic acid, the presence of endotoxins, and autoimmunity. None of these putative agents has been proved. The bulk of cases require no therapy after diagnosis. Occasionally an "anecdotal case" is treated with long-term antibiotics or even steroids, usually to no avail.

PSC is the most common biliary tree disease affecting patients with IBD. This is a slowly progressive disorder of unknown cause that may result in obstruction, biliary cirrhosis, and hepatic failure. Several controversies remain. First, is there true intrahepatic duct involvement? The classic definition of PSC is that of extrahepatic duct involvement, but during the past few years investigators have begun to accept sole or concomitant intrahepatic duct involvement as being true of PSC.

PSC is associated with other underlying diseases. About 1% to 4% of patients with ulcerative colitis have concomitant PSC. If one poses the question differently and studies the association of PSC and ulcerative colitis, about 50% to 75% of all patients with PSC have associated ulcerative colitis, or, in a few cases, Crohn's disease. Looking at this from either side, there is an intimate association between ulcerative colitis and PSC.*

What determines survival in PSC? First, age is very important in that the younger the patient, the better the prognosis. Second, a bilirubin level of 6 mg/dL or greater is ominous and should suggest prompt therapy. Third, the patient's hemoglobin level is an important factor, because anemia is an ominous sign. Fourth, the presence of concomitant IBD is a bad sign. Finally, an important prognostic parameter is the liver biopsy. If cirrhosis is documented, eventual orthotopic liver transplantation is the therapeutic method of choice.

The pathophysiology of PSC is quite interesting. For a while there was great interest in the fact that it could have been a virally induced or viral-associated disease. When pregnant mice were infected with reovirus 3, a condition similar to PSC developed in their offspring. This has not been documented in human beings in whom reovirus titers have been obtained, and there is no greater prevalence of positive findings in people with the disease compared with control subjects.

Genetics may play an important role in the development of PSC. There seems to be an intimate link between HLA-B8 and HLA-DR3 with PSC. The problem is that two HLA types are extremely common and cannot be used as diagnostic tools.

Finally, do immunologic factors play a role? Many researchers say "Yes," but the evidence is lacking.

A very interesting idea raised by the oncologists is that PSC is a vasculitis that may lead to destruction of the biliary tree, with resultant sclerosis and eventual secondary biliary cirrhosis. With intra-arterial 5-

*Editor's Note: See Chapter 2 (p. 9). The majority of patients with PSC tested positive for ANCA.

fluorouridine, a picture identical to PSC can be produced in some patients via a severe arteriolitis.

The diagnosis of PSC is prompted by clinical suspicion and by the use of either endoscopic retrograde cholangiopancreatography (ERCP) or transhepatic cholangiography (THC). ERCP is preferred, but if the patient cannot be cannulated, THC should be used. The main reason for doing this is to rule out cholangiocarcinoma. This tumor can complicate up to 10% to 15% of all cases of PSC.

Many modalities of PSC therapy have been tried, but nothing seems to work except orthotopic liver transplantation. Penicillamine showed promise; recent trials have proved it to be ineffective, and it is now out of favor. Colchicine was also used and discarded. Most recently trials with cyclosporine are underway, but preliminary data are not encouraging. Orthotopic liver transplantation has become the major tool in the management of this disease. The timing for operation is the key and is beyond the scope of this chapter. Occasionally ERCP- or THC-mediated dilatation of isolated ductal structures can be useful, but this is the exception rather than the rule.

Is there a pathophysiologic relationship between PC and PSC? Many pathologists now seem to think there is. They believe that PC has the same morphologic features as PSC, and some will even call PC the "PSC of the small bile duct."

In summary, the liver and the hepatobiliary tree are affected in many places and by many lesions. Ten percent of all patients with IBD have liver involvement, and PC and PSC have emerged as the two most important entities. Further research will clarify their actual pathophysiology, and may show them to be two facets of the same disease.

SUGGESTED READING

1. Helzberg JH, Peterson JM, Boyer JL: Improved survival in primary sclerosing cholangitis: A review of clinicopathological features and comparison of symptomatic and asymptomatic patients. *Gastroenterology* 1987; 92:1869–1879.
2. LaRusso NF. Wiesner RH, Ludwig J, et al: Primary sclerosing Cholangitis. *N Engl J Med* 1984; 310:899–902.
3. Wee A, Ludwig J: Pericholangitis in chronic ulcerative colitis: Primary sclerosing cholangitis of the small bile ducts? *Ann Intern Med* 1985; 102:581–585.
4. Wiesner RH, Grambach PM, Dickson ER, et al: Primary sclerosing cholangitis: Natural history, prognostic factors and survival analysis. *Hepatology* 1989; 10:430–436.

Pregnancy, Fertility, and Contraception in Inflammatory Bowel Disease

Daniel Adler

Estimates of the prevalence of inflammatory bowel disease (IBD) in the United States range between one and two million people. Twenty thousand to 25,000 new cases are diagnosed each year.[19] Because ulcerative colitis and Crohn's disease are predominantly diseases of young persons, with the peak prevalence in the 15- to 30-year-old age group for Crohn's disease and 20- to 35-year-old for ulcerative colitis, both diseases coincide with the most fruitful childbearing years. This concerns both men and women.

For the male patient with IBD, issues regarding fertility arise. These concern the natural course of disease, its medical and surgical treatment, and safety of drug therapy regarding potential damage to the sperm and teratogenicity. For the female patient additional concerns include the effects of the gestational period on the IBD, and vice versa, and the effects on the developing fetus of medications that cross the placenta or the effect of those carried by breast milk on the newborn.

Much of the data available regarding pregnancy in the IBD patient were based on studies and observations from the 1940s and 1950s before the advent of the medical armamentarium with which we now treat these diseases. Although some more recent studies have served to supplement these early observations, many questions still remain unanswered. Earlier reviews of our knowledge on relationships between IBD and pregnancy have been reported.[20, 21]

FERTILITY IN WOMEN

Women with ulcerative colitis were thought to be relatively less fertile compared with the general population.[11, 25] When adjusted for patient age and desire for pregnancy, however, their fertility rate is probably normal.[40] The situation with Crohn's disease, however, is different; fertility is reduced in proportion to Crohn's disease activity, and can be reversed when appropriate drug therapy results in remission. Furthermore, the ovaries and fallopian tubes may be involved in the inflammatory process, especially on the right side because of their proximity to the terminal ileum.[13] One study concluded that fertility is less with colon involvement compared with ileal involvement.[13] Perhaps this relates to the higher prevalence of perianal, perineal, and rectovaginal abscesses and fistulas seen in this distribution, and its resulting poor hygiene, dyspareunia, and decreased libido, either for the patient or her husband. The overall toxicity of Crohn's disease, with its attendant fever, abdominal pain, diarrhea, and suboptimal nutrition, has also been implicated.[18]

Although far more difficult to quantify, we believe that fear of pregnancy is also a major factor reducing fertility in young women with Crohn's disease. This fear has been introduced by the obstetrician or the gastroenterologist by warning the patient that outcome of either the course of the IBD or the condition of the fetus may be unfavorable.

FERTILITY IN MEN

Infertility in men due to sulfasalazine therapy is well documented.[4] Within 2 months of beginning the drug, sperm counts may decrease, abnormal sperm morphology with ballooned, pale-staining head structures may appear, and motility may be reduced.[36] Some or all of these abnormalities appear in 64% of all male patients so treated. Beginning 2 months after withdrawal of the drug, however, there is improvement in semen quality satisfactory for impregnation.[37]

If and when pregnancy becomes a priority for the male patient, withdrawal of the sulfasalazine can result in clinical compromise if a less effective drug must be substituted. The managing gastroenterologist must share with the patient the concerns for using this drug as well as its withdrawal. This problem has now been markedly reduced by the availability of oral aminosalicylic acid (5-ASA), the effective split product of sulfasalazine, which does not cause any damage to the sperm.

After total proctocolectomy in men, neurogenic impotence has been reported; fortunately it is a rare complication of this procedure.[23, 27] To date no studies have examined the issue of infertility directly attributable to Crohn's disease or ulcerative colitis in men.

CONTRACEPTION AND INFLAMMATORY BOWEL DISEASE

Two recent studies examined the absorption and bioavailability of oral contraceptives in patients with ulcerative colitis who had undergone proctocolectomy and ileostomy. The first study examined the serum concentrations of ethinyl estradiol and levonorgestrel after oral administration.[15] The mean serum concentrations in these patients were equivalent to those in a noncolitis control group. A second study examined plasma concentrations of 1-levonorgestrel in colitis patients before and after colectomy and found that the postoperative patients had a slight decrease in serum levels that was statistically significant when compared with control subjects.[29] This suggests that in patients with active colitis or an ileostomy, oral contraceptives can be relied upon, but low-dose "mini-pills" are not dependable.

Two epidemiologic studies have observed the association between oral contraceptives and IBD. A significantly excessive number of women with Crohn's disease of the colon were observed to be taking oral contraceptives in the year before the onset of symptoms.[33] A second study found nearly twice the incidence of both Crohn's disease and ulcerative colitis in women who used oral contraceptives compared with nonusers.[38] No etiologic or pathophysiologic mechanism has yet been revealed to explain these observations.

In contrast to the preceding, a recent study from the University of Chicago Medical Center analyzed, with use of case-matched control techniques, 48 women with ulcerative colitis who were taking oral contraceptives.[24] No association between current or former use of oral contraceptives was found.

MacDougall [21] believed that women need not be advised to discontinue birth control pills when ulcerative colitis is diagnosed. It is our own conviction that patients with IBD should avoid oral contraceptives until their exact influence on normal and diseased bowel is understood.

RISK OF OFFSPRING DEVELOPING INFLAMMATORY BOWEL DISEASE

Both male and female patients with IBD wish to know the chances of having a child who will eventually develop IBD. For Crohn's disease,

30% of patients have at least one blood relative who also has Crohn's disease or (less often) ulcerative colitis. About 20% of patients with ulcerative colitis have blood relatives with that disease. Most gastroenterologists accept the polygenic theory that more genes are likely to lead to Crohn's disease and less genes to ulcerative colitis. Familial groupings have been documented among Jews. The most common relationships have been father-daughter, father-son, brother-sister, and first cousins. Farmer et al.,[12] at the Cleveland Clinic, found that 35% of patients with Crohn's disease and 29% of those with ulcerative colitis had a family history of IBD. Despite these observations, geneticists have not been willing to establish Crohn's disease or ulcerative colitis as inheritable diseases. In giving advice to patients, the preceding statistics and a polygenic type of influence with varying degrees of penetration should be acknowledged.

INFLUENCE OF INFLAMMATORY BOWEL DISEASE ON PREGNANCY AND FETAL OUTCOME

Many studies have examined the effects of ulcerative colitis on pregnancy and the fetus. The largest series examining more than 100 patients have reported normal healthy offspring in 76% to 97%, congenital abnormalities in 0% to 3%, spontaneous abortions in 1% to 13%, and stillbirths in 0% to 3%.[4, 6, 7, 19–23] Each of these figures approximates that of the normal population. Among the most recent data, Baiocco and Korelitz[3] reported that 83% of mothers with ulcerative colitis delivered normal healthy newborns. Premature delivery was seen in 2.5%, spontaneous abortion in 12%, and no stillbirths or congenital abnormalities were observed. Porter and Stirrat[31] found that the birth weights of babies born to mothers with ulcerative colitis were lower than normal, but this did not achieve statistical significance. In addition, the presence of ulcerative colitis did not affect mode of delivery (vaginal vs. cesarean section or spontaneous vs. forceps) or the incidence of preeclampsia/eclampsia during the gestational period.

Fewer large studies exist that focus on the pregnant patient with Crohn's disease. The two involving more than 100 cases reportedly show congenital abnormalities in 0% to 1%, stillbirths in 1% to 4%, and spontaneous abortion in 3% to 9%, respectively, all approximating that of the non-IBD population.[26, 28] In one study involving 38 pregnancies among 30 women, there was a statistically significant decrease in infant birth weights (lower tenth percentile) among the Crohn's disease group compared with the control group.[4]

Baiocco and Korelitz[3] found that, among patients with Crohn's disease whose pregnancies resulted in developmental defects, stillbirth, or spontaneous abortion, active disease was present in 62%. Most of these patients were on one or more medications to control symptoms (most commonly corticosteroids or sulfasalazine), but case analysis revealed that **disease activity** and not the drug treatment was responsible for the increase in complications.

The influence on the pregnancy of drug therapy used in the treatment of IBD must also be considered. Most drugs commonly employed in treatment of the IBD in a pregnant patient are the same as used for treatment of the disease in the patient who is not pregnant; these drugs include corticosteroids, sulfasalazine and its derivative, 5-ASA, and antibiotics.

The sulfonamides have generally been safe medications during all stages of pregnancy and lactation. These medications will cross the placenta and can displace unconjugated bilirubin from albumin, inducing a theoretic risk of drug-induced neonatal jaundice and kernicterus. No study to date has shown this to occur in patients receiving sulfasalazine, however. Sulfasalazine reaches the breast milk at a level equal to 45% of the maternal serum. Neither sulfasalazine nor either of its split products, sulfapyridine or 5-ASA, has been shown to cause harm to the neonate.[16]

Animal studies involving corticosteroids have demonstrated increased spontaneous abortion rates, reduced DNA synthesis, decreased litter size, and increased stillbirths, all possibly due to placental hypoxia.[5, 9, 14] Studies in human beings, however, have failed to demonstrate any deleterious effect.[3, 26]

All antibiotics have been found in breast milk. Tetracycline, when taken by pregnant women, will cause cataracts, can retard skeletal growth and induce fatty necrosis of the liver, and can cause pancreatitis and renal damage. Metronidazole has been shown to be mildly fetotoxic and teratogenic in mice; it may cause carcinomas of the lung, breast, liver, and lymphatic system in animals on long-term treatment. The relevance of these studies to the human patient with IBD has not been clinically determined.

Immunosuppressive therapy with either azathioprine or 6-mercaptopurine is being used with increasing frequency in refractory patients with Crohn's disease and ulcerative colitis. Therapeutic advantages include its ability to induce remission and eliminate steroids in both groups.[1, 32] Experimental studies have implicated these agents in causing low birth weights and congenital abnormalities.[34, 35] Among human renal transplant recipients taking azathioprine (at higher doses than commonly used in IBD), however, birth defects were reported in 7 of 103 births.[8] This question has been insufficiently studied in the patient with IBD. Recently, however, a study of 16 pregnancies in 14 women was reported in patients with IBD treated with azathioprine. A single case of infectious hepatitis B was the only reported complication. No congenital abnormalities or subsequent health problems were reported in the offspring.[2]

Because of the lack of Food and Drug Administration (FDA) approval for using immunosuppressive drugs in patients with IBD and because of the current litigious atmosphere in which we practice, most authors have not used these drugs during pregnancy. We have recommended conscientious birth control for couples when either is taking 6-mercaptopurine. We then recommend waiting 3 months after no longer taking the drug before attempting conception. We also suggest therapeutic abortion if accidental conception occurs while taking the drug.*

EFFECT OF PREGNANCY ON INFLAMMATORY BOWEL DISEASE

In the 1940s and 1950s it was thought that patients with ulcerative colitis had a high risk of exacerbation with pregnancy and that the likelihood of controlling the exacerbation was poor. DeDombal et al.,[11] in 1965, studied 80 patients whose disease was inactive at the time of conception. They found a 34% recurrence rate during a 1-year period beginning with conception. Two other studies have subsequently confirmed an exacerbations rate of 30% and 35%, respectively.[26, 40] These statistics are all similar to a group of nonpregnant patients observed for 12 months. In the largest study to date (55 pregnancies) on the course of active ulcerative colitis during pregnancy, Willoughby and Truelove[40] found that 40% improved, 27% showed no change, and 33% worsened. Therefore, about three of four patients with active disease at conception will continue to have active disease throughout their pregnancy.

Patients who had undergone total proctocolectomy with ileostomy are quite capable of pregnancy and the delivery of healthy children. DeDombal et al.[11] reported six pregnancies in twenty-nine of these patients, with all six women delivering healthy full-term infants, five by the vaginal route and one via cesarean section. Prolapse of the ileal stoma has been a complication reported in two patients in a series of nine deliveries in five patients; all delivered full-term healthy infants.[24]

To date there are little available data on pregnancy in patients who have had subtotal colectomies with either ileoanal anastomosis or a

*Editor's note: The results of the study cited in reference 2 led Lennard-Jones and his colleagues to suggest that azathioprine need not be stopped during pregnancy.

Kock pouch. Eighty-four percent to 90% of female patients who underwent such procedures reported a postoperative increase in frequency of intercourse, mostly attributable to improved general health.[39] Improved self-image resulting from elimination of the external appliance was also reported in about 10% of women after conversion from an ileostomy to a pouch. Both types of procedures also led to a decreased prevalence of dyspareunia, less so in patients with the Kock pouch than in those with the ileoanal pouch anastomosis. Approximately 80% of patients who underwent these procedures have been able to conceive. All have delivered healthy offspring with vaginal or cesarean delivery rated comparable to that of the non-IBD population.[39]

Fewer studies involving patients with Crohn's disease are available for analysis. The two most recent studies of Khosla et al.[18] and Neilson et al.[28] involve 52 and 57 pregnancies showing a 15% and 39% relapse rate, respectively, during pregnancy for those patients in remission at the time of conception. This is again not markedly different from the experience with the nonpregnant population with Crohn's disease.[10] These two studies also conclude that for the patients with Crohn's disease whose disease is active at the time of conception, one-third will improve, one-third will deteriorate, and one-third will remain unchanged.

DeDombal et al.[11] have reported a 50% relapse rate within 3 months after the postpartum period. It is postulated that falling endogenous cortisol levels are responsible for this, but psychologic factors, including postpartum depression, have also been implicated. This high postpartum relapse rate has not been substantiated in subsequent studies.

In some cases ulcerative colitis may be diagnosed for the first time during pregnancy. Early studies reported a poor prognosis for these patients.[10, 29] More recently, however, it had been demonstrated that the outcome need not be any worse than in the patient for whom the diagnosis was previously established. Crohn's disease diagnosed for the first time during pregnancy has also been reported. The prevalence is less than that of ulcerative colitis. This type of presentation is also thought to carry a poor prognosis, but these observations have not been substantiated more recently.[13, 20, 30]

MANAGEMENT OF INFLAMMATORY BOWEL DISEASE DURING PREGNANCY

For both Crohn's disease and ulcerative colitis, if the disease is inactive at the time of conception it is likely to remain inactive, and if active at the time of conception it is likely to remain active. Surgical intervention is appropriate for unequivocal indications such as severe hemorrhage, perforation, and megacolon refractory to medical therapy and nonoperative decompression. It must be appreciated, however, that total colectomy and ileostomy, with attendant manipulation of the uterus at the time of surgery, carry a 60% risk of postoperative spontaneous abortion.[26] It therefore behooves the clinician to attempt aggressive medical management of the patient with IBD to induce remission before or in the early stages of pregnancy.

As mentioned, sulfasalazine, its 5-ASA derivatives, and corticosteroids can be used during pregnancy if clinically warranted. Antibiotics, especially metronidazole, should probably be avoided if possible, particularly in the first trimester, and immunosuppressive drugs should not be used at all starting 3 months before conception. Needless radiographic studies, subjecting the pregnant patient to small but finite doses of radiation, should be avoided; if needed to contribute to important therapeutic decisions, they should not be withheld. Theoretically there is little danger to be expected from diagnostic radiation in the second and third trimesters.

Cesarean section may be the preferred route of delivery for the patient with perianal Crohn's disease, thus avoiding the possibility of involving the episiotomy scar in the fistulous tracts.

General supportive measures, such as control of diarrhea and perinatal vitamin supplements, may be used. The use of total parenteral nutrition in the pregnant patient with IBD has not been studied. It should be reserved at this time for indications similar to those in the nonpregnant patient.

Narcotic analgesics relieve the pain of abdominal cramping and decrease intestinal motility; therefore they decrease diarrhea and impart a sense of well-being and euphoria. The potential for narcotics addiction in the pregnant patient with symptomatic IBD is as real as in the nonpregnant patient, with the added risk of opiate dependence and withdrawal in the newborn. If the underlying bowel disease is treated aggressively and the specific cause of pain is diagnosed and dealt with, the long-term use of narcotic analgesics will not be necessary.[17]

CONCLUSIONS AND RECOMMENDATIONS

IBD is not a contraindication to pregnancy. Sharing legitimate concerns with the patient and the spouse about the variability of IBD and use of drug therapy during the gestational period should be done. Infertility with active Crohn's disease warrants aggressive medical management in the female patient. When infertility is an issue, and the male patient has been taking sulfasalazine, sperm analysis to confirm the source of the problem should be performed before discontinuing the drug, with its attendant risk of exacerbation. An alternative would be to substitute 5-ASA for the sulfasalazine because this drug has been shown to be similarly effective for maintenance of remission without causing damage to the sperm. Sulfasalazine and corticosteroids are safe to use during pregnancy and the postpartum period. Finally, if the IBD is in the active form, we advise patients to delay pregnancy, allowing time for adequate treatment.

REFERENCES

1. Adler DJ, Korelitz BI: The therapeutic efficacy of 6-MP in refractory ulcerative colitis. *Am J Gastroenterol* 1989; 85:717–722.
2. Alstead EM, Ritchie JK, Lennard-Jones JE, et al: Safety of azathioprine in pregnancy in IBD. *Gastroenterology* 1990; 99:443–446.
3. Baiocco PJ, Korelitz BI: The influence of IBD and its treatment on pregnancy and fetal outcome. *J Clin Gastroenterol* 1984; 6:211–216.
4. Birnie GG, McLeod TF, Watkinson G: Incidence of sulfasalazine-induced male infertility. *Gut* 1981; 22:452–455.
5. Blackburn WR, Kaplan HS, McKay DG: Morphologic changes in the developing rat placenta following prednisone administration. *Am J Obstet Gynecol* 1965; 92:235–246.
6. Crohn BB, Yarnis H, Crohn EB, et al: Ulcerative colitis and pregnancy. *Gastroenterology* 1956; 30:391–403.
7. Crohn BB, Yarnis H, Korelitz BI: Regional ileitis and pregnancy. *Gastroenterology* 1956; 31:615.
8. Davidson JM, Lindheimer MD: Pregnancy in women with renal allografts. *Semin Nephrol* 1984; 4:234–251.
9. DeCosta EJ, Abelman MA: Cortisone and pregnancy: An experimental and clinical study of the effects of cortisone on gestation. *Am J Obstet Gynecol* 1952; 64:746–767.
10. DeDombal FT, Burton IL, Goligher JC: Crohn's disease and pregnancy. *Br Med J* 1972; 3:550.
11. DeDombal FT, Watts JM, Watkinson G, et al: Ulcerative colitis and pregnancy. *Lancet* 1965; 2:599–602.
12. Farmer RG, Michner WM, Mortimer EA: Studies of family history among patients with IBD. *Clin Gastroenterol* 1980; 9:271–288.
13. Fielding JF, Cooke WT: Pregnancy and Crohn's disease. *Br Med J* 1970; 2:76–77.

14. Fraser FC, Fainstat TD: Production of congenital defects in the offspring of pregnant mice treated with cortisone. *Pediatrics* 1951; 8:527–533.
15. Grimmer SF, Black DJ, Orme ML, et al: The bioavailability of ethinyloestradiol and levonorgestrel in patients with an ileostomy. *Contraception* 1986; 33:151–159.
16. Kahn AKA, Truelove SC: Placental and mammary transfer of sulphasalazine. *Br Med J* 1979; 2:1553.
17. Kaplan MA, Korelitz BI: Narcotic dependence in IBD. *J Clin Gastroenterol* 1988; 10:275–278.
18. Khosla R, Willoughby CP, Jewell DP: Crohn's disease and pregnancy. *Gut* 1984; 25:52–56.
19. Kirsner JB, Shorter RG: Recent developments in nonspecific IBD. *N Engl J Med* 1982; 306:837–848.
20. Korelitz BI: Pregnancy, fertility and IBD. *Am J Gastroenterol* 1985; 80:365–370.
21. Korelitz BI: Fertility and pregnancy in IBD, in Kirsner JB, Shorter RG (ed): *Inflammatory Bowel Disease.* Philadelphia, Lea & Febiger, 1988.
22. Lashner BA, Kane SV, Hanauer SB: Lack of association between oral contraceptive use and ulcerative colitis. *Gastroenterology* 1990; (Part 2): A184.
23. Lee ECG, Dowling BL: Perimuscular excision of the rectum for Crohn's disease and ulcerative colitis. *Br J Surg,* 1971; 59:29.
24. MacDougall I: Ulcerative colitis and pregnancy. *Lancet* 1956; 2:641–643.
25. Metcalf AM, Dozios RR, Kelly KA: Sexual function in women after proctocolectomy. *Ann Surg* 1986; 204:624–627.
26. Mogadam M, Dobbins WO, Korelitz BI, et al: Pregnancy and IBD; Effect of sulfasalazine and corticosteroids on fetal outcome. *Gastroenterology* 1981; 80:75–76.
27. Morowitz DA, Kirsner JB: Ileostomy in ulcerative colitis. *Am J Surg* 1981; 141:370–375.
28. Neilsen OH, Andreasson B, Bondesen S, et al: Pregnancy in ulcerative colitis. *Scand J Gastroenterol* 1983; 18:735–742.
29. Nilsson LO, Victor A, Kral JG, et al: Absorption of an oral contraceptive gestagen in ulcerative colitis before and after proctocolectomy and construction of a continent ileostomy. *Contraception* 1985; 31:195–204.
30. Norton RA, Patterson JF: Pregnancy and regional ileitis. *Obstet Gynecol* 1972; 40:711–712.
31. Porter RJ, Stirrat GM: The effects of IBD on pregnancy: A case-controlled retrospective analysis. *Br J Obstet Gynecol* 1986; 93:1124–1131.
32. Present DH, Korelitz BI, Wisch N, et al: Treatment of Crohn's disease with 6-MP. A long term, randomized, double blind study. *N Engl J Med* 1980; 302:981–987.
33. Rhodes JM, Cockel R, Allen RN, et al: Colonic Crohn's disease and use of oral contraception. *Br Med J* 1984; 288:595–596.
34. Rosekranz JC, Githens JH: Azathioprine (Imuran) and pregnancy. *Am J Obstet Gynecol* 1967; 97:387–394.

35. Scott RJ: Fetal growth retardation associated with maternal administration of immunosuppressive drugs. *Am J Obstet Gynecol* 1977; 128:676–686.
36. Toovey S, Hudson E, Hendry WF, et al: Sulfasalazine and male infertility: Reversibility and possible mechanism. *Gut* 1981; 22:445–451.
37. Toth A: Reversible toxic effects of salicylazosulfapyridine on semen quality. *Fertil Steril* 1979; 31:538–540.
38. Vessey M, Jewell DE, Smith A: Chronic IBD, cigarette smoking and use of oral contraceptives: Findings in a large cohort study of women of child-bearing age. *Br Med J* 1986; 292:1101–1103.
39. Webb MJ, Sedlack RE: Ulcerative colitis in pregnancy. *Med Clin North Am* 1974; 58:823.
40. Willoughby CP, Truelove SC: Ulcerative colitis and pregnancy. *Gut,* 1980; 21:469–474.

Nonsteroidal Anti-inflammatory Drugs and Inflammatory Bowel Disease

Robert A. Mendelsohn

It has now been generally accepted that the group of agents known as the nonsteroidal anti-inflammatory drugs (NSAIDs) have deleterious effects on the upper gastrointestinal tract, predisposing patients to conditions ranging from mild gastritis to multiple ulcerations and even life-threatening hemorrhage.[1] In recent years there have been an increasing number of case reports demonstrating the deleterious effects of these agents on the colonic mucosa.[4, 5, 8, 13, 15, 16, 21, 25] These lower gastrointestinal effects are less well known, and the effects of NSAIDs on the colonic mucosa of patients with inflammatory bowel disease (IBD) are just beginning to be recognized.

This chapter reviews the entity of NSAID-induced colitis and recent developments in the relationship of the nonsteroidal agents and IBD.

HISTORICAL PERSPECTIVE

In 1966 Debenham[5] first reported a 32-year-old female patient who, while being treated with oxyphenbutazone for postpartum pain, developed severe right lower quadrant pain and abdominal fullness resulting from a ruptured viscus. Subsequent laparotomy revealed a 1 cm punched-out ulcer in the cecum. The histologic specimen was unusual in that it failed to show signs of inflammation. Levy and Gaspar,[14] in 1975, reported a case of rectal bleeding associated with the use of indomethacin suppositories. Subsequently they were able to demonstrate that the rectal involvement and activity were dose related to the indomethacin.

These two reports were the initial reports implicating the nonsteroidal drugs as a cause of colonic damage. In the years after these initial reports, many others have been able to document NSAID-induced colitis and have begun to define the effects of these agents on the colonic mucosa.

ARACHIDONIC ACID METABOLISM

The mechanism of action of NSAID-induced colitis requires understanding the metabolism of arachidonic acid and its role in colonic mucosal physiology.

The metabolic pathways of arachidonic acid metabolism are shown in Figure 7–1. The colon contains membrane phospholipids that are

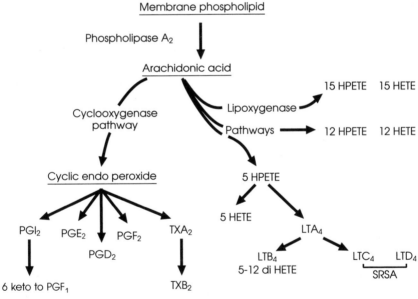

FIG 7–1.
Arachidonic acid metabolism. (Phospholipase A_2 probably is one of several lipases catalysing release of arachidonic acid from membrane phospholipid). *PG* = prostaglandin, *TX* = thromboxane, *LT* = leukotriene, *HPETE* = hydroperoxyeicosatetraenoic acid, *HETE* = hydroxyeicosatetraenoic acid, *SRSA* = slow releasing substance of anaphylaxis. (From Rampton DS, Hawkey CJ: *Gut* 1984; 25:1399–1413. Used by permission.)

catalyzed by phospholipase to arachidonic acid. This is further metabolized via the cyclooxygenase pathway to several prostaglandin compounds. The NSAIDs act by inhibiting cyclooxygenase and thereby preventing the formation of the prostaglandins. The other major metabolic pathway in arachidonic acid metabolism is the lipoxygenase pathway, which results in the formation of several compounds. Most important of these compounds are the leukotrienes. The leukotrienes themselves, namely, LTB_4, have been shown to be active mediators in many inflammatory processes. These important end products of arachidonic acid metabolism are referred to collectively as the eicosanoids. The interrelationship of these pathways and their end products is an important factor in elucidating the cause of NSAID-induced colitis.

ROLE OF PROSTAGLANDINS IN THE COLON

The normal colonic mucus contains arachidonic acid and can synthesize prostaglandin I_2, prostaglandin D_2, prostaglandin F_2, thromboxane B_2, and 12-HETE (12-hydroxy-6,8,11,14-eicosatetraenoic acid; eicosanoids). Eicosanoids have previously been shown to have a protective role in maintaining mucosal integrity in the stomach and duodenum.[1] In the colon, however, there are conflicting reports in the literature. There are several animal studies showing that the eicosanoids can reduce the deleterious effects on the colon by agents such as alcohol or clindamycin.[6, 11, 22]

In contrast, there have been both in vitro and in vivo studies showing that eicosanoids can produce a syndrome that mimics the signs and symptoms of ulcerative colitis.[8, 17, 24] A recent report by Kornbluth et al.[13] demonstrates an exacerbation of Crohn's disease in a patient taking the prostaglandin analog misoprostol. To explain these seemingly contradictory findings, two hypotheses have been proposed. One is that the enhanced production of eicosanoids is actually beneficial in active inflammatory processes. For example, prostaglandin E_2, prostaglandin E_1, prostaglandin A, and HETE have been found both in vitro and in vivo to inhibit the absorption of colonic water and electrolytes as well as to increase colonic secretory activity. These actions produce diarrhea, reducing transit time, which in turn reduces the time toxins are in contact with the colonic mucosa, thereby protecting mucosal integrity. Another explanation is that the increased production of eicosanoids during the inflammatory process is a consequence of the inflammation rather than its cause, and what is seen is simply an epiphenomenon. These two hypothetic considerations help explain why some observers have found the eicosanoids to be a causative factor and others a protective factor.

EVIDENCE IMPLICATING NONSTEROIDAL ANTI-INFLAMMATORY DRUGS IN COLONIC DISEASE

Anecdotal Reports

Hall et al.[9] and Phillips et al.[16] reported independently the association of enteritis and colitis in patients using mefenamic acid. Kaufmann and Taubin[12] reported a case of sigmoiditis after the patient was treated with the nonsteroidal agent piroxicam. Rampton[18] reported the relapse of proctocolitis in patients with ulcerative colitis after they were treated with ibuprofen.

Timing and Recurrence as Implicating Factors

The evidence in implicating NSAIDs in colonic disease is mostly through anecdotal reports, animal studies, and a few human transport studies. Bravo and Lowman[3] first reported NSAIDs associated with sigmoid ulcers, which recurred with drug rechallenge. Tanner and Raghunath,[26] in a study of 43 patients with colitis, found 4 patients with NSAID-induced colitis, all temporally related to drug usage and all with rapid resolution after the drug was withdrawn. Day[4] showed a physical association for evidence of NSAID-induced colitis by describing two patients on a slow-release formulation of indomethacin who developed colonic ulcers and frank perforations. At surgery the indomethacin capsules were found at the site of the ulcerations.

Human Intestinal Transport Studies

Bjarnason et al.[2] compared patients with irritable bowel syndrome, those with rheumatoid arthritis not treated with NSAIDs, and those with rheumatoid arthritis treated with NSAIDs. They showed increased uptake of indium 111 in the area corresponding to the terminal ileum only in the group of patients treated with NSAIDs. There was also a significant delay in the fecal excretion of the indium 111 in the NSAID-treated group. A similar pattern is found in those patients with Crohn's disease.

CAUSE OF NSAID-INDUCED COLITIS

Two possible etiologic factors have been proposed in NSAID-induced colitis. First, NSAIDs, by blocking the cyclooxygenase pathway, decrease prostaglandin production and therefore may disrupt this cytoprotective mucosal barrier that the prostaglandins provide. This appears to be their mechanism of action in the upper gastrointestinal tract. An alternative theory is that by blocking the cyclooxygenase pathway, arachidonic acid is preferentially metabolized via the lipoxygenase pathway, forming an abundance of the leukotrienes. The leukotrienes have been shown to have deleterious effects on colonic mucosa.[23] Either or both, or a still undefined mechanism, can account for NSAID-induced colitis. Studies of leukotriene inhibitors have not been able to show evidence that the leukotrienes are the offending agents, but further studies in this area are needed.[10]

NSAID EFFECTS IN INFLAMMATORY BOWEL DISEASE

Rampton and Sladen,[20] in 1981, reported four patients with known inactive ulcerative proctocolitis in whom, after the administration of NSAIDs, a rapid relapse developed. Rampton et al,[19] were later able to document reversible relapses of the proctocolitis in one patient upon subsequent treatment with NSAIDs. Kaufmann and Taubin[12] found similar results in patients with inflammatory bowel disease (IBD) in a quiescent phase who, when treated with NSAIDs, had exacerbations. Foster et al.[7] also found an association between relapse of proctosigmoiditis and the use of NSAID agents, but were not able to demonstrate statistical significance when compared with a control group. The mechanism of NSAID effects on IBD has not yet been worked out, but it is probably by the same mechanisms proposed in NSAID-induced colitis, as we have discussed previously.

NSAID USE IN INFLAMMATORY BOWEL DISEASE

The extraintestinal manifestations of IBD are numerous, and include arthritis, ankylosing spondylitis, and biliary tract disease.

In addition, many patients have side effects from the medications used in the treatment of IBD. These include headaches from sulfasalazine use and multiple side effects (including arthralgias, myalgias, and edema) from the use of steroids. The NSAID agents are often utilized to treat the preceding symptoms, not recognizing that these agents may indeed exacerbate the underlying bowel disease. The arthritides of IBD, which often express themselves during a flare-up, should not be treated with NSAID agents. Instead, the underlying bowel disease should be treated aggressively, and the arthritic component will usually resolve with control of the bowel disease. Those patients whose arthritic component is out of proportion to their bowel disease can be cautiously treated with an NSAID agent after a failed trial of other analgesic agents (such as acetaminophen) that are not associated with colitis. It must be kept in mind, however, that this treatment could result in a flare-up of apparently quiescent bowel disease. The issue becomes a matter of priorities and often warrants a patient-physician partnership decision.

Those patients with osteoarthritis or rheumatoid arthritis and IBD pose a difficult dilemma. If the patient can be treated without an exacerbation of bowel disease, cautious use of the NSAID agents for incapacitating arthritic pain can be attempted. If the bowel effects from the nonsteroidal agents are seen, however, it would be prudent to use other analgesic agents or to try to taper the NSAIDs to a lower, better-tolerated dose, because it appears that their effects on the bowel are dose dependent.[19, 25] The use of very low dose NSAID agents in combination with other analgesic agents may prove beneficial. Alternative agents, such as gold, may have a role, but caution here must also be observed because gold itself has been rarely implicated as causing colitis.[27]

CONCLUSIONS

Prostaglandins have a role not only in the protection of gastric mucosa but also in the maintenance of colonic mucosa. The prostaglandins also have some role in IBD, although this is not yet well defined.

The NSAID agents definitely can cause a form of colitis. Their mechanism of action is probably the same as that in NSAID-induced gastritis, by depleting mucosal prostaglandins and their cytoprotective effects, or by increasing the mucosal levels of the leukotrienes, thereby amplifying their detrimental effects. The treatment of NSAID-induced colitis is threefold:

1. Discontinuation of the offending agent is paramount.
2. The use of sulfasalazine either orally or in the form of 5-ASA enemas may be effective for the arthritis as well as the colitis.
3. If the colitis is resistant to the preceding treatment, steroids are

effective for acute-phase therapy and can be administered either in enema form or systemically. Immunosuppressive therapy (6-mercaptopurine or azathioprine) might then serve to keep both the primary bowel disease and the arthritis in remission.

The use of NSAID agents in IBD should be avoided if at all possible. Where there is no reasonable alternative, they should be used with caution, perhaps using low doses combined with another analgesic agent that does not affect the bowel.

REFERENCES

1. Bjarnason I, Smethurst P, Fenn CG, et al: NSAID small bowel injury and cytoprotection. *Gastroenterology* 1989; 97:1344–1355.
2. Bjarnason I, et al: Nonsteroidal antiinflammatory drug–induced intestinal inflammation in humans. *Gastroenterology* 1987; 93:480–489.
3. Bravo AJ, Lowman RM: Benign ulcer of the sigmoid colon: An unusual lesion that can simulate carcinoma. *Radiology* 1968; 90:113–115.
4. Day TK: Intestinal perforation associated with osmotic slow release indomethacin capsules. *Br Med J* 1983; 287:1671–1672.
5. Debenham GP: Ulcer of the cecum during oxyphenbutazone (Tandearil) therapy. *Can Med Assoc J*, 1966; 94:1182–1184.
6. Empey LR, et al: Cytoprotective effect of prostaglandin E-2 analog in acetic acid colitis (abstract). *Gastroenterology* 1988; 94(Part 2):A616.
7. Foster PN, Axon ATR, Packman L, et al: Nonsteroidal antiinflammatory drugs and the bowel. *Lancet* 1989; 2:1047–1048.
8. Gould SR, Brash AR, Connelly ME: Increased prostaglandin production in ulcerative colitis. *Lancet* 1977; 2:98.
9. Hall RI, Petty AH, Cobden I, et al: Enteritis and colitis associated with mefenamic acid. *Br Med J* 1983; 287:1182.
10. Hawkey CJ: Benoxaprofen in the treatment of active ulcerative colitis. *Prostaglandins Leukotrienes Med* 1983; 10:405–409.
11. Jones IRG, Psaila JV: Cytoprotection by PGE2 in the rat colon (abstract). *Scand J Gastroenterol 1982;* 78(suppl 17):416.
12. Kaufmann HJ, Taubin HL: Nonsteroidal antiinflammatory drugs activate quiescent inflammatory bowel disease. *Ann Intern Med* 1987; 107:513–516.
13. Kornbluth A, Gupta R, Gerson CD: Life-threatening diarrhea after short-term misoprostol use in a patient with Crohn's ileocolitis. *Ann Intern Med* 1990; 113:474–475.
14. Levy N, Gaspar E: Rectal bleeding and indomethacin suppositories. *Lancet* 1975; 1:577.
15. O'Brien WM, Baagby GF: Rare adverse reactions to nonsteroidal antiinflammatory drugs. *J Rheumatol* 1983; 12:562–567.

52   *Special Considerations in Diagnosis and Management*

16. Phillips MS, et al: Enteritis and colitis associated with mefenamic acid. *Br Med J* 1983; 287:162.
17. Rampton DS: Prostaglandins and ulcerative colitis. *Gut* 1984; 25:1399–1413.
18. Rampton DS: Nonsteroidal antiinflammatory drugs and the lower gastrointestinal tract. *Scand J Gastroenterol* 1987; 22:1–4.
19. Rampton DS, McNeil NI, Sarner M: Analgesic indigestion and other factors preceding relapse in ulcerative colitis. *Gut* 1983; 24:187–189.
20. Rampton DS, Sladen GE: Relapse of ulcerative proctocolitis during treatment with nonsteroidal antiinflammatory drugs. *Postgrad Med J* 1981; 57:197–199.
21. Ravi S, Keat AC, Keat ECB: Colitis caused by nonsteroidal antiinflammatory drugs. *Postgrad Med J* 1986; 62:773–776.
22. Robert A, Nezamis JE, Lancaster C, et al: Prevention through cytoprotection of clindamycin-induced colitis in hamsters with 16, 16-dimethyl PGE2 (abstract). *Gastroenterology* 1980; 78:1245.
23. Sharon P, Stenson W: Enhanced synthesis of leukotriene B4 by colonic mucosa in inflammatory bowel disease. *Gastroenterology* 1984; 86:435–460.
24. Sharon P, et al: Role of prostaglandins in ulcerative colitis. Enhanced production during active disease and inhibition by sulfasalazine. *Gastroenterology* 1978; 75:138–140.
25. Schwartz H: Lower gastrointestinal side effects of nonsteroidal antiinflammatory drugs. *J Rheumatol* 1981; 8:952–954.
26. Tanner AR, Raghunath AS: Colonic inflammation and nonsteroidal antiinflammatory drug administration. *Digestion* 1988; 41:116–120.
27. White RF, Gabor AC: Gold colitis. *Med J Aus* 1983; 1:174–175.

Chapter 8 _____

Collagenous and Microscopic Colitis

Myron D. Goldberg

Collagenous colitis and microscopic colitis are uncommon clinicopathologic syndromes characterized by chronic idiopathic watery diarrhea, mild abdominal pain, and grossly normal colonoscopy and barium enema examination findings. The symptoms begin most often in middle-aged women in the sixth to seventh decades of life.[1, 4, 12, 17]

TERMINOLOGY

The term *collagenous colitis* was coined by Lindström,[21] in 1976, and since then more than 50 cases have been described. Lindström reported the first case of collagenous colitis in a 48-year-old woman with mild, chronic, watery diarrhea and crampy abdominal pain. Rectal mucosal biopsy demonstrated a distinctive, thickened band of collagen beneath the surface epithelial layer of the colon. He called it collagenous colitis because the thickened collagen layer appeared histologically similar to that seen in the jejunal mucosa of the small intestine in patients with collagenous sprue.

RELATIONSHIP OF COLLAGENOUS COLITIS TO COLLAGENOUS SPRUE

Collagenous sprue is a rare form of malabsorption described in 1970 by Weinstein et al.[37] It is thought to represent a resistant form of celiac disease that is unresponsive to dietary gluten withdrawal. Collagenous sprue is characterized by villous atrophy and subepithelial collagen deposition of the small intestine. The collagen deposition in the small intestine in patients with collagenous sprue is similar to the collagen deposition seen in the colon in patients with collagenous colitis. There have been a few case reports of patients with collagenous colitis in whom small intestinal biopsy specimens revealed villous atrophy and variable amounts of subepithelial collagen deposition.[5, 6, 15] There has been one case report of collagenous colitis with collagen deposition of the terminal ileum and concomitant bile acid diarrhea.[25] Most patients with collagenous colitis or microscopic colitis, however, do not develop malabsorption or steatorrhea. When steatorrhea does occur in patients with collagenous colitis it is mild. The severe symptoms of malabsorption and steatorrhea seen in collagenous sprue or celiac disease do not occur in patients with collagenous or microscopic colitis. Malabsorptive studies, such as quantitative fecal fat, D-xylose absorption, and bile acid breath tests, are usually normal, and symptoms are unrelated to gluten or to any other dietary factor.

MICROSCOPIC COLITIS

In 1980 Read et al.[27] reported 27 patients with diarrhea of unknown origin. In 1982 Kingham et al.[18] used the term *microscopic colitis* to describe similar patients with diarrhea. It soon became apparent that collagenous colitis and microscopic colitis represent similar clinicopathologic syndromes that differ in the histologic appearance of colonic mucosa.[14, 31] Microscopic colitis has been referred to by Lazenby et al.[19] as "lymphocytic" colitis because of the distinctive histologic feature of increased intraepithelial lymphocytes. Other features include damage to surface epithelium, chronic inflammation of the lamina propria, goblet cell depletion, and only minimal distortion of the crypts. In microscopic colitis there is no increase in collagen deposition.

The absence of collagen deposition in patients with microscopic colitis who have been observed up to 5 years would imply that it is separate and distinct from collagenous colitis.[14] In collagenous colitis, however, the thickness of the collagen layer may vary throughout the colon. Where collagen deposition is minimal, the histologic appearance of the colonic mucosa resembles microscopic colitis. This has led to the supposition that, at least in some patients, collagenous colitis and microscopic colitis represent a spectrum of the same illness.[14, 31]

PATHOGENESIS

In collagenous colitis the abnormal deposition of subepithelial collagen is thought to result from a defect in the pericryptal fibroblastic sheath.[10, 16] The pericryptal fibroblastic sheath consists of fibroblasts that surround the crypt epithelium and normally produce only minimal amounts of collagen. As these fibroblasts migrate upward from the base of the crypts to the epithelial layer, they mature into functional fibrocytes. The abnormal excess collagen deposition seen in collagenous colitis may result from a disturbance in this maturation process. The cause of this disturbance is unknown. It has been suggested that the excess collagen deposition represents an inflammatory response to an as yet unidentified noxious agent. There has been no consistent association of collagenous colitis or microscopic colitis with any systemic or intestinal disease, drug, food, bacteria, virus, or toxin, and the cause remains unknown.

Diarrheal symptoms in both collagenous colitis and microscopic colitis are thought to be the result of increased fluid secretion from the colon.[2] The chronic watery diarrhea that these patients experience is characterized by increased stool volumes of up to 4 to 5 L/day. The normal stool electrolytes, the absence of an osmotic gap on stool analysis, and the increased stool volumes are consistent with a secretory diarrhea.[26] In addition, fluid absorption may be reduced by collagen deposition.

Evidence to support an autoimmune basis includes female predominance and isolated case reports of collagenous colitis that coexist with diseases considered to be autoimmune, including thyroid disease,[29] rheumatoid arthritis, Raynaud's disease, and seronegative polyarthritis.[7] There have also been cases of collagenous colitis coexisting with celiac sprue,[22] juvenile scleroderma,[8] pulmonary fibrosis,[38] and ileal carcinoid.[23] HLA stereotyping has been done in patients with collagenous and microscopic colitis. In one study nine patients demonstrated an increase in HLA-A1 and a lesser increase of HLA-DRw53 when compared with control subjects.[14] In another report, HLA-A2 antigen was present in four patients from two families.[33] A true autoimmune basis for collagenous colitis or microscopic colitis has not been established. Immune complex deposition is not seen, and serum complement levels are normal.

DIAGNOSIS

Stool analyses in these patients are negative for enteric pathogens and occult blood. Fecal leukocytes may be increased when diarrheal symptoms flare up.

The gross appearance of the colon is normal both endoscopically and radiographically. For this reason it is important to obtain mucosal biopsy specimens at the time of colonoscopy or sigmoidoscopy in any patient with unexplained diarrhea, despite a normal-appearing colon.[30]

The diagnosis of collagenous colitis is made by obtaining a colonic biopsy that demonstrates both diffuse thickening of the subepithelial collagen layer and increased mucosal inflammation (Fig 8–1). The thickness of the collagen band is variable. Collagen deposition may be less apparent in the distal area of the colon and may often spare the rectum. For this reason, whenever possible, multiple colonic biopsy specimens should be obtained at various levels of the colon and should not be limited to the rectum.[32]

Thickening of the basement membrane may be confused with subepithelial collagen deposition and may lead to the erroneous diagnosis of collagenous colitis. Diffuse thickening of the basement membrane may occur in diabetes mellitus, hyperplastic polyps,[34] and also as an artifact from tangential sectioning of normal colonic biopsy specimens.[20] To avoid confusion with these conditions, a prerequisite for the diagnosis of collagenous colitis is the presence of increased mucosal inflammation.[20] The increased mucosal inflammation seen in both collagenous and microscopic colitis is characterized by a predominance of intraepithelial lymphocytes and increased plasma cells in the lamina propria. Eosinophils may be increased, but neutrophilic infiltrates are rare.

In microscopic colitis, or in patients with collagenous colitis whose disease is in remission, histologic features include damage to surface epithelium and chronic inflammation (consisting predominantly of lymphocytes) similar to that seen in collagenous colitis (Fig 8–2). There is a depletion of goblet cells, with only minimal distortion of the crypts. This is easily differentiated from ulcerative colitis, which is characterized by prominent crypt distortion, more active inflammation consisting mostly of neutrophils, and minimal lymphocytic infiltration of the epithelium.

The histologic changes seen with collagenous and microscopic colitis may not be readily apparent, and often the diagnosis is delayed or made in retrospect only after a more careful review of the colonic mucosal biopsy specimens.

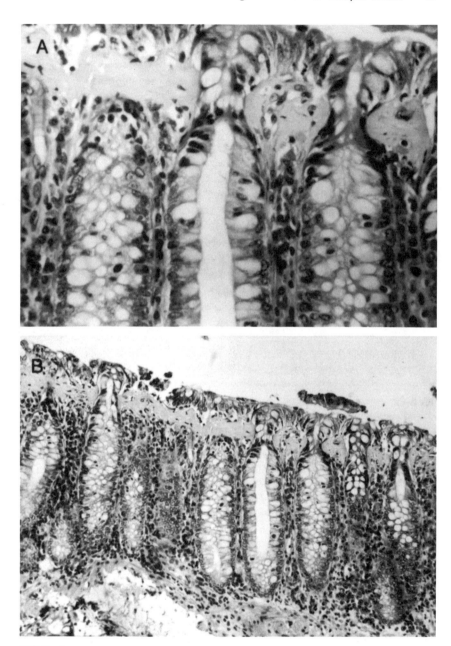

FIG 8–1.
Collagenous colitis. **A** and **B**, note thickened subepithelial band of collagen. (Hematoxylin-eosin stain. **A**, original magnification ×250; **B**, original magnification ×100.)

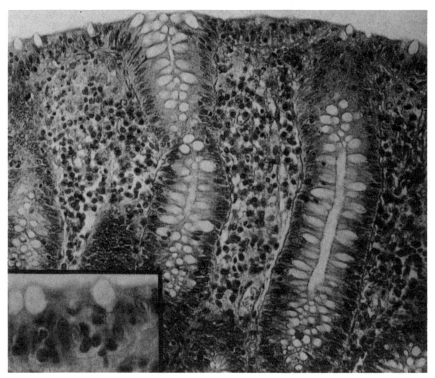

FIG 8−2.
Microscopic ("lymphocytic") colitis. Diffusely increased surface intraepithelial lymphocytes and surface epithelial damage *(inset)* are the major distinguishing features. Increased lamina propria chronic inflammation, prominent crypt lymphocytes, and mild crypt distortion also are seen. (Hematoxylin-eosin stain. Original magnification ×200; inset ×400.) (From Lazenby AJ, Yardley JH, Giardiello FM, et al: *Hum Pathol* 1989; 20:18−28. Used by permission.)

DIFFERENTIAL DIAGNOSIS

As with any patient with unexplained diarrhea, a thorough history and physical examination are essential. A careful drug history will help to exclude antibiotic-associated diarrhea. A stool analysis for enteric pathogens is essential to rule out infectious diarrhea. Inflammatory bowel diseases, such as ulcerative colitis and Crohn's disease, can be excluded after normal colonoscopy and barium enema x-ray examination. Isolated cases of collagenous colitis that coexist with celiac sprue and Crohn's disease[3] have been reported. There has been no consistent association of collagenous colitis or microscopic colitis with inflammatory bowel disease or any other digestive disease, however.[3, 22]

Irritable bowel syndrome (IBS) is the most common diagnosis mistaken for collagenous and microscopic colitis. Both IBS and collagenous/microscopic colitis occur predominantly in female patients, and are characterized by chronic, intermittent diarrhea and abdominal pain. With IBS, however, the onset of symptoms is usually much earlier in life, often beginning in adolescence. In collagenous and microscopic colitis, symptoms usually begin after the age of 50. To distinguish IBS from collagenous and microscopic colitis, sigmoidoscopy or colonoscopy should be done, and mucosal biopsy specimens should be obtained despite a normal-appearing mucosa, to seek the characteristic histologic appearance. All patients with IBS manifested by diarrhea should have one set of colonoscopic biopsies, or at the very least sigmoidoscopic biopsies, to exclude collagenous colitis and microscopic colitis.

TREATMENT

Collagenous colitis and microscopic colitis usually follow a benign course, and spontaneous remission of symptoms often occurs. When necessary, treatment with antidiarrheal drugs, such as loperamide hydrochloride or diphenoxylate, will often improve symptoms. Spontaneous remissions make it difficult to assess the efficacy of medical therapy. If diarrhea persists, however, treatment with sulfasalazine (2 to 3 g/day) or oral 5-aminosalicylic acid has been shown to be effective in many of these patients.[9, 23, 28, 35, 36] With resistant disease, prednisone (20–30 mg/day) may be added for up to 2 to 3 months.[9, 14] Other agents that have been used in those patients with bile acid diarrhea include the bile acid resin cholestyramine.[25]

Collagenous colitis has been reported in two patients after the prolonged use of nonsteroidal anti-inflammatory drugs, specifically indomethacin and ibuprofen, and after short-term use of antibiotics.[13] Nonsteroidal anti-inflammatory drugs or antibiotics should therefore be avoided in these patients, especially during episodes of diarrhea.

PROGNOSIS

Collagenous colitis and microscopic colitis usually follow a benign course, and most patients will respond to antidiarrheal therapy. Recurrence of diarrheal symptoms is common, however. The thickness of the collagen layer varies throughout the colon. This may explain why in some patients the collagen layer appears to regress after subsequent biopsies.[24] For this reason the mucosal biopsy specimens should be obtained from different segments of the colon at the time of sigmoidoscopy or colonoscopy. With prolonged symptomatic improvement the collagen layer will often diminish throughout the colon, but chronic mucosal inflammation persists.

There is a single case report of colon carcinoma coexisting with collagenous colitis.[11] A retrospective review of 100 cases of colon adenocarcinoma demonstrated no other case of collagenous colitis.

REFERENCES

1. Baum CA, Bhatia P, Miner PB Jr: Increased colonic mucosal mast cells associated with severe watery diarrhea and microscopic colitis. *Dig Dis Sci* 1989; 34:1462–1465.
2. Bo-Linn GW, Vendrell DD, Lee E, et al: An evaluation of the significance of microscopic colitis in patients with chronic diarrhea. *J Clin Invest* 1985; 75:1559–1569.
3. Chandratre S, Bramble MG, Cooke WM, et al: Simultaneous occurrence of collagenous colitis and Crohn's disease. *Digestion* 1987; 36:55–60.
4. Coverlizza S, Ferrari A, Scevola F, et al: Clinico-pathological features of collagenous colitis: Case report and literature review. *Am J Gastroenterol* 1986; 81:1098–1103.
5. DuBois RN, Lazenby AJ, Yardley JH, et al: Lymphocytic enterocolitis in patients with "refractory sprue." *JAMA* 1989; 262:935–937.
6. Eckstein RP, Dowsett JF, Riley JW: Collagenous enterocolitis: A case of collagenous colitis with involvement of the small intestine. *Am J Gastroenterol* 1988; 83:767–771.
7. Erlendsson J, Fenger C, Meinicke J: Arthritis and collagenous colitis. Report of a case with concomitant chronic polyarthritis and collagenous colitis. *Scand J Rheumatol* 1983; 12:93–95.
8. Esselinckx W, Brenard R, Colin JF, et al: Juvenile scleroderma and collagenous colitis. The first case. *J Rheumatol* 1989; 16:834–836.
9. Farah DA, Mills PR, Lee FD, et al: Collagenous colitis: Possible response to sulfasalazine and local steroid therapy. *Gastroenterology* 1985; 88:792–797.
10. Fausa O, Foerster A, Hovig T: Collagenous colitis. A clinical, histological, and ultrastructural study. *Scand J Gastroenterol [Suppl]* 1985; 107:8–23.
11. Gardiner GW, Goldberg R, Currie D, et al: Colonic carcinoma associated with an abnormal collagen table. Collagenous colitis. *Cancer* 1984; 54:2973–2977.
12. Giardiello FM, Bayless TM, Yardley JH: Collagenous colitis. *Compr Ther* 1989; 15:49–54.
13. Giardiello FM, Hansen FC III, Lazenby AJ, et al: Collagenous colitis in setting of nonsteroidal antiinflammatory drugs and antibiotics. *Dig Dis Sci* 1990; 35:257–260.

14. Giardiello FM, Lazenby AJ, Bayless TM, et al: Lymphocytic (microscopic) colitis. Clinicopathologic study of 18 patients and comparison to collagenous colitis. *Dig Dis Sci* 1989; 34:1730–1738.

15. Hamilton I, Sanders S, Hopwood D, et al: Collagenous colitis associated with small intestinal villous atrophy. *Gut* 1986; 27:1394–1398.

16. Hwang WS, Kelly JK, Shaffer EA, et al: Collagenous colitis: A disease of pericryptal fibroblast sheath? *J Pathol* 1986; 149:33–40.

17. Jessurun J, Yardley JH, Giardiello FM, et al: Chronic colitis with thickening of the subepithelial collagen layer (collagenous colitis): Histopathologic findings in 15 patients. *Hum Pathol* 1987; 18:839–848.

18. Kingham JG, Levison DA, Ball JA, et al: Microscopic colitis-a cause of chronic watery diarrhoea. *Br Med J* 1982; 285:1601–1604.

19. Lazenby AJ, Yardley JH, Giardiello FM, et al: Lymphocytic ("microscopic") colitis: A comparative histopathologic study with particular reference to collagenous colitis. *Hum Pathol* 1989; 20:18–28.

20. Lazenby AJ, Yardley JH, Giardiello FM, et al: Pitfalls in the diagnosis of collagenous colitis: Experience with 75 cases from a registry of collagenous colitis at the Johns Hopkins Hospital. *Hum Pathol* 1990; 21:905–910.

21. Lindstrom CG: "Collagenous colitis" with watery diarrhoea—a new entity? *Pathol Eur* 1976; 11:87–89.

22. O'Mahony S, Nawroz IM, Ferguson A: Coeliac disease and collagenous colitis. *Postgrad Med J* 1990; 66:238–241.

23. Nussinson E, Samara M, Vigder L, et al: Concurrent collagenous colitis and multiple ileal carcinoids. *Dig Dis Sci* 1988; 33:1040–1044.

24. Prior A, Lessells AM, Whorwell PJ: Is biopsy necessary if colonoscopy is normal? *Dig Dis Sci* 1987; 32:673–676.

25. Rampton DS, Baithun SI: Is microscopic colitis due to bile salt malabsorption? *Dis Colon Rectum* 1987; 30:950–952.

26. Rask-Madsen J, Grove O, Hansen MG, et al: Colonic transport of water and electrolytes in a patient with secretory diarrhea due to collagenous colitis. *Dig Dis Sci* 1983; 28:1141–1146.

27. Read NW, Krejs GJ, Read MG, et al: Chronic diarrhea of unknown origin. *Gastroenterology* 1980; 78:264–271.

28. Rokkas T, Filipe MI, Sladen GE: Collagenous colitis with rapid response to sulphasalazine. *Postgrad Med J* 1988; 64:74–76.

29. Roubenoff R, Ratain J, Giardiello F, et al: Collagenous colitis, enteropathic arthritis, and autoimmune diseases: Results of a patient survey. *J Rheumatol* 1989; 16:1229–1232.

30. Salt WB, Llaneza PP: Collagenous colitis: A cause of chronic diarrhea diagnosed only by biopsy of normal appearing colonic mucosa. *Gastrointest Endosc* 1986; 32:421–423.

31. Sylwestrowicz T, Kelly JK, Hwang WS, et al: Collagenous colitis and microscopic colitis: The watery diarrhea colitis syndrome. *Am J Gastroenterol* 1989; 84:763–768.

32. Teglbjaerg PS, Thaysen EH, Jensen HH: Development of collagenous colitis in sequential biopsy specimens. *Gastroenterology* 1984; 87:703–709.

33. Van Tilburg AJ, Lam HG, et al: Familial occurrence of collagenous colitis. A report of two families. *J Clin Gastroenterol* 1990; 12:279–285.
34. Wang HH, Owings DV, Antonioli DA, et al: Increased subepithelial collagen deposition is not specific for collagenous colitis. *Mod Pathol* 1988; 1:329–335.
35. Weidner N, Smith J, Pattee B: Sulfasalazine in treatment of collagenous colitis. Case report and review of the literature. *Am J Med* 1984; 77:162–166.
36. Wengrower D, Pollak A, Okon E, et al: Collagenous colitis and rheumatoid arthritis with response to sulfasalazine. A case report and review of the literature. *J Clin Gastroenterol* 1987; 9:456–460.
37. Weinstein WM, Saunders DR, Tytgat GN, et al: Collagenous sprue: An unrecognized type of malabsorption. *N Engl J Med* 1970; 283:1297–1301.
38. Wiener MD: Collagenous colitis and pulmonary fibrosis. Manifestations of a single disease? *J Clin Gastroenterol* 1986; 8:677–680.

Discussion

Q: Can the nonsteroidals provoke diarrhea in itself without implicating inflammatory bowel disease? And Dr. Mendelsohn, would you not say that would be true of the majority of cases?

A: *Yes, you do not have to have inflammatory bowel disease to have an NSAID-induced colitis and diarrhea from the nonsteroidals by themselves. How can you tell this isn't a typical inflammatory bowel disease exacerbated by nonsteroidals? I don't think you can definitely tell, with the exception that, by treating the NSAID-induced colitis by withdrawal of the offending agent, if the patients get better and then relapse again without the agent, I think you have to attribute that to inflammatory bowel disease as well.*

Q: Do you think it warrants a workup with colonoscopy and biopsies, or is it better to just stop the drug and see if the problem goes away?

A: *In the short term, stop the offending agent; you can wait and see. I don't think there's any urgency, but I think all colitides should be evaluated colonoscopically.*

Q: Do NSAIDs affect the small bowel?

A: *There have been a few studies showing involvement of ulcerations secondary to the nonsteriodals in the ileum, but there have been no studies showing observations of ileitis per se, other than ulcerations from the actual nonsteroidals. It appears to be mostly the slow-release products that are released at a higher pH and are concentrated in the small bowel.*

Q: When the patient with ileitis calls from the office of the orthopedist and says, "Doctor so and so wants to start me on Indocin; is it okay with you?" I say no.

A: *I would prefer avoiding it in this situation.*

Q: Dr. Adler, what do you feel regarding oral contraceptives?

A: *I don't think we have enough data to make recommendations at this point. We have only two epidemiologic studies. One involved both Crohn's disease and ulcerative colitis. The other involved only Crohn's disease. It seemed by retrospective review that a much higher percentage of patients than would have been expected had been on oral contraceptives in the year prior to the onset of symptoms. Oral contraceptives certainly are a generally safe and widely used method of contraception throughout the world. I don't think we have enough data to make recommendations that they should not be used because of being a potential cause of inflammatory bowel disease at this point. Prospectively, however, we generally recommend that our patients who already have established bowel disease find an alternate method of contraception.*

When pregnancy becomes a priority for a couple and the male patient is on an immunosuppressive, we recommend that the immunosuppressive be stopped 3 months before attempting conception and that a good, reliable method of contraception be continued for that 3-month period.

Dr. Korelitz: *Yes, I believe that there are other easy methods of contraception, especially in an unmarried patient. Practicing in New York City and considering the possibilities of HIV infection, we have many good reasons for recommending alternate contraceptive methods. My attitude, too, is that inflammatory bowel disease is complicated enough. When the question comes up about oral contraceptives, I say no. There are other methods of contraception. Let's be clear enough about what we don't know about Crohn's disease to manage it as best we can.*

Chapter 9 _____

Nutrition in Patients With Inflammatory Bowel Disease

Arthur D. Heller

_____

And this I know, moreover, that to the human body it makes a great difference whether the bread be fine or coarse, of wheat with or without the hull . . . baked or raw . . . whoever pays no attention to these things, or paying attention, does not comprehend them, how can he understand the diseases which befall a man? For by every one of these things, a man is affected and changed this way or that, whether in health, convalescence, or disease. Nothing else, then, can be more important or more necessary to know than these things.

Hippocrates, On Ancient Medicine

With increasing interest in nutrition and with increasing knowledge of such dietary factors as eicosanoids and short-chain fatty acids, the above statement remains relevant even after 2,300 years. For patients with inflammatory bowel disease (IBD) the sentiment is particularly germane.

In general terms there are a number of major nutritional issues dealing with the management of IBD:

1. The role of nutritional screening
2. Treatment of growth failure in children
3. Bowel rest in the management of fistulas
4. Management of the short bowel syndrome
5. Bowel rest and parenteral nutrition as primary or adjunctive therapy
6. Elemental diets as primary or adjunctive therapy
7. Diet and nutrition in the cause and pathogenesis of IBD
8. Future directions for diet and nutrition in IBD

THE ROLE OF NUTRITIONAL SCREENING

Assessment of General Nutrition and Macronutrient Status

The data base concerning the nutritional status of patients with IBD is of somewhat modest size but is ever increasing. Interpretation of the available data can be difficult because many of the studies have methodologic shortcomings; some are retrospective with use of historical controls, others are uncontrolled, and still others concern heterogeneous populations.

Malnutrition may accompany IBD.[16, 36] Although overt manifestations of classical deficiency syndromes may be uncommon, the practitioner should be aware that, just as the underlying disease process can be insidious and difficult to diagnose, so may the concomitant nutritional deficiencies. Weight loss is common in IBD[36]; calorie intake will be addressed in the section on growth failure.

Protein

Hypoproteinemia (hypoalbuminemia) is a well-documented occurrence in IBD.[16] In the absence of edema or ascites, a low serum albumin level may be due to decreased hepatic synthesis, increased protein losses, or increased tissue breakdown. The general adaptive response to simple starvation is to maintain serum albumin by decreasing catabolism more than decreasing synthesis.[125] Numerous studies[15, 16, 51, 80, 168] have demonstrated that patients with active IBD have increased gastrointestinal protein losses that correlate with disease severity, i.e., extent of bowel involvement, number of bowel movements, and volume of blood, exudate, and transudate losses. Even the depleted patients with active disease can be placed in positive nitrogen balance if intake is sufficient; this may require up to 2.0 g/kg or more of protein. Patients with quiescent disease do not have increased needs for protein, calories, and probably trace minerals and other micronutrients after these have been replenished.[12] Reasonable protein intake of 0.8 to 1.25 g/kg of high-quality protein usually suffices for these patients.

Fat

Fat malabsorption, as measured by increased quantitative fecal fat or bile acid output, may lead to significant calorie wasting; the steatorrhea and bile salt catharsis may lead to choleraic diarrhea, with exacerbated fluid, mineral, and electrolyte losses in about 30% of patients with Crohn's disease.[41, 164] The length of diseased or resected ileum appears to be directly proportional to both the degree[58] and the prevalence[43] of steatorrhea, essentially affecting all patients with more than 60 cm of involved bowel; this may be compounded by loss or incompetence of the ileocecal valve, which is both a governor of lumenal transit and some protection against developing bacterial overgrowth of the small bowel. For the patient who compensates for minimal to mild fat losses during quiescent periods, flare-ups of disease activity, with increased losses and decreased intake, may overcome reserve capacity. The bile salt resin cholestyramine may effectively treat choleraic diarrhea, particularly after ileocolic resection and loss of the ileocecal valve; in turn it may serve to worsen steatorrhea and to cause fat-soluble vitamin deficiency. This occurs most commonly with loss of 100 cm of ileum. The usual dose of cholestyramine is 8 to 12 g (2 to 3 packets) daily.*

Patients with symptomatic steatorrhea may benefit from dietary and nutritional adjustment. A low fat (50–70 g) diet, perhaps supplemented with medium-chain triglycerides (MCT oil), may reduce steatorrhea and hyperoxaluria. Studies have evaluated the effects of high- and low-fat diets on short bowel patients[119, 175]; fluid and electrolyte losses were similar on either diet. Increased losses of divalent cations, such as calcium, magnesium, and zinc, have been noted on high fat diets in some studies.[175]

Lactose and Milk

Reports of lactose malabsorption vary from a prevalence of 46% in Jewish and black children with Crohn's disease vs. 15% in white, Gentile patients[79] with Crohn's disease, to 12.5% hypolactasia in a study of English patients with Crohn's disease,[121] to a 9.2% prevalence in a Danish study[21]; these figures appear consistent with figures for normal subjects of similar ethnic types. More recently a high prevalence of lactose intolerance in patients with ulcerative colitis has been demonstrated. Just as hypolactasia may temporarily follow acute gastroenteritis, some investigators,[121] but not all,[21] have noted this during acute flares of ulcerative colitis. Other disaccharidases appear to be unaffected in ulcerative colitis[9]; in Crohn's disease, especially after repeated surgical resections, loss of intestinal surface area and enzyme activity may be noted.†

---

*Editor's Note: Most patients profit with the use of cholestyramine for 2 to 3 months after ileocolic resection if postoperative diarrhea does not subside within a short time.

†Editor's Note It has been my experience that many patients with IBD have had milk and dairy products restricted from their diets without justification. Adequate treatment of the underlying disease is usually accompanied by elimination of any milk product intolerance.

Milk is the food most often indicated in triggering the symptoms of IBD. Truelove[162] noted that 5% of his patients with ulcerative colitis worsened endoscopically, histologically, and clinically when milk products were introduced into their diets. He proposed the possibility of an abnormal response to milk antigens, although follow-up studies were not entirely conclusive.[174] It remains unanswered whether the increase in symptoms sometimes seen in patients with IBD who use dairy products is due to the lactose, protein, or fat/fatty acid content.

It is prudent to document lactose intolerance by hydrogen breath testing or tolerance testing before excluding dairy products from the diet of patients with IBD.[139] Relatively low lactose products, such as yogurt, and lactose-reduced milk, or lactase tablets may allow these important sources of protein and calcium to remain in patients' diets. I emphasize eating no-fat or low-fat dairy products. This rules out most cheeses, because I try to limit excess total and saturated fat and excess omega-6 fatty acid intake. Patients are later advised to restart dairy products slowly, eating small amounts, as part of mixed meals. Lactase tablets can be taken 5 to 10 minutes before eating dairy products.

Assessment of Mineral and Vitamin Status

Micronutrient (vitamins, minerals) deficiency occurs commonly in hospitalized patients with IBD.[36]; diarrheal diseases are characterized by variable water and electrolyte losses.

Potassium

Serum values may not reflect body stores of potassium. Nyhlin et al.[113] documented significantly lower muscle potassium content in patients with Crohn's disease vs. control subjects, although serum values were not significantly different. Potassium depletion with hypokalemia and symptomatic muscle weakness may be common in ulcerative colitis.[97] Poor intake of potassium-rich foods such as fruits and vegetables may contribute to the problem. Intake of foods such as green leafy vegetables, tomatoes, potatoes, bananas, apricots, and oranges should be encouraged through a variety of forms, e.g., juices and soups. Oral potassium supplementation is not usually needed except for some hospitalized patients; often this required intravenous supplementation is part of the fluid resuscitation plan. Liquid potassium preparations, e.g., potassium citrate, given with food, and in split doses, may be less irritating.* Patients with persistent hypokalemia should be checked for con-

---

*Editor's Note: Oral K+ preparation can be irritating to the gastrointestinal tract and can aggravate IBD. Replacement of the potassium by foods high in potassium or by extra potassium given. Intravenously is preferable.

comitant hypomagnesemia, which must be corrected before the potassium depletion can be treated.

Magnesium

Symptomatic hypomagnesemia complete with hyperirritability, paresthesias, weakness, tetany, arrhythmias, and other central nervous system effects have been noted in patients who have Crohn's disease,[54] as well as in those who have active, symptomatic ulcerative colitis[159, 160] and inactive ulcerative colitis.[39] Those with extensive disease or resections are most at risk. As with potassium, normal serum or plasma values may belie the presence of total body deficiency.[16] Low urinary excretion with avid retention of magnesium has been suggested as a relatively sensitive screening test for early depletion. Low magnesium excretion and low excretion of citrate are factors involved with the hyperoxaluria and increased prevalence of renal oxalate stones seen in patients with Crohn's disease who have ileal disease. Supplementation with 16 to 24 mEq magnesium may be needed; small doses taken frequently may minimize osmotic diarrhea. Various formulations may be used, e.g., magnesium chloride, magnesium oxide, or even magnesium sulfate (Epsom salts): one-eighth level teaspoon three to four times per day may suffice.

Calcium

Patients with IBD are at high risk for calcium deficiency. A survey of patients with Crohn's disease revealed decreased intake and absorption of calcium, as well as decreased bone mass.[29] Other risk factors for osteopenia include female sex, positive family history of osteoporosis, cigarette smoking, amenorrhea, and menopause. Corticosteroid treatment decreases absorption, while increasing calcium excretion,[81, 85, 98] and is a major risk factor for osteoporosis. Patients with fat and fat-soluble vitamin malabsorption, i.e., ileal disease with bile salt losses, are at further increased risk.

Given the preceding factors, calcium supplementation is probably indicated for most patients who have IBD. Most healthy women do not meet the recommended daily allowance (RDA) of 1,200 mg (roughly 4 to 6 glasses of milk daily). Good dietary sources of calcium include yogurt (450 mg/C), broccoli, green leafy vegetables, bean curd (tofu), and canned sardines and salmon (with bones). Calcium carbonate (e.g., TUMS) is the least expensive form available. Calcium citrate may cause less bloating and gas, and may improve urinary calcium solubility. All calcium supplements can be constipating; split doses totaling 1,500 mg may be needed.

Renal stones in Crohn's disease are usually due to hyperoxaluria, not hypercalciuria. Calcium supplementation, citrate supplementation as with Polycitra, magnesium repletion and supplementation where indicated, correction of steatorrhea where possible, avoidance of high oxalate foods, and adequate hydration can go far in minimizing stone formation and symptomatic stone disease. Twenty-four-hour urine collections before and during therapy are helpful to monitor effectiveness.

For those patients with ulcerative colitis who have an ileostomy, there is an increased risk of uric acid stones due to a persistent slight metabolic acidosis and dehydration. Ample hydration and alkalinization of the urine with oral citrate again help to minimize stone formation.

Iron

Iron deficiency anemia is common in IBD mainly because of chronic blood loss and poor intake.[13, 40] Patients with acute flare-ups of ulcerative colitis suffer additional iron loss; up to 80% of patients who have colonic Crohn's disease have low hemoglobin and serum iron levels.[69] Female patients have the additional factor of menstrual losses. The end stage of iron deficiency disease is anemia. Earlier iron deficiency in IBD may be difficult to diagnose because inflammation can affect serum iron, transferrin, and ferritin levels.[25] Often the presenting symptom of patients who have IBD is the so-called picture of the "anemia of chronic disease."

Serum ferritin levels are generally good estimates of iron reserves. Usually levels below 12 to 18 ng/ml[30] denote depletion. Inflammation can raise ferritin levels even in the absence of marrow stores. Marrow evaluation is the sine qua non for diagnosis of iron deficiency, but it is invasive and painful; therefore monitoring fecal blood loss and prudent supplementation, i.e., with the RDA of 18 mg daily, seems a reasonable approach to patients with additional menstrual or chronic gastrointestinal losses. Therapeutic oral iron supplements, e.g., iron sulfate, lactate, or gluconate (100 mg elemental iron), one to three times a day, may be needed; often these are poorly tolerated by the gastrointestinal tract even if taken with food or in slow-release forms, and may serve to aggravate symptoms of the underlying IBD. Parenteral iron dextran may be needed on rare occasions.* The calculated dose of iron may be given slowly intravenously, under observation for allergic reactions, in either

---

*Editor's Note: I have often used iron dextran after IBD has been brought under control, and the blood loss is corrected but the anemia persists. In 9 of 10 patients the injections are tolerated; in an occasional patient they are painful; infrequently there are iron stains about the injection site, which persist. A test dose of 0.5 mL is used, and if tolerated I can continue with 2 mL/day for a total of seven to ten injections.

split doses or as total infusion, although the latter has been reported to be associated with increased risk of side effects and toxicity. Side effects are not uncommon, may be delayed by 24 to 48 hours, and include fever, rash, malaise, arthralgias, and joint swelling. These can occur after intramuscular or intravenous administration. Intravenous therapy has the advantages of not causing local pain or staining at the injection site.

Helpful dietary hints for patients include cooking in cast-iron cookware, avoiding tea and coffee, especially at mealtime, because they can inhibit nonheme iron absorption, utilizing lean cuts of red meat, and supplementing the diet with green leafy vegetables, enriched cereals, legumes, and vitamin C–containing foods. For patients suffering from bloating, pain, and flatulence from the undigestible carbohydrates (stachyose and raffinose) found in beans, cereals, and vegetables, relief may be obtained from use of a proprietary liquid preparation of galactosidase (Beano).

Zinc and Other Trace Metals

Zinc and other trace mineral deficiencies may occur in patients who have IBD.[36, 70] Most information on zinc depletion concerns those who have Crohn's disease; low serum levels have been commonly noted.[49, 86, 102, 146–148, 155, 163] Serum zinc levels correlate with serum albumin values, as is the case for calcium levels. Low serum zinc levels may be due to internal redistribution in times of stress, as is the case for iron. Low serum levels are associated with decreased urinary secretion,[147] decreased taste acuity, especially for sweet,[101] and decreased retinal binding protein synthesis. Overt clinical deficiency signs in IBD that have responded to zinc repletion include night blindness,[103] acrodermatitis-type rash, hypogonadism, testicular failure,[136] and growth retardation.[112, 146]

In ulcerative colitis the picture is not nearly as clear.[38, 102, 147] In the study by Dronfield et al.[38] of cases of newly diagnosed ulcerative colitis, plasma levels of zinc in these patients were normal, and oral supplementation was no better than placebo in hastening healing or ameliorating symptoms. The patients, however, may not have been zinc deficient at baseline.

Several mechanisms for zinc depletion in IBD are possible: (1) Intake may be decreased; (2) zinc absorption is decreased in most patients with extensive or severe Crohn's disease, whether in adults[102] or in adolescents[161]; (3) intestinal losses may occur through fistulas, ileostomy drainage (up to 12 mg/L) or diarrhea (up to 17 mg/L)[172]; (4) requirements may increase because of chronic and acute inflammation; and (5) utilization may be impaired. Patients who have Crohn's disease may be in a chronic state of negative zinc balance, with marginal to significant depletion that can be exacerbated by prolonged total parenteral nutrition (TPN) or enteral feeding with inadequate zinc supplementation.[167, 172] Total body stores are only 1.4 to 2.3 g.

The RDA for zinc in healthy adults was recently reduced to 12 mg/day; patients with IBD may need significantly more. Food sources to be encouraged include meat, liver, eggs, seafood (particularly oysters), grains, and wheat germ. Oral supplementation with doses greater than 100 mg zinc may interfere with absorption of other minerals such as copper, iron, and calcium. TPN needs can be met with 3 to 5 mg ZnSO4; up to 12 mg/day or more may be needed in those patients with significant diarrhea.

Other trace mineral depletion and deficiency states have been noted in patients with IBD generally in those on a regimen of TPN. Increased losses of copper (0.3 mg/day) have been noted in patients with Crohn's disease whose total drainage losses from conditions such as fistulas and diarrhea were greater than 300 g/day.[152] Liver copper stores are increased in patients with cholestatic liver disease, including sclerosing cholangitis. Copper is routinely omitted from TPN formulas for these patients. Hepatic copper stores in patients with Crohn's disease without liver complications are apparently normal.[130] Of interest is Reeve's et al.'s[127] recent case report of a young woman with treated but poorly responsive Crohn's disease; she came to the hospital with congestive heart failure because of the cardiomyopathy of selenium deficiency. This patient was not from an endemic region of selenium deficiency nor had she been on a regimen of TPN. Her case illustrates the need for physicians to be vigilant for subtle and novel presentations of micronutrient deficiencies.[144]

Assessment of Vitamin Status

Vitamin B_{12} (B_{12}, cobalamin) is absorbed specifically in the ileum. Up to 50% of patients with Crohn's disease have abnormal Schilling tests[36] and are at increased risk of developing B_{12} deficiency[47, 106, 138]; those with 100 cm or more of ileum affected (or resected) are at highest risk,[55] largely because of the inability of jejunum to adapt to absorb B_{12} or bile salts over time.[47] Although frank B_{12} deficiency is rare in ulcerative colitis, B_{12} malabsorption (by Schilling test) is not uncommon; this may be due to "backwash ileitis" or bacterial overgrowth. Some patients improve with antibiotic therapy; a majority who undergo proctocolectomy normalize their Schilling tests.

It is important to remember that B_{12} deficiency can occur in the absence of the classical hematologic abnormalities, with subtle and vague neuropsychiatric symptoms, as may be seen in patients who have IBD, and with "low-normal" serum B_{12} levels.[29, 149] Serum methylmalonic acid or homocysteine levels may be more sensitive ancillary diagnostic tests in those patients at high risk for deficiency. Parenteral therapy with multiple injections of 1,000 μg doses of B_{12} can be given weekly initially for 6 to 8 weeks[149] until a response is noted (i.e., improvement in peripheral smear, unequivocal and prompt improvement of neuropsychiatric abnormalities, and improvement in serum methylmalonic acid values. Follow-up monitoring and monthly B_{12} injections (1,000 μg) may be needed in a minority of patients who have Crohn's disease after bowel resection.

Folic acid deficiency severe enough to cause megaloblastic anemia has long been noted in IBD.[11, 22, 23] Low serum (or red cell) folate levels vary from 15%[55] to as high as 63% of patients studied[52]; 10% of the patients in the University of Chicago study had macrocytosis.[52] A Danish study of 215 patients with IBD showed that 52% of the 35 patients with Crohn's disease and 59% of those with ulcerative colitis had low serum folate levels.[43]

The mechanisms of folate depletion are complex. First, dietary intake may be inadequate, especially in patients who restrict "roughage" by limiting fruit and vegetable intake. Many,[31, 52] but not all,[57] studies demonstrate impaired folate absorption in patients with small bowel Crohn's disease. Bowel dysfunction and ultrastructural abnormalities have been noted in endoscopically, radiologically, and histologically normal-appearing bowel. This may partly explain the impaired (jejunal) absorption of folate in patients with gross disease limited to the colon. Sulfasalazine interferes with folate absorption by competitive inhibition[52] and interferes with intestinal transport of the vitamin.[143*] Increased cell turnover, as may occur in healing, or acute inflammation increases requirements. The possible role of (local) folate depletion in colonic dysplasia and cancer in ulcerative colitis was addressed preliminarily in a retrospective study by Lashner et al.[88] They recommended supplementation (0.4 mg daily, twice the newly defined RDA) as a "benign and possibly chemopreventive measure for dysplasia and cancer in ulcerative colitis."

Vitamin C (ascorbic acid; AA) intake is commonly low in patients with Crohn's disease, especially those on low residue diets.[56] Several in-

*Editor's Note: This complication of sulfasalazine is probably due to the sulfapyridine component since it has not as yet been observed with the oral 5-aminosalicylic acid products. I routinely prescribe 1 to 2 mg folate daily for patients maintained on sulfasalazine.

vestigators have noted low serum AA[32] (which reflects recent ingestion), low WBC AA[92] (storage depot AA), and decreased tissue AA[58] from resected ileal specimens, particularly in patients with fistulous disease. AA deficiency was postulated as a cause for impaired collagen synthesis in Crohn's disease and thus a cause for fistula formation.[56] Pettit et al.,[124] with use of labeled L-[carboxyl-14C] AA, showed normal AA absorption and body pools of AA in 12 patients with both fistulous and nonfistulous Crohn's disease, compared with 6 control subjects. The majority of patients had AA intake below the RDA (currently 80 mg; 100 mg for smokers). Assessment of AA intake is indicated in all patients with Crohn's disease, and supplements should be given when indicated. Megadoses, i.e., tenfold RDA or greater, are not indicated; there is the potential for increasing urinary oxalate, together with the risk of oxalate stones.

Isolated case reports of other water-soluble vitamin deficiencies have been noted in patients with IBD, notably pellagra (niacin deficiency) and biotin deficiency. Dietary deficiency of niacin or its precursor, tryptophan, is associated with mucosal lesions from lips to anus, including a friable colon. In patients with pure pellagrous bowel disease, treatment with the vitamin alone suffices to reverse the lesion. Clearly this is not the case in the vast majority of patients with IBD. Biotin deficiency, extremely rare in the pre-TPN era, is a possible complication in severely compromised patients with IBD who are maintained on long-term biotin-deficient formulas; those patients with decreased colonic flora due to proctocolectomy or prolonged broad-spectrum antibiotic therapy may be at increased risk of developing this very uncommon deficiency.

Patients with Crohn's disease may be at increased risk of developing vitamin D deficiency and osteomalacia because of altered enterohepatic circulation of fat-soluble vitamins, intake may be low, and malnourished patients who have Crohn's disease may be housebound for long periods of time.[68] As stated earlier, past or current steroid use, tobacco use, and amenorrhea greatly increase the risks for osteoporosis. Surveys from Europe during winter[27-29] and summer[67] and from the United States[35, 37] revealed low 25-hydroxyvitamin D (25-OHD) levels in up to 70% of patients with Crohn's disease studied, together with a high prevalence of secondary hyperparathyroidism; in a significant number of patients studied, histologic examination revealed osteomalacia. This is noteworthy because in many of these patients disease was clinically silent, i.e., there were no musculoskeletal symptoms, and screening serum alkaline phosphatase, calcium phosphorus, and routine radiologic studies revealed normal findings.

Patients with ileal disease or resections, weight loss, general debility, amenorrhea, TPN use, steroid use, hypomagnesemia, renal oxalate stones, or steatorrhea are at especially high risk for the metabolic bone disease complications. Patients at risk should be screened with 25-OH vitamin D levels, perhaps dual photon densitometry or spine computed tomographic (CT) studies, and bone biopsy where indicated. Successful therapy has been initiated with doses of from 4,000 IU vitamin D_2 daily up to 120,000 IU vitamin D_2/week for up to 6 months or more, or 50 μg 25-OH D_3/day given orally for 6 months.[35, 37] Serum hormone, alkaline phosphatase, calcium, and phosphorus levels need to be monitored during therapy; preferably, follow-up bone biopsy specimens should be obtained as well. Daily calcium intake of 1,200 to 1,500 mg should be encouraged. Estrogen replacement is probably indicated for those patients with secondary amenorrhea or (premature) menopause. Patients should be weaned off steroids for this reason, as well as for many other reasons (see Chapter 27).

Because relatively rapid, inexpensive screening tests for functional vitamin A deficiency are available, i.e., dark-adaptation,[24, 134] one should consider testing patients with Crohn's disease who are at risk and giving appropriate supplementation while monitoring liver enzymes and vitamin levels.[99] Although rare, the synthetic analog 13-*cis*-retinoic acid has been reported to induce proctosigmoiditis, which resolved upon withdrawal of the agent and recurred upon rechallenge.[100]

Low levels of carotene (previtamin A) are seen commonly in patients with IBD because of low intake; those with severe small bowel disease or steatorrhea may have impaired absorption or conversion to the vitamin. Carotenoids may indeed play a role in the "chemoprevention" of cancer by exerting an antioxidant effect.[123] The potential of such agents in the colonic dysplasia carcinoma sequence in chronic ulcerative colitis deserves further investigation.

Like other fat-soluble vitamins, malabsorption of dietary vitamin K can occur in IBD. Although prolongation of prothrombin time is not commonly noted in patients with IBD, some investigators have noted subclinical abnormalities of coagulation parameters in patients with Crohn's disease that were correctable with parenteral vitamin K supplementation.[55] The possible effects of sulfasalazine and antibiotic therapy on intestinal flora and endogenous vitamin K production have not been investigated.

In the TPN era, sporadic cases of vitamin E deficiency have been documented. Howard et al.[72] reported a patient with long-term Crohn's disease, multiple bowel resections, and short bowel syndrome who had scotomata, weakness, ataxia, hyperreflexia, and bilateral Babinski responses. Serum vitamin E was low, and in vitro peroxide hemolysis was markedly abnormal. Aggressive supplementation initially with parenteral vitamin E and later with oral water-miscible vitamin E (Aquasol E, 100 mg twice daily) afforded near complete recovery after 2 years of treatment. For those patients with severe malabsorption and weight loss, it is appropriate to screen for vitamin E status and to supplement as indicated.

In summary of this section on nutritional screening, all patients with IBD are at increased nutritional risk for deficiency of calories, protein, vitamins, particularly B_{12}, folic acid, vitamins C and D, and minerals such as iron, calcium, magnesium, and zinc. Clinical assessment by appropriately trained personnel can be as accurate as more technical laboratory evaluation. Relevant indices include height, weight (including recent changes and percent of ideal body weight), anthropometrics measuring subcutaneous fat stores, mid arm circumference, and muscle mass. An individual measuring below 90% of ideal on anthropometric examination is at increased nutritional risk. Laboratory assessment (including hemoglobin, hematocrit, serum albumin, cholesterol, iron, total iron binding capacity, ferritin, calcium, magnesium, alkaline phosphatase, transaminases, vitamin B_{12}, and serum [or red blood cell] folate, serum vitamins A, E, and D, prothrombin time, and zinc levels, absolute lymphocyte count, and anergy status) are relatively easy to obtain and may be pertinent to the individual patient. Interpretation of some results may be more difficult because of complicating factors such as inflammation, infection, and even cigarette smoking. Increased awareness of these factors and specific interventions may decrease the impact of those deficiencies on progression of IBD and the general condition of patients.

TREATMENT OF GROWTH FAILURE IN CHILDREN

IBD can be diagnosed in 15% to 40% of patients during childhood and adolescence; from 30% to 85% of patients with Crohn's disease in this age group may have growth retardation, growth failure, and delayed sexual maturity.[19, 170] Growth retardation is not weight loss, but is a slowing or cessation of linear growth below that expected for a given age and pubertal stage. This may manifest as a decrease in the expected growth velocity or fall off in height percentile. Short stature of itself does not necessarily imply growth retardation. Growth rates slower than 5 cm/yr in prepubertal children should be investigated. Often there is associated delay in skeletal maturation as determined by X-ray study of the hand and wrist.

There are many possible causes for poor growth in children with IBD, including decreased intake, malabsorption, hormonal changes, specific nutrient deficiencies, and increased nutrient losses from the gastrointestinal tract.

With the anorexia, nausea, vomiting, bloating, and pain that commonly occur with symptomatic Crohn's disease, it is not surprising that oral caloric intake may be reduced to almost half the RDA.[78, 79, 89] Because Crohn's disease causes structural damage in the bowel, one might think that malabsorption was the primary cause of malnutrition; for those patients with severe, extensive Crohn's disease or multiple extensive resections, this may be true. Most patients, however, have normal D-xylose tests and no significant steatorrhea.

Growth failure often predates the diagnosis of Crohn's disease. Steroids may either contribute or not be a significant factor in the growth failure; in fact, a relative growth spurt may occur after steroid therapy suppresses inflammation and disease activity. Hormone secretion and levels appear normal and are unlikely to be responsible for the growth retardation. One is unable to sustain growth if any specific nutrient, e.g., zinc, is deficient. No consistent deficiency has been noted in all reported cases.

The caloric (and likely protein) requirements of patients with quiescent IBD are not significantly different from normal, and can be estimated from standard formulas.[12] During disease flare-ups with active inflammation, however, loss of intestinal protein and other nutrients will be associated with loss of blood, pus, loose or watery stool, and exudates. Moreover, general hypercatabolism will increase the metabolic rate and the nitrogen and nutrient losses, leading to further depletion of limited reserves.[14]

The appreciation of the nutritional deficiencies in Crohn's disease coincided with the advent of TPN. Layden et al.[89] demonstrated catch-up growth in four growth-retarded patients after 4 weeks of TPN added to their medical management; their patients did not uniformly have malabsorption, but did uniformly have decreased caloric intake at the outset of the study. Kelts et al.[77] treated an additional seven growth-retarded children with Crohn's disease with TPN combined with oral nutrition for 8 weeks, and induced a growth spurt, weight gain, and improved well-being that continued for 6 months to a year after cessation of TPN without a change in other therapy. Strobel et al.[154] used home TPN as an adjunct to treatment in 17 pediatric patients with Crohn's disease. Serum albumin levels normalized in 10 patients, all 17 gained weight, 10 demonstrated catch-up growth, and appropriate linear growth occurred in another four patients. Catch-up growth induced by TPN has been noted in a 20-year-old patient with Crohn's disease[36] and in a 22-year-old with radiation enteritis.[50] TPN is expensive financially and physiologically, encouraging other approaches to nutritional support.

A maxim of nutritional support is, "If the gut works, use it." Morin et al.[108] reported catch-up growth in four growth-retarded patients with Crohn's disease given 6 weeks of nocturnal infusions of elemental (predigested) defined-formula diets. All of their patients were initially in positive nitrogen balance; two of the four had caloric intakes within the normal range at the start of the study. Kirschner et al.[78, 79] demonstrated, in seven growth-retarded children with Crohn's disease, that daily oral supplementation with 600 to 1,200 kcal/day of an intact protein, polymeric formula (Ensure) increased caloric intake to more than 90% of RDA and induced catch-up growth in five of the seven patients.

The exact protein and energy needs of growth-retarded youngsters with Crohn's disease are unknown. The studies discussed offer us some consistent findings, however. Most groups recommended energy intake of 70 to 80 kcal/kg/day, which is roughly similar to that of normal individuals of comparable age. The method of nutritional support depends on the individual's disease activity and symptoms. Use of the simplest, most palatable supplements is desirable. If patients are not lactose intolerant, a milk-based formula, e.g., Carnation Instant Breakfast, may be helpful. Protein intake in the preceding studies varied from 1.66/kg/day (50 g) to 2.2/kg/day. It is important to emphasize that for oral intake to be adequate symptoms must be controlled with the appropriate drug therapy. On occasion, surgical resection of an inflamed or stenotic segment of bowel may be needed for symptom relief, but postsurgical growth spurts do not occur in most growth-retarded children with Crohn's disease.[71]

BOWEL REST IN THE MANAGEMENT OF FISTULAS

TPN and enteral nutrition have been used to treat all types of fistulas. The reported success of nutritional therapy in healing fistulas is difficult to assess, because there have been no randomized trials comparing nutritional support with standard medical therapy; thus the role of TPN remains controversial. Driscoll and Rosenberg[36] reported a 43% in-hospital healing rate and a 30% long-term (1 year) healing rate with TPN and bowel rest. Subsequent studies[44, 63, 110, 118] have reported roughly similar results. Ultimately, most patients in these studies whose fistulas were due to tight strictures required definitive surgical treatment. The decision as to when to intervene should be individualized; some patients find the preceding results with TPN satisfactory and chances of success worth taking.* There are insufficient data regarding enteral nutrition in the treatment of fistulas to draw conclusions. The role of octreotide (somatostatin analog) in the treatment of fistulas is yet to be determined, but appears promising.

NUTRITIONAL SUPPORT AND THE SHORT BOWEL SYNDROME

Although the majority of patients in home TPN (HTPN) registries have Crohn's disease, the short bowel malabsorption syndrome afflicts only a small minority of patients with Crohn's disease, since enthusiastic and aggressive medical therapy, conservative surgical indications, and conservative surgical techniques can bring the disease into remission in the majority of patients.[173] For the rare occurrence of short bowel in a patient with Crohn's disease, HTPN can be life sustaining; a majority of these patients may be nutritionally rehabilitated to enjoy oral feedings. HTPN can be well tolerated in patients who have Crohn's disease, with an acceptable complication rate,[124, 153] notably the risk of sepsis, and the increased risk of hepatobiliary complications that exists for patients with HTPN who have a diseased or absent ileum.†

TOTAL PARENTERAL NUTRITION, ELEMENTAL DIETS, AND BOWEL REST AS PRIMARY AND ADJUNCTIVE THERAPY IN SEVERE INFLAMMATORY BOWEL DISEASE

Another maxim of nutritional support is that it treats the malnutrition, not necessarily the underlying disease. The most effective way of overcoming the malnutrition induced by these diseases is to treat the underlying disease adequately and appropriately. The appropriate

---

*Editor's Note: It has been my experience that the fistulas of Crohn's disease do heal with TPN, but they also heal with high-dose intravenous adrenocorticotropic hormone followed by 6-mercaptopurine, without requiring prolonged hospitalization, without risk of sepsis starting at the central line site, and without requiring restriction of oral feedings. Therefore I have concluded that TPN is strictly supplementary in Crohn's disease, by replenishing nutrition, to provide for a better response to drug therapy or to prepare for elective surgery.

†Editor's Note: Somatostatin shows promise in treatment of short bowel syndrome as well as multiple abdominal wall fistulas.

means and the role of parenteral and enteral support in IBD, as well as in other diseases, remain controversial.[87, 129, 169] Numerous studies have documented improved nutritional parameters, but the efficacy of these therapies as primary therapy remains unproved.[53, 62, 65]

Just how necessary is bowel rest in the treatment of the severe primary bowel activity of IBD?[107] Many of the early studies predicated the use of TPN in IBD on the concept of bowel rest being beneficial in the acute stages of the disease. Some believed that the absence of dietary protein antigens, or decreased fecal stream, might help abate the inflammation. McIntyre et al.[104] in a controlled trial, looked at 47 inpatients with ulcerative colitis, Crohn's colitis, and indeterminate colitis treated with steroids and either bowel rest or oral diet. There was no significant difference in terms of rapid improvement by day 7 or in the need for surgery. A recent randomized, controlled, prospective multicenter study examined hospitalized patients with Crohn's disease who were receiving steroids and 3 weeks of either TPN (bowel rest), tube-fed intact protein, polymeric diet (partial bowel rest), or partial peripheral parenteral nutrition supplemented by oral intake of hospital food. No significant difference was noted in remission acutely, remission at 1 year, or need for surgery.[64] This study makes one question the role of absorbed food antigens in the inflammatory process, especially while under steroid therapy,[120] and demonstrates that bowel rest is not necessary to quiet the primary bowel manifestations of Crohn's disease.

There have been very few prospective, randomized, controlled trials of TPN or enteral nutrition (EN) as primary treatment for IBD. Most studies use TPN or EN in patients for whom "standard" medical therapy has failed, although this "standard" therapy varied between, and even within, study groups. Often in these studies "standard" medical therapy was continued during the nutritional support phase, and clinical end points were not uniform, thereby adversely affecting interpretation of the data.

A number of retrospective and uncontrolled prospective studies of TPN in Crohn's disease reported in-hospital remission rates from 23% to 100% in patients treated from 3 to 6 weeks with TPN.* To date there have been only two randomized, prospective, controlled trials of TPN in Crohn's disease.[34, 64] Dickinson et al.[34] studied a group of 36 inpatients with acute colitis (both Crohn's disease and ulcerative colitis) for 2 weeks. Because the patients were not stratified, there were three with Crohn's disease in the control (steroids alone) group and 6 in the treat-

---

*References 5, 6, 10, 14, 17, 18, 26, 33, 42, 44, 46, 48, 64, 90, 94, 109, 110, 111, 114, 118, 128, 140, 145, 165.

ment (steroids plus TPN) group. All three patients in the control group with Crohn's disease went into remission; so did four of the six patients in the TPN group. One patient in the TPN group had a long-term remission. Unfortunately, the numbers are too small to draw meaningful conclusions about the efficacy of TPN in patients with Crohn's disease.

Fewer studies have examined the effects of TPN in ulcerative colitis.[33, 34, 44, 46, 48, 75, 109, 128, 165] The studies and populations are not truly comparable insofar as there are significant differences in the patients' level of illness; the wide range of remission (9% to 80%) reflects this. Pooling the data, there is an "overall" remission rate of 41%. In Dickinson et al's study[34] there was no significant difference in remission rate or in the need for surgery. TPN did exert a significant nutritional effect; the "standard" treatment group lost roughly 7% of total body protein, whereas the TPN group maintained lean body mass. In the published reports, TPN has been successful overall for nutritional repletion and as adjunctive therapy to prevent starvation in a patient who may otherwise be non per os, but it does not appear to induce or maintain remission as primary therapy (less than 30% remission induction, 15% to 20% success at 1 year) for ulcerative colitis.

ENTERAL NUTRITION IN ACUTE INFLAMMATORY BOWEL DISEASE

Elemental diets were developed for use by NASA astronauts. These "space age" diets, which are low or no residue and peptide- or amino acid–based, were subsequently used for bowel preparation in patients undergoing gastrointestinal surgery, including patients with Crohn's disease. Some of these patients were noted to improve symptomatically, nutritionally, and radiologically.[61]

A number of uncontrolled, retrospective,[10, 131, 156, 166] and prospective[3, 20, 95, 116, 117, 126, 150] studies suggested induction of (in-hospital) remission in roughly 60% of patients, comparable to reported success with TPN. Based on preliminary or pilot study success noted, a number of prospective, randomized, controlled trials comparing elemental diets with steroids,[79, 93, 115, 117, 135, 137, 141] or nonelemental diets,[56] have been performed. The results are confusing. O'Morain et al.[115] randomized 21 patients to "standard" prednisolone therapy at 0.75 mg/kg/day, or an elemental diet. Assessment at 4 and 12 weeks showed at least comparable improvement with both groups as measured by a "simple activity index," which comprised well-being, number of liquid stools, abdominal mass, tenderness, fistulas, and extraintestinal manifestations. Patients in the EN group were able to add oral intake and stop EN at 4 weeks into the study; at the end of the study the steroid group was still receiving 10 to 20 mg prednisolone daily. In long-term follow-up those with tight strictures needed surgery. O'Morain et al. suggested that those who may benefit the most are those with nonstenosing disease.*

Sanderson et al.[132] confirmed the preceding findings in a randomized control trial comparing an elemental diet with intramuscular adrenocorticotropic hormone at 2 IU/kg/day (and sulfasalazine) followed by oral prednisolone at 2 mg/kg/day. Both were effective in inducing improvement in disease activity, erythrocyte sedimentation rate, C-reactive protein and albumin levels, and body weight. Linear growth velocity was better in the EN group.

Saverymuttu et al.[137] randomized 37 patients to a regimen of elemental diet plus nonabsorbable antibiotics vs. prednisolone in a controlled trial. Both groups showed clinical improvement, with a comparable fall in the Crohn's Disease Activity Index, erythrocyte sedimentation rate, and fecal granulocyte excretion. Logan et al.[96] noted reduced fecal protein, WBC loss, and improved nutritional status in seven patients with Crohn's disease fed an elemental diet.

A series of preliminary reports[73, 93, 95, 142] of controlled studies have been reported recently with variable results. A study of 107 patients in the European Cooperative Crohn's Disease Study showed that the rate of remission in the EN group was significantly worse than in the steroid group.[95] Longer follow-up in two studies did not confirm O'Morain's et al.'s success.[73, 95] Hunt et al.[73] studied 29 adults randomized to elemental diet for a month or prednisolone 0.75 mg/kg for 2 weeks. Their results emphasize the major disadvantage of elemental diets, unpalatability; 40% of the EN group withdrew from the study. They concluded, however, that when it is tolerated EN is as effective as prednisolone in acute exacerbations of new and recurrent Crohn's disease.

There may be a theoretical advantage to the use of elemental diets, but intact protein formulas are more palatable and less expensive. In a controlled study of 30 patients with Crohn's disease, Giaffer et al.[59] found that at 28 days into the study 36% of the patients receiving a polymeric formula were in remission compared with 75% of those receiving an elemental formula. Aside from the difference in protein content, the difference in fat content may play a role in the inflammatory process. There are reports, however, of inducing remission in acute

*Editor's Note: I do not believe that randomization sufficiently identified degree of narrowing in the small bowel so that it was clearly equal in both groups. With obstruction of any degree, a liquid diet, whether elemental or otherwise, is likely to relieve symptoms.

Crohn's disease utilizing a nonelemental formula diet[60] and even a high calorie diet combining whole food and a polymeric formula.[2]

In summary of the consideration for elemental diets in the treatment of the primary bowel manifestations of Crohn's disease, there is evidence that EN can be effective in Crohn's disease, not simply by liquefying intestinal contents and providing symptomatic relief, but by affecting the inflammatory process.[82] Because "standard" steroid therapy is effective and inexpensive, the advantage of elemental diets as primary therapy has not yet been proved. Further studies will probably continue to be aimed at the population refractory to "standard" therapy.

Feeding the patient with nonacute disease can sometimes be a challenge. Many patients with Crohn's disease are maintained on a low fiber diet, even in the absence of severe stenotic disease. Levenstein et al.[91] performed a controlled study in 30 Italian outpatients on a low fiber diet, compared with 28 outpatients on a more liberalized fiber intake; there was no significant difference in outcome. We need not necessarily limit our patients' dietary fiber intake; we may need to advance the diet slowly, on a case-by-case basis, and carefully choose water-soluble vs. water-insoluble foods according to fiber content.

Restricting "provocative" foods may help minimize symptoms but not necessarily reduce the inflammation; in some patients,[4] unfortunately, there is no uniformity in defining these problem foods or provocative factors.[122] A recent study[157] concluded that specific food intolerances do not appear to be an important cause for relapses after diet-induced remission of Crohn's disease.

THE ROLE OF DIET AND NUTRITION IN THE ETIOLOGY AND PATHOGENESIS OF IBD

The hypothetical mechanisms of action regarding nutritional management of disease activity in IBD have recently been reviewed.[141] Although both the etiology and the pathogenesis of Crohn's disease and ulcerative colitis remain unknown, it has been appreciated that some interaction(s) of host responses, perhaps immunologically mediated, perhaps genetically influenced, and exogenous influences, such as infections or dietary factors, may be involved.[76] Allergy to food or food components was considered by an early worker as a possible trigger for two of his patients' symptoms of abdominal cramps, diarrhea, canker sores, and chronic arthritis.[7] The histories of the patients were not inconsistent with Crohn's disease, although no details of histologic diagnosis were given. Rowe[133] and Andreson[8] further surmised that "at least

66% of the cases" of ulcerative colitis were due to food allergy. Other workers through the years have not confirmed such a high prevalence rate.[158]

Several investigators have examined the role of premorbid diet in patients with IBD.[45] Factors studied have included the possible association of infant bottle feeding, early gastroenteritis, and subsequent IBD.[1] Whorwell et al.[171] showed a weak, possible correlation in a minority of patients. James,[74] in an unblinded, biased study, proposed that increased intake of cornflakes in the breakfast diet was an etiologic factor in Crohn's disease. This premise was not confirmed in larger follow-up studies. Other workers investigated the role of dietary fiber intake, specifically low fiber intake, in the etiology of IBD; results have been conflicting.

Several workers noted increased intake of refined sugar in the pre-illness diet of well-established and newly diagnosed patients with Crohn's disease.[101] There are methodologic limitations in all these studies.[122] In any event, the clinical significance of these findings is not known. Mayberry et al.[101] noted dietary abnormalities in their study of 32 patients with recently diagnosed IBD. They hypothesized that this may simply reflect a deficiency in perception of sweet taste in patients with this condition.

FUTURE DIRECTIONS FOR DIET AND NUTRITION IN INFLAMMATORY BOWEL DISEASE

Looking to the future, one may expect further work evaluating the potential role of short-chain fatty acids (SCFAs) in the pathogenesis of IBD, especially ulcerative colitis. The work of Harig et al.[66] in the use of SCFA infusion to treat diversion colitis is exciting (see Chapter 16). These SCFAs are derived from bacterial fermentation of dietary carbohydrate, and are the preferred fuel of colonocytes; enterocytes prefer glutamine. Neither of these nutrients is routinely added into either TPN or most enteral formulas. Also of interest is the ongoing work of Koruda et al.[83] who used a rat model to study the effects of intravenous SCFA infusion. SCFA-supplemented TPN was as effective as intracecal infusion of SCFAs in preventing the usual TPN-associated mucosal atrophy.

Lastly, I refer back to comments of Bayless regarding the Japanese experience with IBD; as meat and dairy intake (total fat intake, saturated fat intake, omega-6 fatty acid intake) have increased in Japan, so apparently has the incidence of IBD, both Crohn's disease and ulcerative colitis (see Chapter 3). In our own country during the past century, total calorie and protein intake have remained fairly stable. The sources of dietary protein have changed from largely vegetable sources (low in fats, high in SCFA precursors) to largely animal sources (high in fats, low in SCFA precursors). It is known that dietary intake of fats can have an effect on the body's mediators of inflammation, e.g., prostaglandins, leukotrienes, and cytokines. Data regarding eicosanoids in IBD[151] are provocative, preliminary, and exciting. These factors, their role in IBD, as well as other nutrients such as glutamine, selenium, vitamin E, and glutathione, need further investigation.

REFERENCES

1. Acheson ED, Truelove SC: Early weaning in the aetiology of ulcerative colitis: A study of feeding in infancy in cases and controls. *Br Med J* 1961; 2:929–935.
2. Afdhal NH, et al: Remission induction in refractory Crohn's disease using a high calorie whole diet. *J Parenter Enter Nutr* 1989; 13:362–365.
3. Alun Jones V: Comparison of total parenteral nutrition and elemental diet in induction of remission of CD. *Dig Dis Sci* 1987; 32:1005–1007.
4. Alun Jones V, et al: Crohn's disease: Maintenance of remission by diet. *Lancet* 1985; 2:177–180.
5. Anderson DL, Boyce HW Jr: Use of parenteral nutrition in treatment of advanced regional enteritis. *Am J Dig Dis* 1973; 18:633–640.
6. Andersen H, et al: Absorption studies in patients with Crohn's disease and in patients with ulcerative colitis. *Acta Med Scand* 1971; 190:407–410.
7. Andresen AFR: Gastrointestinal manifestations of food allergy. *Med J Record* 1925; 122(suppl):271.
8. Andreson AFR: Ulcerative colitis—an allergic phenomenon. *Am J Digest Dis* 1942; 9:91–98.
9. Arvanitakis C: Abnormalities of jejunal mucosal enzymes in ulcerative colitis and Crohn's disease. *Digestion* 1979; 19:259–266.
10. Axelsson C, Jarnum S: Assessment of the therapeutic value of an elemental diet in chronic IBD. *Scand J Gastroenterol* 1977; 12:89–95.
11. Barker WH, Hummel LE: Macrocytic anemia in association with intestinal strictures and anastomoses. *Bull Johns Hopkins Hosp* 1939; 64:215–236.
12. Barot LR, et al: Caloric requirements in patients with IBD. *Ann Surg* 1981; 195:214–218.
13. Barr M, et al: Studies of the anemia in ulcerative colitis with special reference to the iron metabolism. *Acta Paediatr* 1955; 44:62–72.
14. Beeken WL, et al: Intestinal protein loss in Crohn's disease. *Gastroenterology* 1972; 62:207–214.
15. Beeken WL: Absorptive defects in young people with regional enteritis. *Pediatrics* 1973; 52:69–74.

16. Beeken WL: Remediable defects in Crohn's disease, a prospective study of 63 patients. *Arch Intern Med* 1979; 135:686–690.
17. Blair GK, et al: Preoperative home elemental enteral nutrition in complicated Crohn's disease. *J Pediatr Surg* 1986; 21:769–771.
18. Box LP, Weterman IT: Total parenteral nutrition in Crohn's disease. *World J Surg* 1980; 4:163–166.
19. Burbige EJ, et al: Clinical manifestations of Crohn's disease in children and adolescents. *Pediatrics* 1975; 55:866–871.
20. Bury KD, et al: Use of chemically defined, liquid, elemental diet for nutritional management of fistulas of the alimentary tract. *Am J Surg* 1971; 121:174–183.
21. Busk HE, et al: The incidence of lactose malabsorption in ulcerative colitis. *Scand J Gastroenterol* 1975; 10:263–265.
22. Butt HR, Watkins CH: Occurrence of macrocytic anemia in association with lesions of the bowel. *Ann Intern Med* 1936; 10:222–232.
23. Cameron DG, et al: The clinical association of macrocytic anemia with intestinal stricture and anastomosis. *Blood* 1949; 4:793–802.
24. Carney EA, Russell RM: Correlation of dark adaptation test results with serum vitamin A levels in diseased adults. *J Nutrition* 1980; 10:552–557.
25. Chilo JA, et al: The diagnosis of iron deficiency in patients with Crohn's disease. *Gut* 1973; 14:642–648.
26. Christie PM, Hill GL: Effect of intravenous nutrition on nutrition and function in acute attacks of IBD. *Gastroenterology* 1990; 99:730–736.
27. Compston JE, Creamer B: Plasma levels and intestinal absorption of 25 (OH) vitamin D in patients with small bowel resection. *Gut* 1977; 18:171–175.
28. Compston JE, et al: Osteomalacia after small intestinal resection. *Lancet* 1978; 1:9–12.
29. Compston JE, et al: Osteoporosis in patients with IBD. *Gut* 1987; 28:410–415.
30. Cook JD, Finch C: Assessing iron status of a population. *Am J Clin Nutr* 1979; 32:2115–2119.
31. Cox EV, et al: The folic acid excretion test in the steatorrhea syndrome. *Gastroenterology* 1958; 35:390–397.
32. Cox EV, et al: An inter-relationship between ascorbic acid and cyanocobalamin. *Clin Sci* 1958; 17:681–692.
33. Dean RE, et al: Hyperalimentation in the management of chronic IBD. *Dis Colon Rectum* 1976; 19:601–604.
34. Dickinson RJ, et al: Controlled trial of intravenous hyperalimentation and total bowel rest as an adjunct to the routine therapy of acute colitis. *Gastroenterology* 1980; 79:1199–1204.
35. Driscoll RH, et al: Bone histology and vitamin D status in Crohn's disease: Association with nutrition and disease activity. *Gastroenterology* 1977; 77:1051.

36. Driscoll RH, Rosenberg IH: Total parenteral nutrition in IBD. *Med Clin North Am* 1978; 62:185–203.
37. Driscoll RH, et al: Vitamin D deficiency and bone disease in patients with Crohn's disease. *Gastroenterology* 1982; 83:1252–1258.
38. Dronfield MW, et al: Zinc in ulcerative colitis: A therapeutic trial and report on plasma levels. *Gut* 1977; 18:33–36.
39. Duthie ML, et al: Serum electrolytes and colonic transfer of water and electrolytes in chronic ulcerative colitis. *Gastroenterology* 1964; 47:525–530.
40. Dyer NH, et al: Anemia in Crohn's disease. *Q J Med* 1972; 41:419–436.
41. Dyer NH, Dawson AM: Malnutrition and malabsorption in Crohn's disease with reference to the effect of surgery. *Br J Surg* 1973; 60:134–140.
42. Eisenberg HW, et al: Hyperalimentation as preparation for surgery in transmural colitis (Crohn's disease). *Dis Colon Rectum* 1974; 17:469–475.
43. Elsborg L, Larsen L: Folate deficiency in chronic inflammatory bowel diseases. *Scand J Gastroenterol* 1979; 14:1019–1024.
44. Elson CO, et al: An evaluation of total parenteral nutrition in the management of IBD. *Dig Dis Sci* 1980; 25:42–48.
45. Falchuk KR, Isselbacher KJ: Circulating antibodies to bovine albumin in ulcerative Crohn's disease. *Gastroenterology* 1976; 70:5–8.
46. Fazio VW, et al: Inflammatory disease of the bowel. *Dis Colon Rectum* 1978; 19:574–578.
47. Filipsson S, et al: Malabsorption of fat and vitamin B12 before and after intestinal resection for Crohn's disease. *Scand J Gastroenterol* 1978; 13:529–536.
48. Fischer JE, et al: Hyperalimentation as primary therapy for IBD. *Am J Surg* 1973; 125:165–175.
49. Fleming CR, et al: Zinc nutrition in Crohn's disease. *Dig Dis Sci* 1981; 26:865–870.
50. Flombaum C, Berner YN: TPN-induced catch up of growth in a 22 year old male with radiation enteritis. *Am J Clin Nutr* 1989; 50:1341–1347.
51. Florent C, et al: Intestinal clearance of antitrypsin, a sensitive method for the detection of protein-losing enteropathy. *Gastroenterology* 1981; 81:777–780.
52. Franklin JL, Rosenberg IH: Impaired folic acid absorption in IBD: Effects of salicylazosulfapyridine (Azulfidine). *Gastroenterology* 1973; 64:517–525.
53. Gassull MA, et al: Enteral nutrition in IBD. *Gut* 1986; 27:76–80.
54. Gerlach K, et al: Symptomatic hypomagnesemia complicating regional enteritis. *Gastroenterology* 1970; 59:567–574.
55. Gerson CD, et al: Crohn's disease: Small intestine absorptive function in regional enteritis. *Gastroenterology* 1973; 64:907–913.
56. Gerson CD: Crohn's disease: Ascorbic acid deficiency in clinical disease including regional enteritis. *Ann NY Acad Sci* 1975; 258:483–490.
57. Gerson CD, Cohen N: Crohn's disease; Folic acid absorption in regional enteritis. *Am J Clin Nutr* 1976; 29:182–186.

58. Gerson CD, Fabry EM: Ascorbic acid deficiency and fistula formation in regional enteritis. *Gastroenterology* 1974; 67:428–433.
59. Giaffer MH, et al: Controlled trial of polymeric versus elemental diet in treatment of Crohn's disease. *Lancet* 1990; 1:816–819.
60. Ginsberg AL, Albert MB: Treatment of patient with severe steroid-dependent Crohn's disease with nonelemental formula diet: Identification of possible etiologic dietary factor. *Dig Dis Sci* 1989; 34:1624–1628.
61. Giorgini GL, et al: The use of "medical by-pass" in the therapy of Crohn's disease: Report of a case. *Dig Dis Sci* 1973; 18:153–157.
62. Goode A, et al: Use of an elemental diet for long-term nutritional support in Crohn's disease. *Lancet* 1976; 1:122–124.
63. Gouma DJ, et al: Preoperative total parenteral nutrition (TPN) in severe Crohn's disease. *Surgery* 1988; 103:648–652.
64. Greenberg GR, et al: Total parenteral nutrition (TPN) and bowel rest in the management of Crohn's disease. *Gut* 1976; 17:828A.
65. Greenberg GR, et al: Controlled trial of bowel rest and nutritional support in the management of Crohn's disease. *Gut* 1988; 29:1309–1315.
66. Harig JM, et al: Treatment of diversion colitis with short-chain-fatty acid irrigation. *N Engl J Med* 1989; 320:23–28.
67. Harries AD, et al: Controlled trial of supplemental, oral nutrition in Crohn's disease. *Lancet* 1983; 1:887–890.
68. Harries AD, et al: Vitamin D status in Crohn's disease: Association with nutrition and disease activity. *Gut* 1985; 26:1197–1203.
69. Hellberg R, et al: Nutritional and hematological status before and after primary and subsequent resectional procedures for classical Crohn's disease and Crohn's colitis. *Acta Chir Scand* 1982; 148:453–460.
70. Hendrick KM, Walker WA: Zinc deficiency in IBD. *Nutr Rev* 1988; 46:401–408.
71. Homer DR, et al: Growth, course and prognosis after surgery for Crohn's disease. *Pediatrics* 1977; 59:717–725.
72. Howard L, et al: Reversible neurological symptoms caused by vitamin E deficiency in a patient with short bowel syndrome. *Am J Clin Nutr* 1982; 36:1243–1249.
73. Hunt JB, et al: A randomized controlled trial of elemental diet and prednisolone as primary therapy in acute exacerbations of Crohn's disease. *Gastroenterology* 1988; 96:A224.
74. James AH: Breakfast and Crohn's disease. *Br Med J* 1977; 1:943–945.
75. Jarnerot G, et al: Intensive intravenous treatment of ulcerative colitis. *Gastroenterology* 1985; 89:1005–1013.
76. Kasper H, Sommer H: Dietary fiber and nutrient intake in Crohn's disease. *Am J Clin Nutr* 1979; 32:1898–1901.
77. Kelts DG, et al: Nutritional basis of growth failure in children and adolescents with Crohn's disease. *Gastroenterology* 1979; 76:720–727.
78. Kirschner BS, et al: Growth retardation in IBD. *Gastroenterology* 1978; 75:504–511.

79. Kirschner BS, et al: Reversal of growth retardation in Crohn's disease with therapy emphasizing oral nutritional restitution. *Gastroenterology* 1981; 80:10–15.
80. Kirsner JB, et al: Studies on amino acid excretion in chronic ulcerative colitis and regional enteritis. *J Clin Sci* 1950; 29:874–880.
81. Kimberg DB, et al: Effect of cortisone treatment on the active transport of calcium by the small intestine. *J Clin Sci* 1971; 50:1309–1321.
82. Koretz RL: Nutritional support: How much for how long? *Gut* 1986; 51:85–95.
83. Koruda MJ, et al: Parenteral nutrition supplemented with short-chain fatty acids: Effect on the small bowel mucosa in normal rats. *Am J Clin Nutr* 1990; 51:685–689.
84. Koda T, et al: Effects of dietary butter fat on fecal bile acid excretion in patients with Crohn's disease on elemental diet. *Dig Dis Sci* 1984; 29:994–999.
85. Krawitt EL, et al: Calcium absorption in Crohn's disease. *Gastroenterology* 1976; 71:251–254.
86. Lanfranchi GA, et al: Serum zinc concentrations in Crohn's disease (letter). *Dig Dis Sci* 1982; 27:1141–1142.
87. Larson PM, et al: Elemental diet: A therapeutic approach in chronic IBD. *J Intern Med* 1989; 225:325–331.
88. Lashner BA, et al: Effect of folate supplementation on the incidence of dysplasia and cancer in chronic ulcerative colitis. *Gastroenterology* 1989; 97:255–259.
89. Layden T, et al: Reversal of growth arrest in adolescents with Crohn's disease after parenteral nutrition. *Gastroenterology* 1976; 70:1017–1026.
90. Lerebours E, et al: An evaluation of total parenteral nutrition in the management of steroid-dependent and steroid-resistant patients with Crohn's disease. *JPEN* 1986; 10:274–278.
91. Levenstein S, et al: Low residue or normal diet in Crohn's disease: A prospective controlled study in Italian patients. *Gut* 1985; 26:989–993.
92. Linaker BD: Scurvy and vitamin C deficiency in Crohn's disease. *Postgrad Med J* 1979; 55:26–29.
93. Lindenbaum J, et al: Neuropsychiatric disorders caused by cobalamin deficiency in the absence of anemia or macrocytosis. *N Engl J Med* 1988; 318:1720–1728.
94. Lindor KD, et al: Comparison of corticosteroid therapy with vital HN alone or vital HN combined with corticosteroids in patients with active Crohn's disease. JPEN 1990; 14(suppl):165.
95. Lochs H, et al: Enteral nutrition versus drug treatment for the acute phase of Crohn's disease: Results of the European Cooperative Study V. *Gastroenterology* 1988; 98:A267.
96. Logan RFA, et al: Reduction of gastrointestinal protein loss by elemental diet in Crohn's disease of the small bowel. *Gut* 1981; 22:383–387.
97. Lubran M, McAllen PM: Potassium deficiency in ulcerative colitis. *Q J Med* 1951; 20:221–232.

98. Lukert BP, et al: Vitamin D and intestinal transport of calcium: Effects of prednisolone. *Endocrinology* 1973; 93:718–722.
99. Main ANH, et al: Vitamin A deficiency in Crohn's disease. *Gut* 1983; 24:1169–1175.
100. Martin P, et al: Isotretinoin associated proctosigmoiditis. *Gastroenterology* 1987; 93:606–609.
101. Mayberry JT, et al: Diet in Crohn's disease: Two studies of current and previous habits in newly diagnosed patients. *Dig Dis Sci* 1983; 26:444–448.
102. McClain CJ, et al: Zinc deficiency: A complication of Crohn's disease. *Gastroenterology* 1980; 78:272–279.
103. McClain CJ, et al: Zinc-deficiency-induced retinal dysfunction in Crohn's disease. *Dig Dis Sci* 1987; 28:85–87.
104. McIntyre PB, et al: Controlled trial of bowel rest in the treatment of severe acute colitis. *Gut* 1986; 27:481–485.
105. McIntyre RB, et al: Management of enterocutaneous fistulas: A review of 132 cases. *Br J Surg* 1989; 71:293–296.
106. Maynell MJ, et al: Serum-cyanocobalamin level in chronic intestinal disorders. *Lancet* 1957; 1:901–904.
107. Meyers J, Janowitz HD: "Natural history" of Crohn's disease: An analytic review of the placebo lesson. *Gastroenterology* 1984; 87:1189–1194.
108. Morin CL, et al: Continuous elemental parenteral alimentation in children with Crohn's disease and growth failure. *Gastroenterology* 1980; 79:1205–1210.
109. Mullen JL, et al: Ten years experience with intravenous hyperalimentation and IBD. *Ann Surg* 1978; 187:523–529.
110. Muller JM, et al: Total parenteral nutrition as the sole therapy in Crohn's disease—a prospective study. *Br J Surg* 1983; 70:40–43.
111. Nelson LM, et al: Use of an elemental diet (Vivonex) in the management of bile acid–induced diarrhea. *Gut* 1977; 18:792–794.
112. Nishi Y, et al: Zinc status and its relation to growth retardation in children with chronic IBD. *Am J Clin Nutr* 1980; 33:2613–2621.
113. Nyhlin N, et al: Plasma and skeletal muscle electrolytes in patients with Crohn's disease. *J Am Coll Nutr* 1985; 4:531–538.
114. O'Keefe SJD, et al: Steroids and bowel rest versus elemental diet in the treatment of patients with Crohn's disease: The effects on protein metabolism and immune function. *J Parenter Enter Nutr* 1989; 13:455–460.
115. O'Morain C, et al: Elemental diet in acute Crohn's disease. *Arch Dis Child* 1983; 53:44–47.
116. O'Morain C, et al: Elemental diets in treatment of acute Crohn's disease. *Br Med J* 1980; 281:1173–1175.
117. O'Morain C, et al: Elemental diet as primary treatment of acute Crohn's disease: A controlled trial. *Br Med J* 1984; 288:1859–1862.
118. Ostro MJ, et al: Total parenteral nutrition and complete bowel rest in the management of Crohn's disease. *J Parenter Enter Nutr* 1985; 9:280–287.
119. Oversen L, et al: The influence of dietary fat on jejunostomy output in patients with severe short-bowel syndrome. *Am J Clin Nutr* 1983; 38:270–277.

120. Payne-James JJ, Silk DBA: Total parenteral nutrition as primary treatment in Crohn's disease—RIP? *Gut* 1988; 29:1304–1308.
121. Pena ADS, Truelove SC: Hypolactasia and ulcerative colitis. *Gastroenterology* 1973; 64:400–404.
122. Persson PG, et al: Crohn's disease and ulcerative colitis: A review of dietary studies with emphasis on methodologic aspects. *Scand J Gastroenterol* 1987; 22:385–389.
123. Peto R, et al: Can dietary beta-carotene materially reduce human cancer rates? *Nature* 1981; 290:201–208.
124. Pettit SH, et al: Ascorbic acid absorption in Crohn's disease. *Dig Dis Sci* 1989; 34:559–566.
125. Powell-Tuck J, et al: Rates of whole body protein synthesis and breakdown increase with the severity of IBD. *Gut* 1984; 25:460–464.
126. Rees RGP, et al: Elemental diet administered nasogastrically without starter regimens to patients with IBD. *J Parenter Enter Nutr* 1986; 10:258–262.
127. Reeves WC, et al: Reversible cardiomyopathy due to selenium deficiency. *J Parenter Enter Nutr* 1989; 13:663–667.
128. Reilly J, et al: Hyperalimentation in IBD. *Am J Surg* 1976; 131:192–200.
129. Rhodes J, Rosen J: Does food affect acute IBD? The role of parenteral nutrition, elemental and exclusion diets. *Gut* 1986; 27:417–474.
130. Ritland S, et al: Liver copper content in patients with IBD and associated liver disorders. *Scand J Gastroenterol* 1981; 14:711–715.
131. Rocchio MA, et al: Use of chemically defined diets in the management of patients with acute IBD. *Am J Surg* 1974; 127:469–475.
132. Rombeau JL, et al: Preoperative total parenteral nutrition and surgical outcome in patients with IBD. *Am J Surg* 1982; 143:139–143.
133. Rowe AH: Chronic ulcerative colitis—allergy in its etiology. *Ann Intern Med* 1942; 17:83–100.
134. Russell RM et al: Dark adaptation testing for diagnosis of subclinical vitamin A deficiency and evaluation of therapy. *Lancet* 1973; 2:1161–1164.
135. Sanderson IR, et al: Remission induced by an elemental diet in small bowel Crohn's disease. *Arch Dis Child* 1987; 61:123–127.
136. Sandstead HH, Howard L: Zinc deficiency in Crohn's disease. *Nutr Rev* 1982; 40:109–112.
137. Saverymuttu S, et al: Controlled trial comparing prednisolone with an elemental diet plus non-absorbable antibiotics in active Crohn's disease. *Gut* 1985; 26:994–998.
138. Schofield PF: Some aspects of Crohn's disease. *Dis Colon Rectum* 1967; 10:262–266.
139. Sciaretta G, et al: Hydrogen breath test quantification and clinical correlation of lactose malabsorption in adult irritable bowel syndrome and ulcerative colitis. *Dig Dis Sci* 1984; 29:1098–1104.
140. Seashort JH, et al: Total parenteral nutrition in the management of IBD in children: A limited role. *Am J Surg* 1982; 143:504–507.
141. Seidman EG: Nutritional management of IBD. *Gastroenterol Clin North Am* 1989; 17:129–155.

142. Seidman EG, et al: Elemental diet versus prednisone as primary treatment of Crohn's disease. *Gastroenterology* 1986; 90:1625A.
143. Selhub J, et al: Inhibition of folate enzymes by sulfasalazine. *J Clin Immunol* 1978; 316:221–224.
144. Shike M, et al: Copper metabolism and requirements in total parenteral nutrition. *Gastroenterology* 1981; 81:290–297.
145. Shiloni E, et al: Role of total parenteral nutrition in the treatment of Crohn's disease. *Am J Surg* 1989; 157:180–185.
146. Solomons NW, et al: Zinc deficiency in Crohn's disease. *Digestion* 1977; 16:87–95.
147. Solomons NW, et al: Leukocytic endogenous mediator in Crohn's disease. *Infect Immunol* 1978; 22:637–639.
148. Solomons NW, Rosenberg IH: Zinc and IBD (letter). *Am J Clin Nutr* 1981; 34:1447–1448.
149. Stabler SP, et al: Clinical spectrum and diagnosis of cobalamin deficiency. *Blood* 1990; 76:871–881.
150. Steinhardt HJ, et al: Enteral nutrition in acute Crohn's disease: Effect of whole vs. hydrolyzed protein on nitrogen economy and intestinal protein loss. *Gastroenterology* 1988; 94:A443.
151. Stenson WF: Role of eicosanoids as mediators of inflammation in IBD. *Scand J Gastroenterol* 1990; 25(suppl 172):13–18.
152. Stevens RV, Randall HT: Use of a concentrated, balanced, liquid elemental diet for nutritional management of catabolic states. *Ann Surg* 1969; 170:642–667.
153. Stokes MA, Irving MH: How do patients with Crohn's disease fare on home parenteral nutrition? *Dis Colon Rectum* 1988; 31:454–458.
154. Strobel CT, et al: Home parenteral nutrition in children with Crohn's disease: An effective management alternative. *Gastroenterology* 1979; 77:272–279.
155. Sturniolo GC, et al: Zinc absorption in Crohn's disease. *Gut* 1980; 21:387–391.
156. Teahon K, et al: 10 years experience with elemental diets in the management of Crohn's disease. *Gut* 1990; 31:1133–1137.
157. Teahon K, et al: Improved nutrition is not an important mechanism by which elemental diets work in acute Crohn's disease. *Gut* 1990; 31:A624.
158. Teahon K, et al: Significance of food intolerances in patients with Crohn's disease. *Gut* 1990; 31:A624.
159. Thoren L: Magnesium deficiency studied in two cases of acute fulminant ulcerative colitis treated by colectomy. *Acta Chir Scand* 1962; 124:134–143.
160. Thoren L: Magnesium deficiency in gastrointestinal fluid loss. *Acta Chir Scand* (Suppl) 1963; 306:5–65.
161. Thornton JR, et al: Diet and Crohn's disease: Characteristics of the pre-illness diet. *Br Med J* 1979; 2:762–764.
162. Truelove SC: Ulcerative colitis provoked by milk. *Br Med J* 1961; 1:154–160.
163. Valberg LS, et al: Zinc absorption in IBD. *Dig Dis Sci* 1986; 31:724–731.

164. VanPatter WR, et al: Regional enteritis. *Gastroenterology* 1954; 26:350–450.
165. Vogel CM, et al: Intravenous hyperalimentation in the treatment of IBD. *Arch Surg* 1974; 108:460–467.
166. Voitk AJ, et al: Experience with elemental diet in the treatment of IBD: Is this primary therapy. *Arch Surg* 1973; 107:329–333.
167. Weisman K, et al: Zinc depletion syndrome with acrodermatitis during long-term intravenous feeding. *Clin Exp Dermatol* 1976; 1:237–242.
168. Welch CS, et al: Metabolic studies on chronic ulcerative colitis. *J Clin Immunol* 1937; 16:161–168.
169. Whittaker JS: Nutritional therapy of hospitalized patients with IBD. *Dig Dis Sci* 1987; 32(suppl):895–945.
170. Whittington PR, et al: Medical management of Crohn's disease in adolescence. *Gastroenterology* 1977; 72:1338–1344.
171. Whorwell PJ, et al: Bottle feeding, early gastroenteritis, and IBD. *Br Med J* 1979; 1:382.
172. Wolman GL, et al: Zinc in total parenteral nutrition: Requirements and metabolic effects. *Gastroenterology* 1979; 76:458–467.
173. Woolf GM, et al: Diet for patients with short bowel: High fat or high carbohydrate? *Gastroenterology* 1983; 84:823–828.
174. Wright R, Truelove SC: A controlled therapeutic trial of various diets in ulcerative colitis. *Br Med J* 1965; 2:138–144.
175. Young E: Short bowel syndrome: High fat versus high carbohydrate diet (editorial). *Gastroenterology* 1983; 84:872–874.

Chapter 10 _____

Narcotics and Other Supplemental Drug Dependence in Inflammatory Bowel Disease

Marvin A. Kaplan

Abdominal pain is one of the primary symptoms of inflammatory bowel disease (IBD). Narcotics and, to a lesser extent, other supplemental drugs, such as tranquilizers, sedatives, and antidepressants, are prescribed when more specific treatments have not been effective. Because of the persistence of symptoms and the frustration of both the patient and the physician, these supplemental drugs are often continued for longer than intended, leading, with many of these medications, to the risk of drug dependence.

Drug dependence is defined as repeated intoxication with an inability to decrease use for at least 1 month. It is accompanied by an impairment in social functioning as well as evidence of physiologic tolerance or withdrawal.[1, 2] The thesis of this chapter is that iatrogenic drug dependence is an unappreciated, common, and avoidable side effect of IBD. Because narcotics are the most common dependence-producing drugs in IBD, their use will be emphasized.

Early reports suggested a high prevalence of drug dependence in chronically medically ill patients.[9, 11] Porter and Jick,[10] however, reported only four cases of drug dependence among 11,882 nonaddict inpatients who received a narcotic preparation, and a low prevalence has been reported by others.[6, 8] All of these studies have serious methodologic problems (e.g., how is the diagnosis of drug dependence reliably determined?), and these errors tend in the direction of underestimating the prevalence of drug dependence in medically ill patients.

Further, some percentage of medically ill patients have a prior or ongoing drug problem. From a large and recent epidemiologic study,[12, 13] the lifetime prevalence rate for drug abuse/dependence was 5.5% in the general population of three different American communities. The rates were much higher in younger people (aged 18–24), which coincides with the age of many patients with IBD. The prevalence of alcohol abuse/dependence was even higher in this age group, particularly among men. The other major problem with the reports in the literature is that clear distinctions have not been made in the use of narcotics in acute vs. chronic conditions, inpatient vs. outpatient, and in terminal situations vs. nonterminal illnesses. For example, in our study of IBD patients,[7] 85% became drug dependent on an outpatient basis, while the literature is otherwise completely based on inpatients.

The true rate of drug dependence in IBD is unknown. Because the prevalence of drug abuse/dependence in the general population is 5.5% (and more than double this when alcohol abuse/dependence is included), it is highly unlikely that a population often in pain and having access to narcotics would have a lower prevalence than the general population. Therefore, as a conservative estimate, at least 5.5%, or a little more than one of every twenty patients, with IBD, probably becomes drug dependent at some time during life.

Making the diagnosis of drug dependence is difficult because the patient almost always denies it. Multiple lost prescriptions and a preoccupation with pain medications are often clues, but in our experience the most reliable way is to interview the family or friends. Compared with the patient's need to hide the problem, relatives and friends are invariably concerned and report the use of narcotics in the absence of pain, that the patient has multiple prescriptions from different physicians, and signs of repeated intoxications and impairment in functioning. The diagnosis of drug dependence should not be excluded until family or friends of the patient have been interviewed.

CASE REPORT

A 31-year-old woman with a history of Crohn's disease since the age of 13 was admitted because of increasing abdominal pain and bloody diarrhea. Neurologic and psychiatric evaluations were requested because the patient was confused and ataxic on admission. It was found that she was taking 32 to 40 Percocet tablets per day while in the hospital, augmenting her own supply by persuading a house officer to order it for headaches as well as abdominal pain. The patient was indignant when this was brought up to her and adamantly denied that her Percocet use was a problem.

Her husband, however, provided a history of increasing codeine and diazepam (Valium) use during the preceding 5 years. For the past year the patient had been taking four Percocet tablets per dose routinely, and he estimated that she took between 30 and 40 tablets per day. She was not functioning at her job nor at home, and had fallen numerous times, including one time when she lost consciousness. The various drugs had been obtained from different physicians who were unaware that the other physicians were also prescribing them. Subsequently she did well on a coordinated plan in which only one physician prescribed pain medications, and she was seen briefly for psychotherapy.

The other way of making the diagnosis is when patients develop narcotic bowel disease. At first presentation they have puzzling gastrointestinal symptoms, usually constipation and pain or alternating diarrhea and constipation, superimposed on their IBD. [14] Many times this is misdiagnosed as an irritable bowel syndrome. If the patient is hospitalized and treated with a trial of clonidine, however, the symptoms rapidly abate, and the diagnosis of narcotic dependence (with narcotic bowel disease) is established. [5, 14]

Prevention is the key to combating drug dependence because in the large majority of cases it is iatrogenic. [7] Prevention starts with the conviction that these drugs are truly supplemental, and efforts must always be made to find the specific cause of pain and treat it accordingly. Next, take a drug and alcohol history to identify high-risk patients; given the lifetime prevalence statistics of drug and alcohol dependence and their high prevalence in younger patients, roughly one of every nine patients should give a history of prior or current drug or alcohol dependence (or both drug and alcohol dependence). These patients are at high risk of developing drug dependence. In addition, Crohn's disease and borderline personality disorder may also be added risk factors. [7] Finally, there needs to be a familiarity with the pharmacology of common dependence-producing drugs, and some of this information is summarized in Table 10–1.

Once these general steps have been taken, there are specific guidelines that, if followed, seem to prevent iatrogenic drug dependence. The most important is the designation of a single physician to be the only one to prescribe narcotics and other dependence-producing drugs. Rather than have the patient's internist, gastroenterologist, surgeon, and any other specialist prescribe these drugs (too frequently without knowing what the other has done), one physician should be selected as the only one who can write these prescriptions for the patient.* This does

---

*Editors Note: Often the drug-dependent patient rings for the nurse, who in turn sends for the tired house officer who might not be familiar with the case.

TABLE 10—1.

Common Medications Causing Drug Dependence in Patients With IBD

Generic Name	Brand Name	Usual Route	Usual Dosage for Short-term Use/Day	Dependence-Producing Dose/Day*
Oxycodone	Percocet	PO	10−20 mg (2−4 tablets)	30−40 mg (6−8 tablets)
Propoxyphene	Darvon	PO	260−390 mg	260−825 mg
Meperidine	Demerol	IM	250−600 mg	400−800 mg[15]
Morphine		SC	24−60 mg	40−50 mg[1]
Pentazocine	Talwin	IM	180−480 mg	200−600 mg
Codeine[†]		PO	120−600 mg	600−1,800 mg
Diphenoxylate[‡]	Lomotil	PO	5−20 mg (2−8 tablets)	100−300 mg (PDR) (40−120 tabs)
Alprazolam	Xanax	PO	0.5−2.0 mg	2−4 mg
Diazepam	Valium	PO	4−20 mg	100−1,500 mg[15]
Triazolam	Halcion	PO	0.125−0.25 mg	1−2 mg
Secobarbital	Seconal	PO	100−200 mg	400−800 mg[15]
Pentobarbital	Nembutal	PO	90−100 mg	400−800 mg

*The dose at which drug dependence develops is extremely variable, and these doses are only rough guides. It also depends on how dependence is defined (e.g., for narcotics, nalorphine-induced withdrawal gives different results than acute discontinuation. The doses given are for 1−2 weeks for narcotics and 1−3 months for the other drugs. If no specific reference () is given, the range indicated is from clinical experience. PDR = *Physicians' Desk Reference.* Orodell, N.J., Medical Economics Co., 1976.
†Not common to produce dependence alone, but can be part of multidrug abuse.
‡Very rarely produces dependence—included for comparison only.

two things: it highlights the potential problem in the patient's mind and it makes that physician responsible for preventing drug dependence.

Once this system is set up, a sharp distinction is made between acute pain (1–3 weeks) and chronic pain. In acute pain, one can use high doses of narcotics to control pain even in high-risk patients without fear of producing drug dependence. The narcotics should be ordered on a regular schedule rather than on an "as-needed" basis, because there is clinical and experimental evidence that the pain control is better and the total dose of narcotic lower when ordered this way.[3, 4] Medications such as hydroxyzine may be added to each narcotic dose to potentiate its effects. High-risk patients should be completely tapered off narcotics once the acute episode resolves.

In chronic pain the situation is entirely different. The prescribing physician should be convinced that long-term narcotic use can lead to lower pain thresholds,[17, 18] tolerance, and the risks of drug dependence (particularly in high-risk patients). The focus remains on finding specific treatment for the patient's underlying illness while attempting to increase the patient's pain tolerance. Both anxiety and depression can dramatically lower pain tolerance, and the first approach is to treat these with appropriate anxiolytics, antidepressants, or psychotherapy. Buspirone is a nondependence-producing anxiolytic that can be used if there is concern about developing dependence on benzodiazepines. If these measures do not succeed in eliminating long-term narcotic use, relaxation training, hypnosis, biofeedback, group therapy (with other patients with pain or IBD), or family therapy is effective at times. If patients prove refractory to all of these, they should be referred to specialized pain treatment centers.

CASE REPORT

A 50-year-old man with Crohn's disease diagnosed at the age of 42 was seen on an outpatient basis because of chronic abdominal pain and increasing narcotic use. He was angry and depressed about how his illness dominated his life. For the preceding 2 years he had the symptoms of major depression with severe insomnia, anorexia with trouble maintaining his weight (which may have been due to his Crohn's disease), trouble concentrating, and a diurnal mood variation in which he felt worse in the morning and better as the day went on. He was taking varying amounts of pentazocine (Talwin), propoxyphene (Darvocet), codeine, diazepam (Valium), and flurazepam (Dalmane), in addition to sulfasalazine, with little benefit. Although quite skeptical, he was started on an antidepressant and short-term once-per-week psychotherapy. His depression decreased during the next month, with a marked decrease in all his symptoms, including the severity of his pain. He was able to stop all narcotics and tranquilizers except for codeine used for control of the diarrhea. He has been kept on a maintenance dose of an antidepressant drug for the past 6 years, with good pain control and no need for increased use of narcotics.

Use of narcotics prescribed for diarrhea should be mentioned. In general, codeine and diphenoxylate with atropine sulfate (Lomotil) very rarely produce drug dependence when prescribed for this purpose. When codeine is prescribed for both pain control and diarrhea, however, it can produce dependence.[7]

If patients have an iatrogenic single drug dependence without major psychopathology, they can often be treated without psychiatric intervention. They need firm confrontation about their drug dependence and gradual detoxification. The patient who has prescriptions from multiple physicians may need to be hospitalized to be detoxified, and the various physicians need to be coordinated in a therapeutic plan. Generally these patients have a good prognosis as long as their access to supplemental drugs is carefully controlled.

Patients with iatrogenic multiple drug dependence or noniatrogenic drug dependence almost always need specialized psychiatric treatment.

Usually psychiatric hospitalization is necessary in the beginning of therapy.[16] Their prognosis is generally poorer.

REFERENCES

1. Adriani J: Drug dependence in hospitalized patients, in *A Treatment Manual for Acute Drug Abuse Emergencies*, Washington, D.C., U.S. Department of Health, Education, and Welfare, 1976.
2. *Diagnostic and Statistical Manual of Mental Disorders*, ed 3. Washington, DC, American Psychiatric Association, 1980.
3. Foley K: The practical use of narcotic analgesics. *Med Clin North Am* 1982; 66:1091–1104.
4. Fordyce W, et al: Operant conditioning in the treatment of chronic pain. *Arch Phys Med Rehabil* 1973; 54:399–408.
5. Gold M, et al: Opiate withdrawal using clonidine: A safe, effective and nonopiate treatment. *JAMA* 1980; 243:343–346.
6. Kanner RM, Foley KM: Patterns of narcotic drug use in a cancer pain clinic. *Ann NY Acad Sci* 1981; 362:161–172.
7. Kaplan M, Korelitz BI: Narcotic dependence in IBD. *J Clin Gastroenterol* 1988; 10:275–278.
8. Marks R, Sachar E: Undertreatment of medical patients with narcotic analgesics. *Ann Intern Med* 1973; 78:173–181.
9. Pescor M: The Kolb classification of drug addicts, in *Public Health Report Supplement 155*. Washington, D.C., U.S. Public Health Service, 1931.
10. Porter J, Jick H: Addiction rate in patients treated with narcotics. *N Engl J Med* 1980; 302:123.
11. Rayport M: Experience in the management of patients medically addicted to narcotics. *JAMA* 1984; 156:684–691.
12. Regier DA, et al: The NIMH Epidemiological Catchment Area program: Historical context, major objectives, and study patient characteristics. *Arch Gen Psychiatry* 1984; 41:934–941.
13. Robins LN, et al: Lifetime prevalence of specific psychiatric disorders in three sites. *Arch Gen Psychiatry* 1984; 41:949–958.
14. Sandgren J: Narcotic bowel disease treated with clonidine. *Ann Intern Med* 1984; 101:331–334.
15. Shader E (ed): *Manual of Psychiatric Therapeutics*. Boston, Little, Brown, 1975.
16. Streltzer J: Treatment of iatrogenic drug dependence in the general hospital. *Gen Hosp Psychiatry* 1980; 2:262–266.
17. Wolff BB, et al: Response of experimental pain to analgesic drugs (I). Morphine, aspirin, secobarbital and placebo. *Clin Pharmacol Ther* 1966; 6:224–238.
18. Wolff BB, et al: Response of experimental pain to analgesic drugs (III). Codeine, aspirin, secobarbital and placebo. *Clin Pharmacol Ther* 1969; 10:217–228.

Chapter 11 _____

Appropriate Use of Radiologic Techniques in Inflammatory Bowel Disease

Bette Harig

What contribution can radiology make in the management of inflammatory bowel disease (IBD)? A practical approach to the workup of patients with IBD must include an eye to the monetary and time constraints of current medical practice. Initially, radiology should be used to characterize the disease and evaluate the extent of disease. Subsequently, contrast examinations should generally be limited to instances in which the patient's symptomatology has changed. In complex settings imaging techniques frequently provide more complete information.

Colonoscopy has replaced the air contrast enema in many centers.* Flexible sigmoidoscopy combined with the air contrast enema, however, does provide similar accuracy in the assessment of bowel disease at less cost and with no sedation. In ulcerative colitis, of course, the low sensitivity of x-ray examination in assessing dysplasia and even in cancer detection makes colonoscopy mandatory.

Small bowel studies are only as good as the radiologist performing them. Enteroclysis is a sophisticated examination. It is the study of choice for patients who have multiple skip lesions, multiple areas of stenosis, and excessive secretions.[11, 15] These patients tend to have very slow transit and poor definition of the underlying disease on routine small bowel studies. The procedure does involve more physician time to allow for positioning of the tube, more radiation because of increased

*See Discussion by Present, following Chapter 13.

fluoroscopy, and extra ancillary help. The Maglinte enteroclysis tube, which is recommended for one-time use, costs more than $100. An electric pump for the infusion is also useful. In the community hospital or in a private office, other practical approaches exist. The detailed small bowel study with compression films and fluoroscopic palpation still provides excellent definition of the disease and should be the procedure of choice for routine screening.[2, 16] The peroral pneumocolon, which is designed specifically to evaluate the last 20 to 40 cm of ileum, gives excellent detail of the mucosal surface in almost 90% of patients.[5] This is also useful to evaluate the anastomosis in patients postoperatively. Preferably the patient receives a bowel preparation to eliminate fecal artifact. When barium reaches the hepatic flexure air is introduced via the rectum after the patient receives intravenous glucagon.

Because of its availability and the lack of radiation, ultrasound evaluation is frequently used as a screening procedure for right lower quadrant pain, especially in children and young women.[7] Today abnormal bowel is routinely visualized with state of the art equipment. One study detected abnormal bowel in 85% of patients with Crohn's disease.[16] The involved segment is described classically as having a target or pseudokidney appearance produced by lumenal echoes contrasted with a surrounding edematous wall that is usually hypoechoic. Response to treatment can be monitored without radiation by following bowel wall thickness. Complications such as an abscess can be similarly detected and followed.[3a] Transvaginal ultrasound is generally available in even the smallest departments. This can be extremely useful in evaluating the lower portion of the abdomen in women when bowel has obscured detail or when symptoms mimic gynecologic pathology. Transrectal ultrasound is found more often in larger centers, which limits its usefulness to some degree. It has been used to judge the extent of perineal disease, but experience is somewhat lacking.

Indium leukocyte scanning has a major advantage over gallium because of its lack of excretion in normal bowel. Any uptake is abnormal, although not diagnostic for IBD. This is an expensive procedure (about $300) for labeling. Approximately 50 to 60 mL of blood is needed. In New York City practically all specimens are sent to an outside laboratory and returned the next day for injection. Time constraints as a result of this can affect the timing of the studies. A three-phase study is thought to be most sensitive for IBD.[1, 4a, 12] Immediately after injection you may see a transient uptake because hyperemia in either mild or treated disease can be seen. After 4 hours, optimal opacification of the diseased bowel takes place. In small departments, however, there may be no coverage after work hours, and this phase may be difficult to obtain. Most scans at Lenox Hill Hospital are done at 24 hours. Because of peristalsis the extent of disease is difficult to evaluate. This is useful, however, for evaluation of the presence or absence of abscesses. The role of indium in IBD is controversial. Reported accuracy ranges from 50% to 95% with the three-phase technique. In patients with known disease, it may prove to be a useful tool for following the extent of activity on a long-term basis.[14]

Magnetic resonance imaging (MRI) is finding more and more of a niche in abdominal conditions. No radiation is involved. Unfortunately it is still expensive; in New York City it averages about $800 for MRI of the pelvis and another $800 for the abdomen. More powerful units and faster scanning sequences are available to suppress respiratory motion and bowel artifact. Oral contrast agents are being developed to improve detail. The differences in the characteristic signals seen with tumor, edema, blood, and fibrosis may in the future allow us to evaluate the bowel without resorting to more invasive studies.[6]

With the spatial resolution of MRI, direct coronal and sagittal images allow for accurate assessment of the rectum and the perineum and their relationship to the levator ani muscle, which can affect surgical planning.[9]* Although computed tomography (CT) does have good innate contrast in the perineum, reconstructions in different planes are rather crude. Partial volume averaging on axial scans through the levator ani muscle may mimic inflammatory changes.

CT is still the gold standard of imaging. In one study CT findings in symptomatic patients with IBD altered clinical management in 25% of cases.[4] Intravenous contrast should be used routinely to better assess tissue characteristics.

Mucosal disease cannot be evaluated. Mural disease is readily apparent as marked thickening of the bowel wall. With intravenous contrast there may be a ring or halo effect of the bowel wall. Initially believed to be quite suggestive of IBD, it can be seen in many mural diseases.[8]

In the patient with a palpable mass, CT will show not only the diseased bowel but also the adjacent mesentery and retroperitoneum. Fibrofatty proliferation or creeping fat, represented by increased density and infiltration around the bowel, is frequently seen and readily distinguished from an underlying abscess.[13] Although contrast may not enter a fistula, air bubbles may be apparent. The fistulas themselves are seen as linear soft tissue densities. Extension to the adjacent muscles will

*See Chapter 15. The MRI is being utilized in the preoperative screening of Crohn's disease complex perirectal fistulas for complicating carcinoma.

cause swelling and surrounding edema, which may also be seen clinically as a mass. Mildly enlarged lymph nodes are common. Numerous nodes more than 1 cm in size should raise the possibility of lymphoma. Perianal and perineal disease can be evaluated with CT and MRI. Fistulas may not be visualized with routine contrast studies, because of pain, swelling, or positioning of the catheter tip. CT can better delineate the extent of disease because of the innate tissue differences between fat and soft tissue. Many CT scans routinely finish at the level of the pubic symphysis. Because approximately 30% of patients with Crohn's disease may have inflammatory changes below this point, the examination should continue through the entire perineum.[17]

CT scanning can be further tailored to assess other complications. Evaluation of bladder fistulas or renal disease, such as oxalate stone formation, may necessitate both precontrast and postcontrast scans. Postoperatively, because of bandages and bowel gas, patient evaluation is difficult with ultrasound. Complications are readily visualized with CT. With use of CT guidance, diagnostic aspiration or drainage of collections can be performed at the same time.[3, 10]

REFERENCES

1. Becker W, et al: Three-phase white blood cell scan: Diagnostic validity in abdominal inflammatory disease. *J Nucl Med* 1986; 27:1109–1115.
2. Carlson H: Perspective: The small bowel examination in the diagnosis of Crohn's disease. *AJR* 1986; 147:63–65.
3. Casola G, et al: Abscess in Crohn's disease: Percutaneous drainage. *Radiology* 1987; 163:19–22.
3a. DiCandido G, et al: Sonographic detection of postsurgical recurrence of Crohn's disease. *AJR* 1986; 146:523–526.
4. Fishman E, et al: CT evaluation of Crohn's disease: Effect on patient management. *AJR* 1987; 148:537–540.
4a. Froelich J: Nuclear medicine imaging of IBD. *Radiol Clin North Am* 1987; 25:133–141.
5. Glick S: Crohn's disease of the small intestine. *Radiol Clin North Am* 1987; 25:45.
6. Goldberg H: MRI of the gastrointestinal tract. *Radiol Clin North Am* 1989; 27:805–812.
7. Gore R: Cross sectional imaging of the inflammatory bowel disease. *Radiol Clin North Am* 1987; 25:115–131.
8. Gore R: CT of inflammatory bowel disease. *Radiol Clin North Am* 1989; 27:717–729.
9. Koelbel G, et al: Diagnosis of fistulae and sinus tracts in patients with Crohn's disease: Value of MRI. *AJR* 1989; 152:999–1003.

10. Lambiase R, et al: Percutaneous drainage of abscesses in patients with Crohn's disease. *AJR* 1988; 150:1043–1045.
11. Maglinte D, et al: Small bowel radiography: How, when and why? *Radiology* 1987; 163:297–305.
12. Navab F, et al: Early and delayed indium 111 leukocyte imaging in Crohn's disease. *Gastroenterology* 1987; 93:829–834.
13. Orel S, et al: Computed tomography vs. barium studies in the acutely symptomatic patient with Crohn's disease. *J Comput Assist Tomogr* 1987; 11:1009–1016.
14. Park R, et al: Can indium 111 autologous mixed leukocyte scanning accurately assess disease extent and activity in Crohn's disease? *Gut* 1988; 29:821–825.
15. Theoni R: Small bowel. *Curr Opin Radiol* 1989; 1:60–65.
16. Worlicek H, et al: Ultrasound findings in Crohn's disease and ulcerative colitis: A prospective study. *J Clin Ultrasound* 1987; 15:153–163.
17. Yousem D, et al: Crohn's disease: Perirectal and perianal findings at CT. *Radiology* 1988; 167:331–334.

Chapter 12 _____

X-Ray or Endoscopic Examination for Initial Evaluation and Follow-Up in Patients With Colonic Inflammatory Bowel Disease

Jerome Waye

The diagnosis and therapy of inflammatory bowel disease (IBD) are usually established by clinical parameters to which are added radiology, sigmoidoscopy, and rectal biopsy. Most patients will not require colonoscopy at any time during the course of their disease. The barium enema has long been accepted as the major imaging procedure in IBD. This x-ray examination is readily available, a standard technique is used, it is noninvasive, is well tolerated, and results in a set of films for study, review, and comparison with subsequent examinations.[1, 24]

On the other hand, while colonoscopy in patients with IBD may be quite valuable, the specific indications are relatively limited. In most instances the colonoscopic examination is properly the last step in a succession of diagnostic examinations performed during evaluation of a specific problem arising in a patient with colitis.

Colonoscopy is not performed routinely in patients with ulcerative colitis because management decisions are rarely made on the basis of an endoscopic examination.*[5, 7, 35] The endoscopic examination of the large bowel should follow the barium enema x-ray examination, except in a few selected situations such as the postoperative evaluation of pa-

*Editor's Note: From my perspective as a clinician specializing in IBD, this is no longer true. The endoscopic picture does not always coincide with the clinical picture. What I have seen through the scope now often influences my change in management and a favorable outcome.

tients and during screening for premalignant conditions. When difficulty arises in the interpretation of a barium enema, colonoscopy becomes a valuable complementary investigation in the patient with IBD, especially for obtaining biopsy specimens or evaluating strictures, filling defects, and mass lesions. Specific histopathologic lesions are not usually found during endoscopic biopsy, and when the differential diagnosis between normal and idiopathic colitis depends on the microscopic interpretation of a series of tissue samples,[5] the astute clinician will realize that often biopsy specimens of normal colonic mucosa will be reported as containing "acute and chronic inflammation." Colonoscopy and biopsy can be of value in the differential diagnosis between IBD and other kinds of colitis (see Chapter 13).

ULCERATIVE COLITIS

Ulcerative colitis is a mucosal disease with the pathologic abnormalities occurring primarily in the mucosal layer.[34] Secondary changes in the configuration of the bowel wall may occur because of alteration in the smooth muscle tone.

Erythema

Erythema is the first sign of colitis, resulting in loss of the normal vascular markings. This change is discernible only endoscopically, and cannot be identified radiographically.

Granularity

Granularity is the earliest mucosal abnormality that can be detected radiologically.[27] It is caused by diffuse mucosal edema. The granular quality of the surface is related to multiple minute depressions where crypt penetration occurs. The texture of granularity can vary considerably, with fine granularity apparent in the earliest stages of ulcerative colitis, before the development of ulceration or erosion. On the double-contrast barium enema, the smooth, even texture of the barium coating is lost, becoming amorphous or finely stippled. Seen tangentially, the fine mucosal line is slightly thickened and indistinct. The earliest changes of colitis on the single-contrast barium enema are an abnormal mucosal fold pattern on the postevacuation film.[32] Endoscopically, granularity is identified when the reflection of light from the colon wall is broken into multiple highlights representing the surface edema punctuated by each colon crypt.

Friability

Friability is the tendency for the colon wall to bleed spontaneously or bleed readily when the surface is touched or rubbed. This property is a visual phenomenon, and is identified only endoscopically. The bleeding of ulcerative colitis is frequently from mucosal oozing related to diffuse friability. Spontaneous bleeding is usually related to multiple tiny or microscopic mucosal ulcerations, with edema and hyperemia.

Ulcerations

Ulcerations develop from erosions that become deeper or coalesce into large ulcers. The ulcers in ulcerative colitis invariably occur on a background of mucosal inflammation, detected radiologically as surrounding granularity and endoscopically as ulcers amidst an area of erythema, friability, and granularity.

CROHN'S DISEASE

Crohn's disease may affect every part of the gastrointestinal tract with transmural inflammation. It is characterized by marked thickening of the bowel wall and involvement of regional lymph nodes. There is a tendency toward the formation of deep ulcers, abscesses, and fistulas. In most cases the involvement with Crohn's disease is discontinuous rather than contiguous. In its early stages this may be manifested by discrete small ulcers in an area of normal mucosa. In later stages, total colon involvement may occur, or segments containing severe disease may be separated by intervening normal mucosa.[33, 34]

Aphthous Ulcers

Aphthous ulcers are the earliest radiographic finding in Crohn's disease, and are demonstrated as small central collections of barium surrounded by a radiolucent halo.[25] These lesions have no predilection for any portion of the colon or rectum, and are frequently found in a background of normal mucosa. The precursor lesions to these small ulcers are areas of focal inflammation in submucosal lymphoid nodules, which then ulcerate through the mucosa to become the "aphthae" with a small collar of edema (the "halo").[37] These small ulcers can be visualized endoscopically. Biopsies of ulcers in Crohn's disease characteristically yield a low prevalence of granulomas (about 5%–10%), since the enlarging ulcer tends to engulf and destroy the initial focal inflammatory response. The greatest possibility for demonstrating the presence of granulomas with histopathologic examination occurs when the tissue specimen is taken from small aphthous ulcers.[14, 15]

Discontinuous Involvement

Skip lesions, or areas of diseased bowel interspersed with normal segments, are one of the major hallmarks of Crohn's disease. In the earliest stages the aphthous ulcers are separated by normal mucosa. As the ulcers enlarge, patches of normal mucosa can usually be identified between them. The pattern of discontinuous involvement has been demonstrated in 90% of patients with Crohn's disease.[26] When ulcers coalesce to create a totally denuded surface, the disease may be indistinguishable from ulcerative colitis. In Crohn's disease, however, the intervening mucosa tends to be normal and is not granular, a feature common to both radiographic and endoscopic study. Endoscopic biopsy specimens obtained from visually uninvolved mucosa are characteristically normal.

Asymmetry

Asymmetry is another characteristic feature of Crohn's disease. Involvement of one portion of the bowel wall may occur, while the opposite wall appears normal both radiographically and endoscopically. This tendency causes the x-ray appearance of ballooning and sacculation of the large intestine, a feature not frequently recognized endoscopically.[4]

Cobblestoning

Cobblestoning of the mucosa is one of the diagnostic features in granulomatous colitis, and is described differently by radiologists and pathologists than by endoscopists. The classic description of cobblestoning is that of nonulcerated mucosa separated by serpiginous longitudinal and transverse ulcers in distinct isolated segments of mucosal islands. Each of these edematous portions of wall has a relatively flat surface with peripheral depression at their edges. When viewed en masse this repetitive pattern is reminiscent of cobblestones. The deep ulcerations around cobblestones are rarely seen endoscopically, because these patients are usually acutely ill with a severe episode of colitis and endoscopy with air insufflation is contraindicated. A different but equally pathognomonic type of cobblestone pattern is recognized endoscopically when areas of normal-appearing mucosa are thrown into multiple regular bumpy elevations by the submucosal involvement. Endoscopically the borders of each "cobblestone" may or may not be ulcerated. Cobblestones are distinguished from pseudopolyps by their low height (usually not taller than 2 mm), the tendency for uniformity of nodulations, and because the base diameter is greater than the height of each elevation.

OTHER MAJOR CONSIDERATIONS

Extent of Disease

Although easily performed, it is unusual to require colonoscopy for evaluation of the extent of colitis, since that information is rarely vital in determining the clinical approach to the patient. Most treatment decisions are based on the clinical course of the disease regardless of how much of the large bowel is involved. There is a specific instance when colonoscopy can be quite useful in assessment of disease extent, however; when "proctitis" does not respond to local therapy with medication, suppositories, or cortisone enemas, the clinician should consider that the disease extends more proximally than the rectosigmoid region, and, under these circumstances, colonoscopy and multiple proximal biopsies may provide the desired information.[8, 21]

Both the barium enema and the visual endoscopic estimate of disease extent will be less than that shown on microscopic examination of biopsy samples.[17] Fifty percent of patients with treatment-resistant proctitis and a proximal x-ray film showing negative findings will have proximal inflammation in colonoscopic biopsy specimens in the absence of gross mucosal abnormalities. The barium enema tends to underestimate the extent of involvement as judged by histology, and total colitis is usually found with histologic examination of endoscopic biopsy specimens in almost every case in which the disease appeared to extend to the hepatic flexure radiographically.[3] When the extent of the disease is questioned, biopsies may double the yield of pathology when compared with the endoscopically visible amount of inflammation, and may be threefold more informative than the barium enema x-ray examination.[16] Radioactive scanning methods with use of indium- 111 or gallium- 67 may be of benefit in delineating the extent of colon involvement when colonoscopy cannot be performed.[22, 28, 39]

Barium Enema Following Colonoscopy

The performance of a barium enema x-ray examination is safe after colonoscopy or flexible sigmoidoscopy and biopsy because the endoscopic forceps takes only a superficial tissue specimen.[2] The deep biopsy specimens obtained through a rigid sigmoidoscope should probably not be followed by a contrast enema examination because this may lead to extravasation of barium. According to a recent study, however, this note of caution may be unnecessary.[48]

Secondary Changes in Chronic Ulcerative Colitis

The radiographic signs include an increase in the postrectal space.[9] The valves of Houston are obliterated in about half of the patients. There may be symmetric complete loss of haustral patterns. The colon may become narrowed and shortened, with depression of the flexures.[31]

Endoscopically the colon in chronic colitis is tubular in configuration, and changes in the vascular pattern are common, with neovascularization resulting in isolated vascular tufts without cross branches or communications.

STRICTURE AND MASS LESIONS

Strictures occur with equal frequency in patients with ulcerative and granulomatous colitis,[31] and may be the result of fibrosis, muscular hypertrophy and spasm, or carcinoma. Most strictures in patients with ulcerative colitis are either fibrous or inflammatory,[38] but carcinoma must be ruled out, although malignancy may account for less than 20% of these narrowed segments.[29] Radiographically, malignant strictures occurring with colitis have an irregular contour with uneven narrowing or shouldering, an eccentric lumen, and irregularity of part or all of the mucosa.[29] The best method for investigation of strictures is colonoscopy,[38] which permits direct inspection of the segment and allows biopsy specimens and cytologic samples to be taken. The colonoscope can be passed up to and often through a stricture to determine its precise nature. Many strictures demonstrated on barium enema x-ray examination can be successfully negotiated with the standard-sized colonoscope, since air insufflation during endoscopy may distend the narrow lumen, especially when the cause is muscle hypertrophy or spasm.[19, 26] Fibrotic strictures appear thin, short, and weblike, while inflammatory strictures are notable for the presence of ulcers, friability, and mucosal erythema.[27] A carcinomatous stricture should be suspected endoscopically when the stricture is rigid, has an abrupt "shelf-like" edge, or cannot be intubated with the colonoscope.[29]

When evaluating each case of stricture, a visual diagnostic impression is insufficient to provide the correct differential diagnosis, and must be supplemented by biopsies at the edge of, and within, the strictured segment, as well as with brush cytology.

Although carcinoma originates from the mucosal surface of the colon, it may spread submucosally, resulting in negative findings in surface mucosal biopsy specimens.[6, 29] For this reason, strictures that appear malignant endoscopically should always be referred for surgery rather than repeatedly monitored by colonoscopic reevaluations. Narrowed strictures that do not accept an adult colonoscope may often be successfully intubated with use of a pediatric instrument, an upper gastrointestinal endoscope, or a small-caliber colonoscope. Even if a stricture can be successfully intubated, the necessity for biopsies and brush cytology remains equally important. The colonic wall in patients with ulcerative colitis is usually thinned and the mucosa friable, which does not permit the longitudinal stretching tolerated by the normal, noncolitic bowel. Because of this the endoscopist should exert only minimal pressure when attempting to pass through strictures in patients with ulcerative colitis, lest the bowel wall be traumatized and perforation result.

Mass Lesions

Mass lesions found on barium enema x-ray examination may range in significance from carcinoma to the nonneoplastic inflammatory polyp. The term *pseudopolyp* should be replaced by the term *inflammatory polyp*, since they are truly polyps, although their genesis is inflammation. Inflammatory polyps are usually small, glistening, and multiple throughout the colon, being found in both ulcerative colitis and Crohn's disease.[23] They may consist of regenerative epithelial islands that remained relatively uninvolved amidst the surrounding destructive ulcerations, or, alternatively, they may be composed of granulation tissue or inflammatory nodules.[34] Whatever their etiology, they have no malignant potential, and a mass lesion, once definitely identified as an inflammatory polyp, can be safely ignored.[20, 40] Occasionally inflammatory polyps may become very large and almost occlude the lumen of the narrowed colon in chronic IBD, and may be a cause of intussusception.[10-12] When solitary and large, inflammatory polyps may mimic a carcinoma, not only on barium enema x-ray examination but also during colonoscopy. A biopsy specimen from any portion of an inflammatory polyp, however, will establish its histologic nature and render the correct diagnosis. Whether sessile or pedunculated, most inflammatory polyps may be removed endoscopically, but resection is not usually required unless they are causing symptoms of partial obstruction or bleeding. Healing of the polypectomy site may be delayed in the presence of surrounding inflammation. When multiple inflammatory polyps are encountered, biopsy of all of them is not possible, and in most instances biopsy is not needed. Histologic sampling should be reserved for those inflammatory polyps that are larger than 1.0 cm in diameter, have spontaneous bleeding, or have an irregular surface configuration. When inflammatory polyps with these features are encountered, they may be confused with carcinoma.

Adenomatous polyps occur in 5% of patients with ulcerative colitis.[40] Adenomas in patients with colitis more frequently resemble inflammatory polyps instead of having the more typical appearance of adenomas occurring in the noncolitic bowel. Adenomas in the bowel afflicted with colitis can be removed endoscopically with use of the snare-cautery technique, as in the normal colon. All adenomas have varying amounts of dysplasia, and the presence of single adenomas should not be considered a marker for carcinoma unless a biopsy specimen was taken from a mass lesion or from a very flat but slightly irregular mucosal surface.

Dysplasia

Dysplasia in chronic ulcerative colitis apparently may be detected with x-ray examination, although this modality is not very effective. Radiographic evidence of dysplasia may be found in 14% of patients harboring this cellular abnormality. The roentgenologic appearance is of a close grouping of multiple adjacent nodules with apposed, flattened edges.[18] The basic tool for discovery of dysplasia is the microscope. The tissue samples are readily obtained via colonoscopy, but dysplasia may not be visually apparent, but found in routine follow-up colonoscopies performed on a regular basis in patients considered to be at high risk for the development of colon cancer (those patients whose disease involves the entire colon (universal disease) for more than eight years). Flow-cytometry may be valuable in studying patients with total ulcerative colitis of more than 9 years' duration, since findings of an abnormal DNA pattern may be seen in patients with dysplasia.[30] When a change in DNA pattern (aneuploidy) is detected, it is not necessarily associated with dysplasia in that same biopsy specimen. Flow-cytometry may be worthwhile for evaluation of biopsy specimens in patients requiring surveillance for chronic ulcerative colitis, but it is not currently an everyday practical tool.

Differential Diagnosis

The differential diagnosis between ulcerative and granulomatous colitis (Crohn's disease) is usually made with the aid of the history, sigmoidoscopy, rectal biopsy, and barium enema x-ray examination.[13, 36, 41] Occasionally differentiation between these two forms of colitis may be difficult, and direct colonoscopic visualization of the entire bowel along with biopsies may provide an accurate diagnosis.[42, 43, 46] An 89% accuracy in the endoscopic differential diagnosis of IBD can be achieved by strict attention to diagnostic criteria.[43, 45, 47]

1. Ulcers may occur in segments of diffusely abnormal mucosa in both forms of colitis, but, when present in an area of otherwise normal mucosa, are characteristic of granulomatous colitis:
2. Aphthous ulcers are pathognomonic of Crohn's colitis:

TABLE 12–1.
Differential Diagnosis of Ulcerative Colitis

	Ulcerative Colitis	Crohn's Disease
Rectum involved	Radiography Endoscopy	
Erythema	Endoscopy	
Granularity	Radiography Endoscopy	
Friability	Endoscopy	
Ulcers		
Normal mucosa*		Radiography Endoscopy
Linear		Radiography Endoscopy
Involved mucosa	Radiography Endoscopy	
Cobblestoning*		Radiography Endoscopy
Asymmetry		Radiography Endoscopy
Discontinuous disease		Radiography Endoscopy

*Pathognomonic finding.

3. Cobblestoning is pathognomonic of Crohn's colitis:
4. Granularity and friability are both common in early ulcerative colitis, but may be late findings in granulomatous colitis.

Inflammatory polyps are present in both types of colitis, and their presence does not assist in the differential diagnosis. Biopsy demonstrates granulomas in approximately 5% of patients with Crohn's colitis.[45–47] Although multiple biopsy specimens should be taken throughout the colon (cecum, ascending colon, hepatic flexure, transverse colon, splenic flexure, descending colon, sigmoid, and rectum) to assist in the differential diagnosis, the most important factor leading to the correct diagnosis may be the pathologist's ability to differentiate microscopically discontinuous mucosal involvement (Crohn's disease) from a pattern of increasing severity distally (ulcerative colitis). Crypt abscesses are not specific for ulcerative colitis, occurring in 25% of patients with ulcerative and in 13% of patients with granulomatous colitis.[34]

The major differential points on x-ray and endoscopy are noted on Table 12–1.

Gastroduodenal Crohn's Disease

Some studies have reported gastroduodenal involvement in 2% to 3% of patients with Crohn's disease.[44] However, these invariably represent advanced disease, characterized clinically by gastric outlet obstruction and radiographically by deformity and narrowing of the antrum and proximal duodenum. Early lesions may be found on biopsy material in as many as 25% to 50% of samples taken from the upper intestinal tract in patients with known Crohn's colitis.

REFERENCES

1. Bartram C: Radiology in the current assessment of ulcerative colitis. *Gastrointest Radiol* 1977; 1:383.
2. Bartram CI, Hall-Craggs MA: Interventional colorectal endoscopic procedures: Residual lesions on follow-up double-contrast barium enema study. *Radiology* 1987; 152:835–838.
3. Bartram CI, Walmesley K: A pathological and radiological correlation of the mucosal changes in ulcerative colitis. *Proc R Soc Med* 1965; 58:713.
4. Berridge FR: Two unusual radiological signs of Crohn's disease of the colon. *Clin Radiol* 1971; 22:444.
5. Blackstone MO: Endoscopy in IBD—how useful? *Curr Gastroenterol* 1987; 7:344–349.

6. Crowson T, Ferrante W, Gathright J: Colonoscopy: Inefficacy for early carcinoma detection in patients with ulcerative colitis. *JAMA* 1976; 236:2651–2652.

7. Edwards F, Truelove S: The course and prognosis of ulcerative colitis. III and IV. *Gut* 1964; 5:1.

8. Elliott P, Williams C, Lennard-Jones J, et al: Colonoscopic diagnosis of minimal change colitis in patients with a normal sigmoidoscopy and normal air-contrast barium enema. *Lancet* 1982; 1:650–651.

9. Endling NPG, Eklof O: The retrorectal soft tissue space in ulcerative colitis. *Radiology* 1963; 80:949–953.

10. Ferguson CJ, Balfour TW, Padfield CJ: Localized giant pseudopolyposis of colon in ulcerative colitis—report of a case. *Dis Colon Rectum* 1987; 30:802–804.

11. Forde K, Gold R, Holck S, et al: Giant pseudopolyposis in colitis with colonic intussusception. *Gastroenterology* 1978; 75:1142.

12. Forderaro AE, Barloon TJ, Murray JA: Giant pseudopolyposis in Crohn's disease with computed tomography correlation. *J Comput Tomogr* 1987; 11:288–290.

13. Freeny PC: Crohn's disease and ulcerative colitis. Evaluation with double contrast barium examination and endoscopy. *Postgrad Med* 1986; 80:139–146.

14. Geboes K, Desmet V, DeWolf-Peters C, et al: The value of endoscopic biopsies in the diagnosis of Crohn's disease. *Am J Proctol Gastroenterol Colon Rect Surg* 1978; 29:21.

15. Geboes K, Van Trappen G: The value of colonoscopy in the diagnosis of Crohn's disease. *Gastrointest Endosc* 1975; 22:18.

16. Holdstock G, DuBoulay C, Smith C: Survey of the use of colonoscopy in IBD. *Dig Dis Sci* 1984; 29:731–734.

17. Holmquist L. Rudic N, Ahren C, et al: The diagnostic value of colonoscopy compared with rectosigmoidoscopy in children and adolescents with symptoms of chronic IBD of the colon. *Scand J Gastroenterol* 1988; 23:577–584.

18. Hooyman JR, MacCarty RL, Carpenter HA, et al: Radiographic appearance of mucosal dysplasia associated with ulcerative colitis. *AJR* 1987; 149:47–52.

19. Hunt R, Teague R, Swarbrick E, et al: Colonoscopy in the management of colonic strictures. *Br Med J* 1975; 2:360.

20. Jalan K, Sircus W, Walker R, et al: Pseudopolyposis in ulcerative colitis. *Lancet* 1969; 2:555.

21. Jenkins D, Goodall A, Drew K, et al: What is colitis? Statistical approach to distinguishing clinically important inflammatory change in rectal biopsy specimens. *J Clin Pathol* 1988; 41:72–79.

22. Jones B, Abbruzzese A, Hill T, et al: Gallium-67-citrate scintigraphy in ulcerative colitis. *Gastrointest Radiol* 1980; 5:267–272.

23. Kelly JK, Gabos S: The pathogenesis of inflammatory polyps. *Dis Colon Rectum* 1987; 30:251–254.

24. Laufer I: *Double Contrast Gastrointestinal Radiology With Endoscopic Correlation.* Philadelphia, WB Saunders, 1979.

25. Laufer I, Costopoulos L: Early lesions of Crohn's disease. *AJR* 1978; 130:307.

26. Laufer I, Hamilton JD: The radiologic differentiation between ulcerative and granulomatous colitis by double contrast radiology. *Am J Gastroenterol* 1976; 66:259.

27. Laufer I, Mullens JE, Hamilton J: Correlation of endoscopy and double contrast radiology in the early stages of ulcerative and granulomatous colitis. *Radiology* 1976; 118:1.

28. Leddin DJ, Paterwon WG, DaCosta LR, et al: Indium-111 labelled autologous leukocyte imaging and fecal excretion—comparison with conventional methods of assessment of IBD. *Dig Dis Sci* 1987; 32:377–387.

29. Lictenstein JE: Radiologic-pathologic correlation of IBD. *Radiol Clin North Am* 1987; 25:3–24.

30. Lofberg R, Tribukait B, Ost A, et al: Flow cytometric DNA analysis in long standing ulcerative colitis: A method of prediction of dysplasia and carcinoma development. *Gut* 1987; 28:1100–1106.

31. Margulis A: Radiology of ulcerating colitis. *Radiology* 1972; 105:251.

32. Marshak RH, Lindner AE: Ulcerative and granulomatous colitis, in Margulis AR, Burhenne HJ (eds): *Alimentary Tract Roentgenology*, vol 1, St. Louis, Mosby–Year Book, 1973, pp 963–1013.

33. McGovern V, Goulston S: Crohn's disease of the colon. *Gut* 1968; 9:164.

34. Morson BC, Dawson IMP: *Gastrointestinal Pathology.* Oxford, Blackwell Scientific, 1972, pp 458–470.

35. Newman SL: Ileoscopy, colonoscopy and backwash ileitis in children with IBD: Quid pro quo. *J Pediatr Nutr* 1987; 6:325–327.

36. Pera A, Bellando P, Caldera D, et al: Colonoscopy in IBD. Diagnostic accuracy and proposal of an endoscopic score. *Gastroenterology* 1987; 92:181–185.

37. Rickert R, Carter H: The "early" ulcerative lesion of Crohn's disease: Correlative light and scanning electron-microscopic studies. *J Clin Gastroenterol* 1980; 2:11–19.

38. Simpkins KC, Young AC: The differential diagnosis of large bowel strictures. *Clin Radiol* 1971; 22:449.

39. Stein D, Gran G, Gregory P, et al: Location and activity of ulcerative and Crohn's colitis by indium 111 leukocyte scan. A prospective comparison study. *Gastroenterology* 1983; 84:388–393.

40. Teague R, Read A: Polyposis in ulcerative colitis. *Gut* 1975; 16:792.

41. Teague R, Waye J: Endoscopy in IBD, in Hunt R, Waye J (eds): in *Colonoscopy: Techniques, Clinical Practice and Colour Atlas.* London, Chapman and Hall, 1981.

42. Waye J: Endoscopy in IBD. *Clin Gastroenterol* 1980; 9:279–284.

43. Waye J, Braunfeld S: Colonoscopy and the indications for surgery in ulcerative colitis, in Salmon P (ed): *Gastrointestinal Endoscopy. Advances in Diagnosis and Therapy.* London, Chapman and Hall, 1984, pp 248–262.

44. Wilder WM, Davis WD: Duodenal enteritis. *South Med J* 1966; 59:884.

45. Williams C: Diverticular disease and strictures, in Hunt R, Waye J (eds): *Colonoscopy: Techniques, Clinical Practice and Colour Atlas.* London, Chapman and Hall, 1981.
46. Williams C, Teague R: Progress report: Colonoscopy. *Gut,* 1973; 14:990–1003.
47. Williams C, Waye J: Colonoscopy in IBD., *Clin Gastroenterol* 1978; 7:701–717.
48. Wytock DH, Baybick J: Depth of colorectal biopsies with proctoscopic forceps. *Gastrointest Endosc* 1987; 33:15–17.

Chapter 13 _____

Appropriate Use of Biopsy in Inflammatory Bowel Disease

Burton I. Korelitz

This chapter deals with the biopsies themselves. It is a topic that is not generally covered, but I have had a special interest in it for some time. In this regard I wish to acknowledge the contributions of the distinguished pathologist, Sheldon C. Sommers, with whom I have had a long association at Lenox Hill Hospital. He has examined, grossly and microscopically, countless biopsy specimens from patients with inflammatory bowel disease (IBD) and has made many of the observations and suggestions that guide me in management. In thinking about biopsy in IBD, a few basic points are clear, as outlined in the next section.

GENERALITIES ABOUT DIAGNOSIS

1. *Biopsy does not secure the diagnosis of ulcerative colitis.* This is true whether specimens are taken from the rectum or from the colon, or whether they are taken at sigmoidoscopy or colonoscopy. Biopsy criteria are very nonspecific, and they can be utilized only in relation to the clinical picture without being diagnostic for their own sake.

2. *Biopsy can confirm the diagnosis of Crohn's disease*, but the frequency of finding diagnostic features is small even though diagnostic features are found more often than in ulcerative colitis.

3. *Biopsy can make the diagnosis of other forms of colitis.* These include:

1. Parasitic
2. Pseudomembranous

3. Ischemic
4. Radiation
5. Cystoplasmic inclusion body
6. Collagenous
7. Microscopic
8. Solitary rectal ulcer syndrome

4. Site of the biopsy can be important. In most instances the site of marked inflammation should be avoided. This is particularly true in Crohn's disease where the yield of granulomas and microgranulomas is the highest in biopsy specimens from normal-appearing mucosa.[6] In fact, sigmoidoscopic biopsy specimens have been more productive than specimens from normal-appearing mucosa located more proximally.[2] In other conditions with gross endoscopic findings, sites of mild but definite inflammation should be favored.

DIFFERENTIAL DIAGNOSIS OF INFLAMMATORY BOWEL DISEASE FROM SELF-LIMITED COLITIS

1. Infectious colitis can sometimes simulate IBD by initial presentation with bloody diarrhea and can give a nonspecific inflammatory picture on sigmoidoscopy. The most common disease entities that do this are *Campylobacter, Salmonella, Amoeba* and *Shigella,* as well as *Clostridium difficile* postantibiotic colitis.

2. Other diagnostic methods are far more dependable than biopsy in recognizing infectious or self-limited colitis. These include historical factors, Gram's stain, direct examination looking for *Amoeba,* and cultures, including the use of specific culture media for certain organisms.

3. No histologic features favor infectious colitis. Histologic features that favor the diagnosis of IBD include the following[9]:

1. Distorted crypt architecture
2. Increased numbers of both round cells and neutrophils in lamina propria
3. Villous surface
4. Epithelioid granuloma
5. Crypt atrophy
6. Basal lymphoid aggregates
7. Basally located giant cells

As many pathologists, particularly Yardley at Johns Hopkins, have emphasized, unless these features are found within the first 4 days, for all practical purposes no histologic findings are specific.[10] Furthermore, workup in most people with acute colitis is not done in this way, they do not have a rectal biopsy performed during the first 4 days, and therefore any value for differential histologic diagnosis will pertain to very few patients.

DIFFERENTIAL DIAGNOSIS OF CROHN'S DISEASE FROM ULCERATIVE COLITIS

Differential Diagnosis

The differential diagnosis is primarily clinical with the support of the x-ray examination, which provides us with distribution, configuration and baseline studies. When we examine endoscopically, confluence of inflammation favors ulcerative colitis, and rectal sparing is going to favor Crohn's disease.

Figure 13-1 shows a radiologic diagram of a barium enema x-ray examination with reflux into the distal aspect of the ileum, demonstrating a variety of features characteristic of Crohn's disease. If we find any of these, we do not need a biopsy. I am referring to the asymmetry of involvement, the strictures, the skip areas, the transverse fissures or rose-thorn lesions, as the British describe them, the involvement of the terminal portion of the ileum with characteristic features of Crohn's disease and sparing of the rectum, the perirectal abscesses, and the fistulas. This makes the role of the biopsy much easier in the sense that we do not have to depend on it. There are no x-ray features characteristic of ulcerative colitis, although confluence of inflammation and loss of haustra in a symmetric distribution with rectal involvement strongly favor that diagnosis.

Indeterminate Colitis

This term refers to IBD limited to the colon that looks characteristic either of ulcerative colitis or of Crohn's disease. Under these circumstances biopsy becomes more valuable. Serial biopsies should be done at the time of first examination. If there are no findings to confirm the diagnosis of Crohn's disease but there is still an index of clinical suspicion, subsequent serial biopsies should be performed at later examinations. At any time biopsy of specific lesions suggestive of Crohn's disease or patches of normal-appearing mucosa in the area of inflammation should be performed, and a diagnosis can be confirmed or altered.

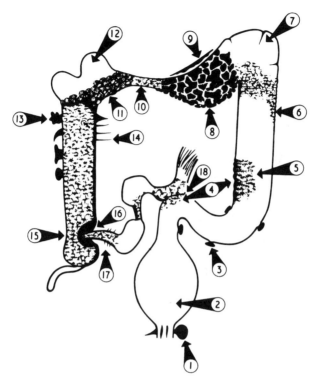

FIG 13–1.
Indicators of Crohn's disease. *1,* Anal lesions; *2,* normal rectum; *3,* ulcers; *4, 7,* and *12,* patches of inflammation surrounded by normal mucosa; *5* and *6,* eccentric involvement; *8,* serpiginous ulceration; *9,* intramural linear ulcerations; *10,* stricture; *11,* cobblestones; *13,* deep ulcerations; *14,* transverse fissures; *15,* right-sided disease; *16,* prominent ileocecal valve; *17,* small bowel involvement; *18,* ileosigmoid fistula. (From Simpkins KC: The barium enema in Crohn's colitis, in Weterman IT, Peña AS, Booth CC (eds): *The Management of Crohn's Disease.* Proceedings of Workshop on Crohn's Disease, Leyden, Oct 23–25, 1975. Amsterdam, Excerpta Medica, 1976. Used by permission.)

Specific Histologic Features

When we find an obvious granuloma the diagnosis is easy. This does not happen very often. We have also learned to recognize the microgranuloma, which was first described at Lenox Hill Hospital.[8] It is a loose collection of histiocytes and lymphocytes far less compact than the mature granuloma. This, too, is diagnostic of Crohn's disease. When the cells in a crypt abscess are mostly eosinophils rather than neutrophils, this finding is characteristic of Crohn's disease. In my studies with Sommers, the diagnostic lesions that we found most frequently were granulomas and microgranulomas in 11%. Edema and fibrosis are of little help, but other areas that are rather unique to Crohn's disease are the lymph follicles and lymphangiectasia which occur in only about 3%.[6]

Other clinical pearls have come from research data on biopsies. We have learned that mature granulomas are found mostly in clinically active cases and that microgranulomas occur in mostly clinically inactive cases. This is not foolproof, but nevertheless is statistically valid. Crypt abscesses, when we find them, are most likely to occur in clinically active cases, as do acute and chronic inflammation.[7]

Other histologic criteria for the diagnosis of Crohn's disease include the following:

1. Focal inflammation (microscopic skip areas)
2. Submucosal inflammation
3. Preservation of goblet cells
4. Ulcerating lymphoid follicles (aphthous ulcers)
5. Lymphangiectasia
6. Granulomas and microgranulomas
7. Eosinophils and macrophages in crypt abscesses
8. Knife-shaped fistulas

It has been shown that ulceration of the lymphoid follicles is the histologic lesion that becomes the aphthous ulcer. Focal inflammation is interesting; Dr. Sommers has emphasized its value in identifying Crohn's disease and differentiating it from ulcerative colitis. These areas of focal inflammation are like skip areas in a microscopic field, and are characteristic of Crohn's disease, similar to the gross skip areas seen in an x-ray film.

Cell Counts

Dr. Sommers introduced this innovation. He very systematically counted cells in rectal biopsy specimens from patients with ulcerative colitis and Crohn's disease, and from that we learned the following[4-7]:

1. Eosinophils were increased in ulcerative colitis but not in Crohn's disease.
2. Mast cells, plasma cells, and neutrophils were increased in ulcerative colitis but not in Crohn's disease.

3. In Crohn's disease there was a statistically significant increase in macrophages, which was not true in ulcerative colitis.

Occasionally we resort to this research technique even for clinical purposes. Of course, pathologists in general do not want to be bothered with cell counts, which are time-consuming, particularly in this day when clinical pathologists are so overworked. Nevertheless, occasionally cell counts will prove to be of clinical value.

Index of Disease Activity

Biopsy is not of great value as an indicator of activity. This is particularly true in ulcerative colitis where you can look at the rectal mucosa directly and easily with a scope. If one sees that the process has been reduced or has disappeared, biopsy is not necessary. Occasionally there will be clinical discrepancies when we might want to resort to biopsy for response to therapy. Of course, the biopsy will always be important for research purposes if not for clinical purposes.

SPECIAL SITUATIONS IN WHICH BIOPSY IS HELPFUL

1. When there is a discrepancy between clinical and endoscopic data, with *suspicion of IBD in a patient with diarrhea of undetermined origin*, biopsy is helpful. This will not happen very often, but rectal biopsy can reveal granulomas even when roentgenograms are entirely normal. Rectal biopsy might provide the only indication of IBD, specifically, Crohn's disease.[2] The same situation pertains to collagenous and microscopic colitis, where the mucosa appears normal and diagnosis is dependent on biopsy.[1,3]

2. When ulcerative colitis appears radiologically or endoscopically to be limited to the rectum (proctitis), but clinically the symptoms are out of proportion, biopsy specimens can be taken endoscopically from multiple more proximal sites; sometimes the degree of inflammation in comparison with the minimal findings grossly can be quite remarkable and can change the thinking about management of the case.

3. When the sigmoidoscopic or flexible sigmoidoscopic examination provides observations that look entirely normal after earlier involvement but the symptoms persist, biopsy of normal areas sometimes reveals activity; often the proximal area is the only area involved with the inflammatory process. This is particularly true in elderly patients.

4. The rectum can look very normal after steroid or 5-aminosalicylic acid enemas. Still, that might be the only segment that looks normal, while a more proximal level can still be the site of active disease.

RESPONSE TO THERAPY

I already stated that one really does not need a biopsy to indicate the degree of activity or the response to therapy. Nevertheless, I do have some data that are interesting. In patients with ulcerative colitis who are converted from positive to negative sigmoidoscopic findings, histologic features before and after were noted.[7] On a statistical basis, crypt abscesses decreased, edema increased, and *no* major lesion increased. With epithelial and connective tissue cell counts done under the same circumstances, mucus goblet cells increased, fragmented nuclei decreased, and eosinophils in the lamina propria decreased. We tried then to see if the manner of response differed with the kind of therapy, and we learned that it did not. As long as the patients responded to therapy it did not make any difference in histologic findings or cell counts if they did so in response to sulfasalazine, steroids, or 6-mercaptopurine; if they responded clinically, the histologic responses were equivalent.

SURVEILLANCE FOR DYSPLASIA AND CANCER

This is one of the most important roles for mucosal biopsies in IBD, and will be covered in separate chapters (see Chapters 13, and 20 to 22). Sometimes surveillance is done in the presence of active disease, sometimes when disease is inactive, and occasionally the disease will be clinically inactive and surprise the examiner when patches of active disease are found with endoscopy. Surveillance in Crohn's disease is also covered elsewhere (see Chapter 22).

BIOPSIES OF SPECIFIC LESIONS

This is where the yield from biopsy has the greatest potential. In IBD sometimes it is difficult to recognize if a polyp is a true polyp or a pseudopolyp. We should biopsy those pseudopolyps that have variations in size, color, hue, configuration, and just look different. An obvious carcinoma may be confronted; sometimes a mass seen at surveillance colonoscopy will be suspicious for carcinoma and the biopsy will settle it. Dysplastic mucosa is an ill-defined situation, but is best represented by a mamillated appearance. We rarely see anything that we can be certain is dysplastic mucosa. It is important to take biopsy specimens from strictures, particularly in ulcerative colitis, where about 20% to 30% of strictures will mask carcinoma. The edge of an aphthous lesion is an important site for diagnosis of Crohn's disease. It is a place where the yield of granulomas is relatively high. In my experience the best area for biopsy in patients with Crohn's disease is the spared or relatively spared rectal segment. Our yield of granulomas and microgranulomas in the rectum has been higher than in any more proximal area. In biopsy of nodules or pseudopolyps associated with friability and exudate, the yield of granulomas is practically nil.

REFERENCES

1. Bo-Linn GW, Vendrell DD, Lee E, et al: An evaluation of the significance of microscopic colitis in patients with chronic diarrhea. *J Clin Invest* 1985; 75:1559–1569.
2. Fochios SE, Korelitz BI: The role of sigmoidoscopy and rectal biopsy in diagnosis and management of inflammatory bowel disease: Personal experience. *Am J Gastroenterol* 1988; 83:114–119.
3. Giardiello FM, Bayless TMJ, Jessurun J, et al: Collagenous colitis: Physiologic and histopathologic studies in seven patients. *Ann Intern Med* 1987; 106:46–49.
4. Korelitz BI, Sommers SC: Differential diagnosis of ulcerative and granulomatous colitis by sigmoidoscopy, rectal biopsy and cell counts of rectal mucosa. *Am J Gastroenterol* 1974; 61:460–469.
5. Korelitz BI, Sommers SC: Responses to drug therapy in ulcerative colitis. Evaluation by rectal biopsy and histopathological changes. *Am J Gastroenterol* 1975; 64:365–370.
6. Korelitz BI, Sommers SC: Rectal biopsy in patients with Crohn's disease. *JAMA* 1977; 237:2742–2744.
7. Korelitz BI, Sommers SC: Responses to drug therapy in Crohn's disease: Evaluation by rectal biopsy and mucosal cell counts. *J Clin Gastroenterol* 1984; 6:123–127.
8. Rotterdam HZ, Korelitz BI, Sommers SC: Microgranulomas in grossly normal rectal mucosa in Crohn's disease. *Am J Clin Pathol* 1977; 67:550–554.
9. Surawicz CM, Belic L: Rectal biopsy helps to distinguish acute self-limited colitis from idiopathic IBD. *Gastroenterology* 1984; 86:104–113.
10. Yardley JH: Pathology of idiopathic IBD and relevance of specific findings, in Bayless TM, *Current Management of IBD*. Toronto, BC Decker, 1989, p 16.

Discussion

Dr. Present: The topic is experience and controversy, and I love to participate because of the controversy. I would like to raise a few controversial issues and make some comments.

I get upset with Dr. Harig about referring to the endoscopist in terms of diagnosis and management, because the endoscopist defers to the x-ray for the initial diagnosis and management. Dr. Marshak would turn over in his grave—or he probably did—if he heard we left the diagnosis to the endoscopist.

I think you have to think of IBD in terms of endoscopy and x-rays as a clinician. You can do it as a researcher, which a lot of us do, but you can think of it as a clinician, and as such my impression is that indium is a waste of time, does not help in the management, and is too expensive. I would get rid of it totally. Just because it is new does not mean it is any better. Aphthous ulcerations seen on barium enema or on colonoscopy are a waste of time; don't go looking for them. Patients with IBD do not come back to see you again if you use double-contrast enemas. They prefer colonoscopy because they are knocked out. The radiologists should stop doing double-contrast barium enemas in IBD because they are a waste of time.

Dr. Waye did not allude to Dr. Modigliani's last study, published recently in *Gastroenterology*, where he has taken it a step further. Not only is there difficult correlation between endoscopists, but also colonoscopy does not add anything to clinical management. There is no correlation between an endoscope and how the patient is clinically. I defy you to make that correlation. I will let you do a double-blind colonoscopy and you cannot tell me how the patient is doing because the colonoscopy can look terrible and the patient could be fine, and vice versa. You can't see fistulas on colonoscopy. The only indication I can see for colonoscopy in Crohn's disease is, as Dr. Waye says, you do not have to be certified; you can get as much money as he can.

First, as far as ulcerative colitis is concerned, contrasting barium enema and colonoscopy, yes it can indicate activity, but I would also bet there is only about a 70% correlation between activity and what you see on colonoscopy. I will show you patients with active colitis on colonoscopy and the patient has only one bowel movement a day. You cannot tell clinically how the patient is doing. It is an excellent test in that we do get to the cecum all the time we do barium enemas, it is very helpful in strictures, and it is most important before you take out a patient's colon to do a barium enema because I can tell you in chronic patients it is helpful in the differential diagnosis, better than colonoscopy, for picking up a case of Crohn's disease that may be difficult to find. I know of three to four cases when surgery was performed and the patient had Crohn's disease. Barium enema will differentiate.

Second, if you distend the rectum you may have another option that we will talk about later today, ileorectal anastomosis. I feel a barium study is a much better study than colonoscopy in Crohn's disease, and in ulcerative colitis you take your choice. I would be interested in comments of the endoscopists and the radiologists.

DR. WAYE: I think you know my point of view. I agree with Dr. Present that in general we do not need to do colonoscopy in the vast majority of patients with IBD. But I think for surveillance for carcinoma it is absolutely necessary. It certainly is not very helpful to use it following therapy, although a lot of colonoscopists feel they have to do a colonoscopy to see how the patient is doing. I think you have to talk to the patients to see how they are doing.

DR. KORELITZ: A lot of people would be disappointed if you did not look.

DR. HARIG: I like the appearance of doing air contrast enemas or regular barium enemas, but I guess practically, at least in the hospital setting, we do not see a lot of early bowel disease. We see the patients with long-standing disease; I think part of it is the fact that people are getting colonoscopy fairly routinely. I do not know that there is an actual drop in NYC or if it is being siphoned off to private offices, but it is an inflammatory topic.

DR. KORELITZ: I certainly agree that indications change, and we utilize barium enemas and small bowel x-rays for a different set of indications than we used to. But they both have their role, even if totally not as much as they are probably being used.

A PHYSICIAN: Question for Drs. Korelitz and Waye: I am trying to learn about this disease, and when I do a colonoscopy on a patient with IBD I try to go into the ileum to look at it and usually take a biopsy. Not infrequently, I find the patient endoscopically has ulcerative colitis but the ileal biopsy shows moderate inflammation. Then I don't know where I am. Any thoughts?

Dr. Korelitz: I don't think it can be settled that way because nonspecific inflammation can occur anywhere in the colon and in the terminal ileum. Furthermore, even though it seems to be lost by the wayside, there is an entity called reflux ileitis that is part of ulcerative colitis. Grossly there is no evidence of its being Crohn's disease. So I would not let that alter your judgment. I think you have to think of it as an indeterminate colitis and use whatever means we have to separate them, whether it is serial biopsies on the first round or subsequent serial biopsies on the second round in a case like that.

Q: What is the significance of eosinophils in the crypt abscesses in Crohn's disease? A comment was made about that and I am interested, especially since eosinophils seem to be prevalent in the biopsies in ulcerative colitis.

Dr. Korelitz: I cannot offer you an explanation; I can only reiterate that it is a confirmed finding, both in the increase in eosinophils in cell counts of ulcerative colitis and in the crypt abscesses of Crohn's disease.

Dr. Waye: There are no statistics concerning the correlation between reflux findings in the terminal ileum with small ulcers and colonoscopy. However, I can tell you that I have a collection of patients who do not have diarrheal illnesses, in whom I have entered the terminal ileum and found that they have tiny aphthous ulcerations. I do not know what to do with these patients. We discuss them at endoscopy breakfast conference with Dr. Present all the time, and it has come to be such a common finding—the tiny aphthous ulcers—that I would hesitate to put any significance on those in a patient with diarrhea. In fact, I would rather not even report them because I think they are relatively nonspecific, and we are going to end up making a label of Crohn's disease in patients who do not have that entity. Dr. Present, what do you think?

Dr. Present: It is a very important issue and it comes up, for example, when I talk about patients in research—the use of colonoscopy to diagnose recurrence in Crohn's disease—when you put a scope in at 1 year over 90% of patients have abnormal findings. But they are not correlated with clinical symptoms. What I was getting to is that an x-ray is a much better test of indication of actual disease. Sedimentation rate may be 30, and if you do not see it on x-ray and you see it just on biopsy, I do not think you can conclude this is IBD yet. It is likely, but I don't think you should treat it until you really have a definite diagnosis. I see patients with biopsied disease treated with steroids all the time, and they do not really have IBD. I would treat these symptomatically.

Dr. Korelitz: The opposite end of the spectrum in answer to the question of barium enema vs. colonoscopy for the terminal ileum—if the patient really does have ileitis it is not so likely that the barium will reflux into the terminal ileum. If there is no reflux you still have a dilemma. The problems can remain unsolved because we have to get into the terminal ileum one way or the other to determine whether the patient has ileitis or not. It will probably take a small bowel series to resolve it.

Dr. Waye: I think the terminal ileum has lots of lymphoid follicles, and one of the roles is to contain cells that will eat up foreign bodies that will get down there. I think that is a normal wear and tear phenomenon of the lymphoid tissue, which is to ingest foreign materials, phagocytize them, and then ulcerations develop. I don't think that is Crohn's disease at all. When you get into the terminal ileum of someone who has carcinoma of the sigmoid colon and you are doing recreational ileoscopy, it is amazing how many people have these tiny ulcerations, and I do not feel you should put a lot of emphasis on it. The reason I say this is because if the patient has diarrhea you would say this is Crohn's disease, which is not necessarily true. I think wear and tear, the little aphthous erosions, look like the aphthous erosions you see in Crohn's disease, but I feel they are nonspecific.

Dr. Korelitz: And still, Dr. Waye, I think you have written that the best place to find granulomas is when you biopsy the edge of an aphthous lesion.

Dr. Waye: If you are looking for granulomas in IBD, you must biopsy the small aphthous ulcer before that ulcer enlarges and it actually scoops out the granuloma as the ulcer gets larger. So the smaller the ulcer the more chance you have of finding a granuloma in it in Crohn's disease. But I biopsy the aphthous ulcers in the small bowel that I find in what I call "normal ileum," and we just don't see granulomas. I don't know if there is a granuloma down there, but I doubt it.

Dr. Korelitz: I think the appropriate comment which will always prove true is that in IBD the doctor has to be a clinician and be able to utilize all of these observations which have been represented and still make the correct decision in the management of that particular patient.

Dr. Margolin: You have two camps—the endoscopists and the radiologists—and I feel it is misleading that it is one or the other. I have found particularly useful the small bowel series and colonoscopy. That complementary set of examinations basically gives the information about the disease.

Dr. Korelitz: Yes, Dr. Margolin, I found in my own office in appropriate cases I do colonoscopies followed by small bowel series so the whole workup is finished in one day, and this has worked out very well.

Dr. Bayless: Microscopic or lymphocytic colitis is probably seen throughout the colon. The aspect that varies is the thickness of the collagen band in collagenous colitis, and that seems to be thickest in the right and in the transverse colon. We reported two to three patients who had lymphocytic colitis but no collagen in the rectal biopsies, while elsewhere they had collagen. So we would like to biopsy the sigmoid if we can, trying not to rely entirely on rectal biopsies.

Comment: Concerning barium enemas and colonoscopy which one does, one of the points brought out is that it is all nice when you have sharp x-ray people, the sharpest probably at Lenox Hill Hospital or Mount Sinai Hospital, but it should be noted that throughout the country all radiologists are not necessarily the sharpest, and you miss an awful lot of carcinoma. It should not be who makes the money on what procedure, but who will do the job best and use both of them properly in determining which test you want done first—if both have to be done, which is first. An awful lot of early lesions were missed that should have been cured. We have these discussions and forget the small cities and towns where we come from, but remember, all our x-ray people are not sharp enough that x-ray can be used as the only means of diagnosis.

Dr. Korelitz: What this means to me is that when you know where the weak link is you have to be stronger or, an old Mount Sinai expression, in the land of the blind the one-eyed man is king.

PART 3

Considerations of Rectal and Perirectal Disease

Chapter 14_____

Antimicrobial Therapy in Inflammatory Bowel Disease

Michael S. Frank

Patients with inflammatory bowel disease (IBD) often receive antibiotics in the course of their treatment. Some patients with colitis may even receive antiprotozoal agents early in their treatment to eradicate a possible pathogen mimicking ulcerative colitis, particularly in certain areas where amebiasis is endemic.*

Patients with Crohn's disease, more commonly than with ulcerative colitis, receive antibiotics to eradicate pyogenic complications of the disease, to treat bacterial overgrowth, or even as primary therapy. Once initiated, broad-spectrum antibiotics may be continued for prolonged periods of time, particularly if they appear to provide relief of symptoms.

Metronidazole is a potent antianaerobic antibiotic that has received much attention in the treatment of Crohn's disease in the past two decades. It has been tried as a primary agent in Crohn's disease, or for prolonged periods of time in the management of the perineal complications of Crohn's disease.

Recently, even antituberculous drugs have been reintroduced as possible therapeutic agents in the treatment of Crohn's disease. This renewed interest is based on the possibility that mycobacteria can actually cause Crohn's disease. Thayer et al.[9] have isolated a strain of mycobacteria from a few patients with Crohn's disease. This agent has been transmitted to animals, who then developed an ileitis-like illness.

*Editor's Note: See Korelitz BI: When should we look for *Amebae* in patients with inflammatory bowel disease? *J Clin Gastroenterol* 1989; 11:373–375.

PRIMARY THERAPY

Broad-Spectrum Antibiotics

In an attempt to demonstrate that broad-spectrum antibiotics are effective in Crohn's disease, Moss et al.[6] conducted a clinical and radiographic study of 44 patients with Crohn's disease, most suffering from ileocolitis for longer than 7 years. Their patients were treated with the antibiotics, some even for long periods of time; some were even maintained for longer than 5 years. Radiographic improvement of disease was seen in 23% of patients, some within weeks of therapy. Ten patients failed to improve, and in five the Crohn's disease progressed despite antibiotic therapy. This prospective, uncontrolled study failed to demonstrate convincingly the role of antibiotics as primary therapy in Crohn's disease. Yet many have had the experience, particularly in patients with ileitis, of rapid and convincing response of clinical symptoms to either ampicillin or tetracycline.* Ambrose and coworkers, in Birmingham, nevertheless studied the efficacy of broad-spectrum antibiotics in 72 patients with Crohn's disease and found that antibiotics were no better than a placebo.[1]

Metronidazole

Metronidazole, a potent antianaerobic agent and well-accepted antiprotozoal agent, is rapidly absorbed orally and has good penetration into inflamed tissues. Ursing and Kamme[12] first investigated its efficacy in high doses; initially they reported promising results, but an unacceptable side effect profile, including nausea, dizziness, fatigue, and peripheral neuropathy, limited its usefulness.

In a carefully designed multicentric prospective study by Ursing et al.,[11] 78 patients with Crohn's disease in six centers in Sweden were studied during a 2½ year period. Patients were randomized to receive either sulfasalazine (3 g/day) or metronidazole (800 mg/day) for a 4-month course and then were crossed over to receive the alternate drug. The authors' conclusion was that both drugs were equally effective.†

Ursing[10] later reported that more than 100 patients with Crohn's disease have been successfully treated with metronidazole at doses

*Editors Note: Both Dr. Present and I, and probably others, have seen remission of active Crohn's disease coincident with the introduction of antibiotics, particularly ampicillin and cephalexin (Keflex), and in some, long-term remission on maintenance therapy thereafter. There is as much justification for trials of broad-spectrum antibiotics in Crohn's disease as there is for some of the newer agents.

†Editors Note: This study emphasized the response of the primary bowel symptoms of Crohn's disease as opposed to the perirectal complications. Metronidazole was slightly better than sulfasalazine for Crohn's colitis.

ranging from 800 to 1,000 mg/day with fewer side effects and efficacy approaching that of sulfasalazine therapy.

These results, however, have not been everyone's experience. Ambrose et al.,[1] in a trial, could not confirm the benefit of metronidazole therapy in Crohn's disease.

Blichfeldt et al.,[3] in Norway, found no statistically significant improvement in 22 patients treated with 1,000 mg of metronidazole per day for a 2-month period. In six patients with colitis only, however, there was striking improvement in diarrhea, pain, and general well-being. This subjective improvement was also associated with improvement in multiple laboratory parameters.*

Antimycobacterial drugs have been widely studied as primary therapy in Crohn's disease because of a postulated pathogenesis of Crohn's disease and its resemblance to mycobacterial infections. Even early negative reports have not discouraged others from multidrug trials, often with medications whose toxic side effect profiles limited their usage.[8] The results from both preliminary studies and well-controlled studies, however, remain unconvincing that antimicrobial therapy is effective in Crohn's disease.

Nonabsorbable Antibiotics.—Although absorbable antibiotics have not been proved useful as primary therapy in Crohn's disease, it was postulated that nonabsorbable antibiotics might remain in the intestine longer and therefore perhaps be more beneficial. Some have suggested that nonabsorbent antibiotics and sulfa drugs are effective when added to other conventional therapies, but their conclusions are in question because of problems with study design. A prospectively controlled study in 40 patients with oral vancomycin demonstrated that this agent offered little to improve the condition of patients with colitis.[5]

Perineal Disease

While the efficacy of broad-spectrum antibiotic therapy in inflammatory bowel disease is limited, antibiotics can be useful in specific situations such as abscesses and perineal Crohn's disease. In 1980 Bernstein et al.[2] reported on prospective studies of metronidazole in more than 30 patients with stubborn perineal Crohn's disease. While initially most patients showed some improvement and others even healed with

---

*Editors Note: In my own experience, metronidazole has infrequently been effective in improving Crohn's disease of any distribution. It has had a supplementary role in those who can tolerate the drug for long-term therapy.

long-term therapy, almost half of the patients required additional intervention to promote healing. High-dose metronidazole (20 mg/kg) was used with a troublesome side effect profile. Most patients developed a furry tongue and metallic taste, while others complained of nausea and decreased appetite. Almost half of the patients developed paresthesias, which usually resolved when the dose was lowered.[4]

Published reports are enthusiastic about metronidazole, and claim that the drug is effective in the management of debilitating perineal complications of Crohn's disease. Yet reports fall short in answering the questions addressed by Sachar[7] in his editorial. Particularly unclear is whether the drug is better than other antibiotics and by what mechanism the drug works.

I have found that metronidazole on rare occasions can be dramatic in its effect, and then serves as the easy answer to a stubborn and painful perineal problem. Unfortunately, this is too rarely the case. More commonly the drug offers initial improvement, but then other agents are needed (i.e., immunosuppressive drugs) or surgery is "required" (see Chapter 15).

In the 10 years since the initial enthusiastic report, many patients have been treated with lower doses of metronidazole with perineal Crohn's disease than initially proposed.

Conclusion

Antibiotics can be effective in IBD when used for specific indications. The use of broad-spectrum antibiotics as primary therapy in IBD seems to be justified only in select cases, mostly involving the small bowel. Metronidazole can be effective in Crohn's colitis and plays a role in the therapy of its perineal complications. In general, antibiotics are useful only for specific pyogenic complications, or in pouchitis and unusual situations of bacterial overgrowth. Antimycobacterial agents do not seem to be effective.

Studies on the effects of more potent antibiotics that have been introduced recently and studies on their use in the management of fistulous and perineal Crohn's disease are eagerly awaited.

REFERENCES

1. Ambrose NS, Allan RN, Keighley MR, et al: Antibiotic therapy for treatment in relapse of intestinal Crohn's disease. A prospective randomized study. *Dis Colon Rectum* 1985; 28:81–85.

2. Bernstein LH, Frank MS, Brandt LJ, et al: Healing of perineal Crohn's disease with metronidazole. *Gastroenterology* 1980; 79:357–365.
3. Blichfeldt P, Blomhoff JP, Myhre E, et al: Metronidazole in Crohn's disease. *Scand J Gastroenterol* 1978; 13:123–127.
4. Brandt LJ, Bernstein LH, Boley SJ, et al: Metronidazole in Crohn's disease. A follow-up study. *Gastroenterology* 1982; 83:383–387.
5. Dickinson RJ, O'Connor HJ, Pinder I, et al: Double blind controlled trial of oral vancomycin as adjunctive treatment in acute exacerbations of idiopathic colitis. *Gut* 1985; 26:1380–1384.
6. Moss AA, Carbone JV, Kressel HY: Radiologic and clinical assessment of broad spectrum antibiotic therapy in Crohn's disease. *AJR* 1978; 131:787–790.
7. Sachar DB: Metronidazole for Crohn's disease—breakthrough or ballyhoo (editorial). *Gastroenterology* 1980; 79:393–395.
8. Shaffer JL, Hughes S, Linaker BD, et al. Controlled trial of rifamicin and ethambutol in Crohn's disease. *Gut* 1984; 25:203–205.
9. Thayer WR, Coutu JA, Chiodini RJ, et al: Possible role of mycobacteria in inflammatory bowel disease. *Dig Dis Sci* 1984; 29:1080–1085.
10. Ursing BO: Metronidazole therapy, Bayless TM (ed): in *Current Management of Inflammatory Bowel Disease*. Toronto, BC Decker, 1989.
11. Ursing BO, Alm T, Barany F, et al: Comparative study of metronidazole and sulfasalazine for active Crohn's disease: The Cooperative Crohn's Disease Study in Sweden. *Gastroenterology* 1982; 83:550–562.
12. Ursing BO, Kamme C: Metronidazole for Crohn's disease. *Lancet* 1975; 1:775–777.

Surgical Considerations in Anorectal Crohn's Disease

Michael A. Weinstein
Norman Sohn

There are a myriad of manifestations of Crohn's disease in the anorectal area. The anorectal complications of Crohn's disease can be a cause of significant morbidity. There are many cases in which the anorectal area is the major cause of symptoms that may be present in a patient with Crohn's disease. Anorectal Crohn's disease can be defined as anorectal abnormalities in a patient in whom Crohn's disease is present anywhere in the gastrointestinal tract or in whom the anorectal findings are typical of Crohn's disease, but in whom there is no other objective evidence to establish that diagnosis. Shortly after Crohn's disease was first described, the importance of the anorectal manifestations was appreciated.[3, 6] Descriptions of cases of probable anorectal Crohn's disease appeared in 19th century textbooks of proctology in which many of the patients described may have suffered from Crohn's disease.[1]

The proportion of patients in any given population who are reported to have anorectal Crohn's disease will vary. These statistics may merely reflect the referral pattern of the reporting author or group of authors rather than the actual prevalence of these complications. It is generally agreed that the prevalence of the anorectal complications increases as the segment of bowel affected by the primary Crohn's disease process approaches the anus. In an occasional patient the initial or sole manifestation of Crohn's disease can be a perianal disorder.

The etiology and pathogenesis of Crohn's disease remain to be elucidated. The same can be said of most of its anorectal complications. Crohn's disease is known to have a predilection for areas of the bowel that contain large amounts of lymphoid tissue. It may well be that through an immunologic, bacteriologic, or other mechanism the pockets of lymphocytes surrounding the crypts of Morgagni may hold a clue to the cause for these complications. Once infections are established they seem to follow the principles of infections in this area that occur in patients with no known Crohn's disease.

According to Hughes',[7] anorectal Crohn's disease can be classified into what he considered to be primary and secondary lesions. He regards the anal fissure, ulcerated edematous pile, and cavitating ulcer as primary lesions, with other complications resulting from them. Crohn[2] believed that diarrhea was responsible for the anorectal complications of Crohn's disease. We have believed that the fecal stream usually contributes very little to an infection that in reality is occurring in the deep perirectal tissues and often not in intimate contact with the bowel lumen. Consequently, my efforts have always been toward local operative therapy without resorting to fecal diversion. Others[9] believe that the fecal stream is responsible for the perpetuation of many cases of Crohn's perirectal infections, and they consequently believe fecal diversion may have a salutary effect. There are many cases in which patients with totally diverted fecal streams have a progressively severe perirectal infection.

The anorectal examination is important in the evaluation of patients with suspected or documented IBD. The presence of a normal anorectum in the face of significant proctocolitis is not the common pattern one sees in Crohn's disease. This is more characteristic of other forms of nonspecific or specific colitides. A careful anorectal examination is thus very important in the assessment of patients with proved or suspected Crohn's disease. These observations of necessity include a meticulous inspection and digital examination with anoscopic as well as rigid proctoscopic or sigmoidoscopic examinations. If necessary these can be performed with the aid of local, regional, or general anesthesia. Biopsy of anorectal lesions or rectal mucosa may be diagnostic of Crohn's disease, but findings may be normal in up to 80% of cases.

Those anorectal findings that should alert the examiner to the possibility of Crohn's disease include anal skin tabs, anal ulcers, anal fistulas, perianal lymphangiomas, perianal erythema, and anorectal strictures at or proximal to the dentate line.

Anal skin tabs tend to be large, edematous, nontender and have a cyanotic hue. These have been termed "elephant ears." Many of the anorectal complications, particularly abscesses and fistulas, appear to exist, independent of the severity of the Crohn's disease elsewhere in the gastrointestinal tract. There are occasional cases in which this may not be true, and the anorectal problems may seem to parallel the Crohn's disease activity. It is difficult to define or quantify an index of Crohn's disease activity, and this area remains unclarified. One anorectal condition that seems to parallel Crohn's disease activity, however, is the anorectal skin tab. These skin tabs can act as a true barometer of Crohn's disease activity, becoming large and edematous when the disease is clearly active, and subsiding with remission or response to medical therapy. These changes can be rapid and dramatic in degree. Tremendous resolution can occur during a period of 4 to 5 days.

Anorectal ulcerations or fissures can be identical to typical anal fissures that occur in the absence of Crohn's disease. They are usually painless, however (although occasionally they may be painful). Their relative painlessness is a prominent and occasionally dramatic clue to Crohn's disease as a cause. They may be surrounded by edematous sentinel piles forming a "hood" over the ulcer. While idiopathic anal fissures are usually located in the posterior or anterior midline, those that occur in the patient with Crohn's disease may be located anywhere on the circumference of the anus. The latter tend to be situated in the typical midline position, anteriorly or posteriorly or both anteriorly and posteriorly. When ulcers are not midline in location or when they are multiple, Crohn's disease as a cause must be sought for.

Anal fistulas may be identical to those prevalent with no known Crohn's disease, but fistulas that tend to be high, complex, recurrent, associated with large areas of infected buttock or perirectal skin resembling hidradenitis suppurativa are more likely to be related to Crohn's disease. A rectovaginal fistula, particularly one arising spontaneously, with no prior obstetric or operative trauma, is also frequently due to Crohn's disease.

Postpartum perineal complications of episiotomies in the form of infections or poor wound healing, with the development of rectovaginal fistulas or anal incontinence, are more common in patients with Crohn's disease, albeit mild or heretofore undiagnosed.

A peculiar diffuse, painless, nonpruritic perianal erythema can occur. This is of no known cause. Perianal lymphangiomas also occur in Crohn's disease. The latter appear as small, bubbly types of lesions that at first glance may be confused with typical anal condylomas. On closer inspection their distinction from condylomata acuminata becomes readily apparent. It is interesting to speculate on the pathogenesis of these lesions, which probably result from lymphatic obstruction.

Anorectal strictures can occur in the patient with Crohn's disease, and these are usually different from the anal strictures that occur in its absence.[5] The kinds of strictures seen may or may not be related to

Crohn's disease. The common strictures seen in the absence of Crohn's disease are usually at the anal verge. These can occur in patients who have or have not had an anal fissure. Many occur with no obvious cause. Long-term use of mineral oil has been suspected of causing these stenoses. The strictures in patients with Crohn's disease, however, usually occur more proximally than the anal verge, usually 1.5 to 4 cm proximal to the anal verge. The reason for this can only be hypothesized. It may be that most of these strictures occur in patients with abscesses or fistulas, and prolonged suppuration around the rectum with scarring are the factors that produce strictures at these high levels. We approach these by judicious use of drainage of the abscess, dilatation of the stricture, and partial internal anal sphincterectomy.*

It had been believed by some authors that therapy, operative or nonoperative, directed toward Crohn's disease situated in the ileum or colon would have a beneficial effect on anorectal complications of Crohn's disease. It has been our experience that these anorectal complications occur and progress independently of the activity of the disease proximally. Therefore I believe that efforts directed toward the more proximal Crohn's disease should proceed, but its successful treatment would not be expected to improve the anorectal situation.

Treatment strategy of the anorectal complications of Crohn's disease should be directed toward symptomatic relief. This is most important because gross anorectal pathology may be present in an asymptomatic patient. It is difficult to justify taking risks, no matter how small, in most asymptomatic patients. Cosmetic anorectal surgery in the patient with Crohn's disease is taboo. Conversely, the older, outmoded concept of never operating on patients with anorectal Crohn's disease also must be discarded. The life of the symptomatic patient with anorectal Crohn's disease can often be significantly enhanced and improved by a simple and safe operation.

The most important symptom is pain. In most patients with Crohn's disease, rectal pain, when present, will be attributable to an incompletely drained rectal abscess. It is important to remember that the patient with Crohn's disease who has rectal pain has a rectal abscess unless proved otherwise. Fissures typically are painless, and infrequently cause rectal pain. Hemorrhoids rarely cause pain in patients with Crohn's disease, and when they do, spontaneous resolution within a few days is expected. (Remission, without any operative intervention,

---

*Editor's Note: Careful digital dilatation, or dilatation performed under direct vision with increasing diameter sigmoidoscopes, can often be done by the managing physician.

from pain caused by hemorrhoids is also expected in patients who do not have Crohn's disease.) Rectal abscess may be difficult to appreciate. If an abscess cannot be readily diagnosed, either because the patient's pain does not permit adequate investigation or because an abscess cannot otherwise be appreciated, rectal examination under anesthesia may be productively employed.

Patients with Crohn's disease have a reputation for poor healing of perirectal wounds. The exact cause for this has not been defined. Diarrhea, perirectal maceration resulting from persistent rectal discharge, as well as nutritional or immunologic factors may contribute. Compulsive, persistent, postoperative wound care, sometimes continued for many months, can affect wound healing. Nevertheless, the patients' wounds may not heal satisfactorily. The specter of a nonhealing wound looms over every anticipated anorectal incision. Sulfasalazine, metronidazole, 6-mercaptopurine, and various broad-spectrum antibiotics have each appeared to facilitate perirectal wound healing in individual patients.

Satisfactory treatment of the perirectal complications can alleviate, in some patients, the major source of their symptomatology. Therapeutic nihilism should be discouraged because a vigorous, enthusiastic, therapeutic regimen, incorporating nonoperative and operative modalities, is often beneficial and very rewarding.

The perirectal complications requiring treatment can be divided into painful and nonpainful conditions. Among the nonpainful conditions are skin tabs. In general they should not be excised. Medical therapy directed toward the underlying Crohn's disease itself may have a salutary effect. These tabs may interfere with personal hygiene. This would require additional efforts to maintain one's personal cleanliness, which is usually readily achievable. The skin tabs may also be unsightly. Cosmetic perirectal surgery in the patient with Crohn's disease is to be discouraged, however, because ulcers, consequent to excisional anal surgery if complicated by impaired wound healing, can produce greater problems than the skin tabs for which the excisions were performed.

Fistulas are believed to arise from an intersphincteric abscess.[10] Lining the rectum, there are about six or eight tiny glands that originate in the crypts of Morgagni. Normally the internal sphincter acts as a barrier to infection. The route to the intersphincteric space is via these crypts, which course through the internal sphincter and thereby gain access to the intersphincteric region, where they may develop the abscess. From the intersphincteric space the abscess can extend throughout the perirectal spaces and follow the classic routes of spread, but the initial point of origin is always the intermuscular abscess.

Parks[10] developed a conservative operation for fistulas. A conservative operation involves not making long tracts that lay open the entire fistulous tract. The basic principle behind this operation involves removal of the cryptoglandular epithelium and opening up the intermuscular plane by removing a portion of the internal sphincter muscle. This drains the intermuscular abscess. Nothing much need be done with the fistulous tract itself. In a period of time the inside wounds will heal, and then after a period of many months the fistula will heal.

Painless anal fistulas can generally be ignored. An adequately drained fistula will paradoxically drain very small amounts of material and be painless. Operation can and should be deferred.

A rectovaginal fistula is a difficult problem. If the symptoms are slight and tolerable, an operative approach should be deferred. A direct repair of the rectovaginal fistula can be undertaken successfully when the condition of the rectal mucosa is satisfactory. More commonly, fecal diversion in the form of an ileostomy or colostomy, in association with a direct repair of the rectovaginal fistula, would be prudent. The recent application of gracilis muscle or inferior gluteal muscolofascial flaps to the correction of rectovaginal fistulas has been found to be practical. This may have a role in the patient with Crohn's disease who has rectovaginal fistulas. Painless anal fissures should not be treated surgically. Their painlessness should make the need for operation unnecessary.

Anal incontinence in the patient with Crohn's anorectal disease is likely to be of iatrogenic origin, often occurring postoperatively. Direct repair of the anal sphincters usually is not practical because of the common association of perirectal infections and fistulas. A Thiersch wire may have a role here. The gracilis muscle transposition may be relevant in this situation, but its use in this clinical setting has not yet been reported. The common association of perirectal infectious processes, which are usually the precipitating factors in those patients who have become incontinent after fistula or abscess surgery, as well as the possibility of impaired perirectal wound healing common to the patient with Crohn's disease, tempers my enthusiasm for this approach. A complementary fecal diversion procedure also is advised if this operative strategy is employed.

Anorectal strictures are often due to chronic ischiorectal abscesses that may have been partially but incompletely drained. The relative proximal location of the abscess, and its partial drainage probably combine to result in a painless condition. Their correction involves correction of this presumed abscess by means of a partial internal anal sphincterectomy. The stricture will then usually respond to simple dilatation. Rectal bleeding in the patient with Crohn's disease often results from mucosal inflammation. There are occasional patients, however, who have rectal bleeding originating from their hemorrhoids. Often it is not possible to discern whether the bleeding is hemorrhoidal or due to the mucosal inflammation. Under these circumstances hemorrhoid injection sclerotherapy may be both therapeutic and diagnostic.

The hemorrhoids are injected in each of three to four quadrants with 0.5 phenol-in-oil preparation. Cessation of bleeding within 3 to 5 days can indicate that the bleeding was of hemorrhoidal origin, and was successfully treated by means of the injection sclerotherapy. Failure to respond to a trial of two or three injections usually indicates that the bleeding is not hemorrhoidal, and further attempts at injection sclerotherapy are not likely to be productive. A positive response to injection sclerotherapy, albeit temporary, usually indicates that further benefit from additional injections is likely to result. These can be repeated at suitable intervals, as required, to eliminate the symptom of rectal bleeding. Very large internal hemorrhoids that cause bleeding are infrequent in the patient with Crohn's disease. In that group, rubber band ligations could be safely attempted. The possibility of a resultant nonhealed ulcer consequent to an elastic band ligation must be considered in assessing the potential benefit of elastic band ligations. Other forms of hemorrhoid destruction, such as infrared photocoagulation, laser destruction, or hemorrhoid electrocoagulation by various devices, have not been reported. Their advantage over hemorrhoid rubber band ligation is not apparent, and the resultant larger wounds could be troublesome if anorectal wound healing is impaired. This same strategy could be applied to the patient with Crohn's disease who has the infrequent occurrence of hemorrhoidal protrusion.

The painful conditions include hemorrhoids, fissures, and abscesses. Hemorrhoids should be treated nonoperatively by the usual conservative modalities because spontaneous resolution is the usual outcome. An anal fissure that is painful and has failed to respond to local therapy should be managed successfully initially by anal dilatation. The technique employed incorporates a precise degree of dilatation. One of two techniques is employed. The procedure is done under local anesthesia after first applying conscious sedation. A careful examination is performed to exclude the possibility of an underlying intermuscular abscess. Either a Parks retractor is placed in the anal canal and opened to a width of 4.8 cm or a balloon 40 mm in diameter inflated to a pressure of 20 psi is used. The dilatation is maintained for exactly 5 minutes.

Most patients with Crohn's disease and rectal pain will have a rectal abscess. A rectal abscess occurring for the first time in a patient with

Crohn's disease can usually be treated by simple incision and drainage. An intermuscular abscess is best treated by means of a partial internal anal sphincterotomy. Parks[10] promoted the concept of the partial internal anal sphincterectomy in the treatment of fistulous abscesses in general. He believed that the primary event in the development of a perirectal abscess was the intersphincteric abscess. Adequate treatment of an intersphincteric abscess consists of a partial internal anal sphincterectomy.[11] By unroofing the intersphincteric component the abscess is adequately treated, and healing of the fistulous abscess is likely to ensue. This concept has been of particular applicability to the patient with Crohn's disease. Small, predominantly intrarectal incisions are utilized. This avoids the problem of the nonhealed perirectal wound. By restricting the excision to the internal sphincter, avoiding incisions in the external sphincter, interference with anal continence is minimized. Partial incontinence might not be a problem to the normal patient, but could be a dreadful complication in the patient with Crohn's disease and consequent diarrhea.

The patients are operated on in the lithotomy or prone position, and usually general anesthesia is employed. In an occasional patient local anesthesia may be utilized. Even when general anesthesia is used, local anesthesia (bupivacaine 0.5% and hyaluronidase and injection of epinephrine [1:200,000]) supplement the general anesthesia. This serves to effect complete sphincteric relaxation, the epinephrine serves to reduce bleeding, and the anesthesia maintains the patient pain free for a few hours postoperatively. Parks or other suitable retractors are utilized. The intersphincteric origin of the fistula is identified by following the principles set forth in Goodsall's rule, probing the crypts of Morgagni or probing the external orifice of the fistula. Utilizing these maneuvers, the intersphincteric origin of the fistulas can be identified in more than 90% of cases. In most of the others the possibilities of the origin can be narrowed down to two possible sites. A 1 $\times$ 1 cm segment of skin and mucosa is then excised. The lower border of the excision is at the intersphincteric groove, the upper border is 3 mm above the dentate line, and the excision is 1 cm wide and centered on the presumed origin of the fistula. The internal sphincter is then dissected off the underlying external sphincter with a hemostat within the same borders and excised. The fistulous tract can then be identified. Occasionally a ¼ in. Penrose drain is brought from the internal origin out through the fistulous tract. This serves to unroof the intersphincteric abscess, which theoretically is the basis for the acute or chronic fistula or fistulous abscess. This alone should result in healing of the fistulous tract. By limiting the excision to the internal sphincter and by avoiding incisions in the external sphincter, interference with continence is minimized. Furthermore, by utilizing a 1 cm square, predominantly intrarectal incision, problems associated with poor healing of perirectal wounds are minimized.

More than 275 patients have been treated in this fashion. There was one case of partial anal incontinence. Approximately 85% of fistulas have healed, although the far-advanced complex fistulas may not heal completely. The goal of alleviating pain, allowing the patient to function, and avoiding recurrent abscess formation almost always can be accomplished. Since embarking on this approach more than 12 years ago, only two patients have come to stoma or resection as a result of the perirectal complications.*

There are patients who have extensive infection of the skin and subcutaneous tissues of the buttocks and perianal region. After the partial internal anal sphincterectomy is performed to treat the underlying intersphincteric abscess, the affected skin is excised. This is performed in stages, excising two or three segments 1 to 2 in. in diameter at each stage. In this fashion the involved skin can be totally removed in two or more stages. The need for skin grafts is eliminated by avoiding massive defects and allowing these to epithelialize before performing additional skin excisions. Nonhealing of these wounds, while theoretically possible, has not yet been a problem.

Metronidazole has been reported to be beneficial in patients with Crohn's disease. An abscess with obvious undrained pus requires operative incision and drainage. Metronidazole or other antibiotics cannot be expected to improve this particular clinical situation. It can, however, be adjunctive, and in the questionable case a trial of metronidazole can be offered with the decision regarding operation deferred. Other broad-spectrum antibiotics or combinations of antibiotics also can have a beneficial effect on the rectal abscess. In addition, 6-MP has been found to be effective in healing patients who have undergone surgery and who have had persistent nonhealed perirectal wounds.

The underlying treatment of Crohn's disease in general should be continued. 6-MP in particular has been helpful in controlling Crohn's disease in general and has affected its perirectal infectious complications in particular.[8]

The goal of treatment of anorectal Crohn's disease should be palliation of symptoms. Operation should be deferred if the patient is having few or no symptoms. It is possible that early operation, effecting early

*Editor's Note: 6-Mercaptopurine (6-MP) was often introduced during the postoperative period for treatment of Crohn's disease, and has contributed to this success.

prompt and adequate drainage, could prevent some of the far-advanced complex fistulas that are known to occur in patients with Crohn's disease. These fistulas have also been seen in other patients who have been identified as belonging to population groups that do not have ready access to sophisticated medical care.

Cancer probably occurs with increased frequency in the patient with Crohn's disease. Cancer can also occur in a chronic anal fistula. Cancers can arise in the anal fistula accompanying Crohn's disease. Both squamous carcinoma and adenocarcinoma have been seen in this setting. In many cases the underlying cancer was never appreciated or even suspected until the tissue obtained at operation was examined microscopically. One of our five cases occurred in a 29-year old patient who had Crohn's disease and an anal fistula for 1½ years. One should always be aware that there is a potential for cancer in the anal fistula occurring with Crohn's disease. The clinician thus has a difficult problem in making this diagnosis. Magnetic resonance imaging of the pelvis has been helpful in evaluating these patients. Magnetic resonance imaging scans are usually obtained in the preoperative evaluation of the patient with a complex anal fistula for a possible complicating carcinoma. This, however, must be considered for nonoperative patients as well.

The treatment of these carcinomas follows the usual principles for the treatment of neoplasms in this area in the absence of Crohn's disease.[4] Adenocarcinoma is treated operatively, perhaps with preoperative adjuvant radiation therapy or chemotherapy. Squamous carcinomas in this location are treated with combination chemotherapy and radiation therapy, with operation reserved for those few in whom residual tumor persists despite this combination therapy.

CONCLUSION

The main emphasis in approaching the patient with Crohn's disease who has accompanying anorectal disease should be relief of pain. It is true that we do not cure all fistulas, and it is true that abscesses can recur even under medical therapy. These patients with anorectal disease can be severely symptomatic. They often require narcotics. This can affect bowel function. If one can control the anorectal disease by local therapy, narcotics can be eliminated, and the patient's bowel condition and symptoms may improve.

An operative approach to Crohn's disease with accompanying anorectal disease has been reported to be satisfactory by several authors. From a review of the literature it may be apparent that there are enthusiasts for operation and those who caution against operation. When the cases are analyzed, it is obvious that there are asymptomatic or mild cases that do not progress, that may not progress, or that even may heal after a period of years, and in whom a vigorous operative approach is contraindicated. It is also apparent that the patient with persistent undrained abscesses without adequate operation is likely to get into difficulty, with incontinence, stricture formation, or persistent sepsis. Conservatism is important but a conservative approach should not deprive a patient of an indicated and required operation. The patient with Crohn's disease and a fistulous abscess must be individualized.

REFERENCES

1. Allingham W: *Diseases of the Colon and Rectum.* New York, Bermingham and Co., 1882.
2. Crohn B: *Regional Ileitis.* Philadelphia, Grune & Stratton, 1949.
3. Crohn B, Ginzburg L, Oppenheimer GD: Regional ileitis: A pathological and clinical entity. *JAMA* 1932; 99:1323–1328.
4. Cummings BJ: Anal cancer. *Int J Radiat Oncol Biol Phys* 1990; 19:1309–1315.
5. Greenstein AJ, Sachar DB, Kark AE: Stricture of the anorectum in Crohn's disease involving the colon. *Ann Surg* 1975; 181:207–212.
6. Homans J: Regional ileitis: A clinical not a pathological entity. *N Engl J Med* 1933; 209:1315–1324.
7. Hughes LE: Surgical pathology and management of anorectal Crohn's disease. *J R Soc Med* 1978; 71:644–651.
8. Korelitz BE: Perianal Crohn's disease, in Bayless IM (ed): *Current Therapy in Gastroenterology,* ed 3. MC Decker, 1990, pp 351–353.
9. Lee E: Split ileostomy in the treatment of Crohn's disease. *Ann R Coll Surg Engl* 1975; 56:94–102.
10. Parks AG: Pathogenesis and treatment of fistula in ano. *Br Med J* 1961; 1:463–469.
11. Sohn N, Korelitz BI, Weinstein MA: Anorectal Crohn's disease: Definitive surgery for fistulas and recurrent abscesses. *Am J Surg* 1980; 139:394–397.

Chapter 16 _____

Implications of Diversion Proctitis in Crohn's Disease

Michael Krumholz

Nonspecific diversion colitis developing in portions of the large bowel excluded from the fecal stream is a phenomenon that has received relatively little attention. It is unclear when this entity was first recognized. The first formal description appeared in 1981. The clinical course and pathologic findings in ten patients who had undergone fecal diversion at the Beth Israel Hospital in Boston were reported.[6]

Most of the patients in this series had required diversion because of complications related to diverticular disease; none had symptoms suggestive of inflammatory bowel disease (IBD). Nine underwent loop or end colostomy; one had an end ileostomy. The four patients in whom sigmoidoscopy was done before or at the time of the diversionary procedure were all noted to have a normal-appearing mucosa. However, all of the patients were found on subsequent examination to have inflammation in the excluded segment, usually within 6 months of the diversion.

The gross sigmoidoscopic appearance was described as being indistinguishable from that of mild ulcerative colitis; histologic alterations were nonspecific, consisting of combinations of acute and chronic inflammation in the lamina propria, crypt abscesses, epithelial cell degeneration, and crypt regeneration. In most, however, the findings were incidental and not clinically significant.

The fate of the rectal segment of these patients varied dependent on whether or not intestinal reanastomosis was performed. Five had restoration of intestinal continuity within 6 months; all did well clinically and developed normal-appearing mucosa on subsequent sigmoidos-

copy. Reanastomosis was not done in the other five. Two of these patients developed a purulent rectal discharge and abdominal cramps after several years, and all five had evidence of continued mucosal
inflammation in the excluded segment. The conclusion was that the observed inflammation in the excluded colonic segments resulted directly
from diversion of the fecal stream, was distinct from other known
causes of colitis, and was reversible with restoration of intestinal continuity.

There have, in addition, been a few case reports in which diversion-
related inflammation may have been present but was not specifically
recognized. Instances of clindamycin-induced pseudomembranous colitis requiring subtotal colectomy have been described in which the rectal stump later had to be resected because of persistent proctitis.[7] One
patient with amoebic colitis who underwent subtotal colectomy and ileostomy has been reported in whom a nonspecific proctitis persisted
until reanastomosis was performed.[16] Recently there have been a few
reports of rectal bleeding due to diversion colitis, including patients
who had undergone diversion for complications of diverticular disease,
neurogenic fecal incontinence, rectal irradiation, and traumatic perineal
lacerations.[2, 8, 17, 20]

Special problems might be expected in patients with underlying
IBD who develop superimposed diversion-related inflammation. In patients with preexisting disease in the excluded segment, the development of diversion colitis might lead to clinical deterioration. In patients
with minimal or no disease, the inflammation may be mistakenly diagnosed as an extension of the underlying IBD; misdiagnosis may in turn
lead to inappropriate therapy and delay in restoration of intestinal continuity.

Since most patients with ulcerative colitis who require surgery undergo proctocolectomy, diversion-related inflammation should rarely
present a clinical problem. Of interest, however, is a study that reviewed
the Mount Sinai Hospital experience with 136 patients with ulcerative
colitis who underwent subtotal colectomy and ileostomy with the rectum left in situ; virtually all of them had persistent inflammation in the
rectal stump, and 94% eventually needed abdominoperineal resection.[13]
The relative contribution of diversion proctitis in this patient population
is purely speculative.

Crohn's disease of the colon characteristically spares the rectal segment. Thus the surgical procedure of choice for these patients will often be resection with anastomosis. However, when this is not possible
because of rectal involvement, fistula or abscess formation, or severe underlying systemic disease, for example, diversion of the fecal stream has

long been believed to have a favorable effect on the course of the disease.[1, 4, 14, 19, 24, 25] Distinction has not been made, however, between the effect of fecal diversion on overall clinical activity and its effect on mucosal inflammation in the distal excluded segment.

A study by Korelitz et al.[10] in the late 1960s suggested that the disease in the distal segment may occur in such patients. Of 39 patients with presumed Crohn's colitis initially sparing the rectum who underwent ileostomy and subtotal colectomy, 34 developed progressive involvement of the rectum, and most eventually required resection of the excluded segment. Interestingly, although the initial resected specimens usually showed pathologic features characteristic of Crohn's disease, such as transmural inflammation and granulomas, the findings in the later resected rectums were often nonspecific. Others have shown that despite overall clinical improvement after diversion in patients with Crohn's colitis, there may be persistent and progressive disease in the rectal segment.[4, 14, 19]

Korelitz et al.[12] recently reviewed their experience during a 10-year period with 32 patients with Crohn's disease who underwent an operation that included an ileostomy or a colostomy with the rectal segment left in place. In 9 patients the ileostomy was a temporary diverting stoma that was closed within 3 months; all of these patients had a normal-appearing rectal mucosa at the time of reanastomosis. The remaining 23 patients had a diverting stoma for a minimum of 6 months. In 3 inflammation was already present, and in 4 the sigmoidoscopic appearance was unknown. The remaining 16 all had a normal-appearing rectal mucosa at the time of diversionary surgery; the course of these latter patients in whom changes caused by diversion should have been most apparent was recently reported.[12]

All 16 had active Crohn's disease. The distribution of disease was primarily colonic in 11 patients, and mostly ileal in 5. Specific complications that served as the ultimate indication for surgery included actual or threatened colonic perforation (3), recurrent small bowel obstruction, large bowel obstruction due to stricture (3), fistula formation (4), and perirectal abscess. Most patients underwent ileostomy with either an ileocolic resection or subtotal colectomy; one had an ileostomy without resection, and two underwent colostomy.

When the rectal segments of these 16 patients were later examined they all showed evidence of inflammation at some time between 3 months and 3 years after diversion (Fig 16–1). Early sigmoidoscopic findings included friability, erosions, and, in two patients, aphthous ulcers. Although aphthous lesions are suggestive of distal extension of Crohn's disease they are not diagnostic, and have recently been re-

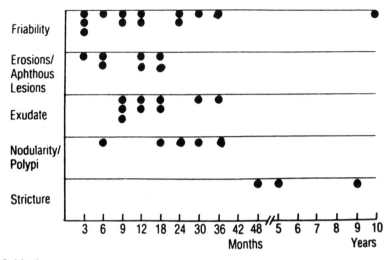

FIG 16–1.
Time of sigmoidoscopic abnormalities in 16 patients with Crohn's disease with normal-appearing rectum at time of diversion. (From Korelitz BE, Cheskin LJ, Sohn N, et al: *J Clin Gastroenterol* 1985; 7:37. Used by permission.)

ported in several non-IBD patients with diversion proctitis.[8, 15, 17] At 9 months to a year exudate, nodularity, and inflammatory polyps were observed, and, in 3 patients, progressive narrowing and stricture formation developed after several years. Most patients were asymptomatic although some with more severe disease did pass blood, mucus, and exudate from the rectum. Clinically, the presenting signs and symptoms of diversion colitis may thus include incidental sigmoidoscopic finding and/or rectal bleeding, purulent discharge, and abdominal cramps.

Histologic findings on rectal biopsy were also generally nonspecific, and included mixed acute and chronic inflammatory infiltrate, fibrosis, crypt abscesses, and large lymphoid follicles; the latter finding has been noted in several other reports.[2, 8, 17]Only two biopsies revealed microgranulomas specific for Crohn's disease.

The subsequent course of these 16 patients is outlined on Figure 16–2. Eight patients continued to have mild to moderate inflammation on sigmoidoscopy; the other 8 developed progressively severe changes. Four patients were given a trial of hydrocortisone enemas, and there was noted sigmoidoscopic improvement in only 1; success with topical corticosteroids in other reports has also been variable.[2, 6] One patient with mild inflammation improved coincident with 6-mercaptopurine therapy for more proximal disease. In 4 patients with mild proctitis reanastomosis was performed despite persistent inflammation in the rec-

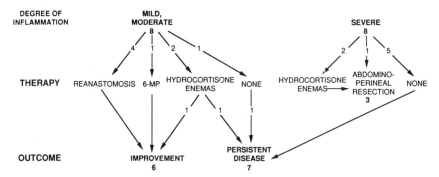

FIG 16—2.
Course of 16 patients with Crohn's disease and diversion-associated proctitis. (From Korelitz BE, Cheskin LJ, Sohn N, et al: *J Clin Gastroenterol* 1985; 7:37 Used by permission.)

tal segment. In all 4 the rectal mucosa returned to normal within 2 to 3 months, and remained normal on periodic sigmoidoscopic examination.[11] In 3 of the 8 patients with severe inflammation, abdominoperineal resection eventually was needed because of persistent purulent discharge and stricture formation. The remaining 7 patients had persistent, and in some progressive, inflammation in the rectum several years after diversion.

Until recently the pathogenesis of diversion-related inflammation was not well understood. Initially it was suggested that fecal diversion might lead to stasis and subsequent emergence of bacterial strains harmful to the colonic mucosa. Bacterial overgrowth has been postulated to account for the enteritis seen in patients bypassed for the treatment of morbid obesity.[5, 21]

Another possible explanation is that the fecal diversion deprives the mucosa of essential nutrients or disturbs symbiotic bacterial mucosal relationships. Recent in vitro studies have emphasized, as noted by Dr. Bayless (see Chapter 3), that short-chain fatty acids, such as acetate and especially butyrate, may serve as the major source of energy for colonocytes.[22] In the absence of these nutrients somehow there may be a compromise of the mucosal integrity.

Recent work by Harig et al.[8] lends support to the latter, nutritional deficiency, theory. They examined 4 patients with diversion colitis, and none were believed to have IBD. Initially levels of short-chain fatty acids, including acetic, proprionic, and *n*-butyric, were measured in the excluded segments of these patients and found to be negligible. The patients then received twice-daily instillations of short-chain fatty acid solutions for a 2- to 4-week period; all had significant clinical, endoscopic, and histologic improvement. Interruption of treatment for 2 weeks resulted in worsening of endoscopic scores, and substitution of saline enemas led to little or no improvement. Maintenance therapy with twice-weekly enemas was effective in sustaining remission in 1 of 2 patients. Utilizing breath hydrogen testing, absence of carbohydrate fermenting anaerobic bacteria was demonstrated in the diverted segments of these patients, and this was postulated to represent the underlying cause of the short-chain fatty acid deficiency.

This hypothesis was supported by the findings of an even more recent report by Neut et al.[18] These investigators compared the rectal microflora in 16 patients who had undergone fecal diversion with 16 controls. The cause of the diversion was IBD in 10 patients. Colonoscopy revealed evidence of diversion colitis in most of the patients. Significantly less anaerobic bacteria were found in the diverted segments, and the ability of these isolates to produce short-chain fatty acids in vitro was impaired.

Local nutritional deficiencies have also been postulated perhaps to underlie other forms of colitis. Interestingly, patients with ulcerative colitis have been shown to have reduced lumenal concentrations of short-chain fatty acids, and mucosal utilization of butyrate in ulcerative colitis may be impaired.[23, 26] Encouraging results were recently reported with use of short-chain fatty acid enemas in patients with ulcerative colitis refractory to other standard treatment.[3] Hoverstad et al.[9] described significantly less fecal excretion of short-chain fatty acids in patients receiving ampicillin and clindamycin, and postulate that this and the associated suppression of the colonic flora may in part be responsible for the development of antibiotic-associated colitis.

CONCLUSIONS

1. Fecal diversion itself is responsible for a nonspecific inflammatory process in the excluded distal aspect of the colon, usually the rectum; previously normal-appearing mucosa becomes inflamed after surgical diversion, and mucosa already abnormal may worsen.

2. Diversion colitis has been seen after ileostomy and colostomy performed for a variety of conditions, such as diverticular disease, colorectal carcinoma, and neurologic disorders, in addition to IBD.

3. The pathogenesis may be related to nutritional deficiency of short-chain fatty acids produced by depleted anaerobic flora.

4. The gross and microscopic pathology are usually nonspecific, although certain features such as aphthous ulcers and nodular lymphoid hyperplasia appear to be common.

5. The inflammation in the excluded segment usually begins as early as 3 months after diversion and may be progressive.

6. Most patients are asymptomatic; however, in some, especially if diversion has been prolonged, there may be rectal bleeding, purulent rectal discharge, and abdominal cramps.

7. In patients with preexisting IBD, extension of inflammation to the excluded segment is most likely due to diversion itself, although there may also be acceleration of the underlying disease. In most patients the characteristic pathology of Crohn's disease is not found in the rectal segment.

8. The role of medical therapy is still unknown. Enemas consisting of solutions of short-chain fatty acids may be effective therapy for individuals who are poor surgical candidates.

9. Inflammation due to diversion is preventable, and thus continuity of the intestinal tract should be maintained whenever feasible; if diversionary surgery is performed, reanastomosis should be carried out as soon as possible despite the presence of inflammation in the excluded segment. Delay may lead to progressive disease, at which time reanastomosis would not be feasible.

10. When intestinal continuity is reestablished, most patients with diversion-related inflammation will have restoration of normal-appearing mucosa within several months.

REFERENCES

1. Aufses AH Jr, Kreel I: Ileostomy for granulomatous ileocolitis. *Ann Surg* 1971; 173:91–96.
2. Bosshardt RT, Abel ME: Proctitis following fecal diversion. *Dis Colon Rectum* 1984; 27:605–607.
3. Breuer RI, Buto SK, Christ ML, et al: Short chain fatty acids for distal ulcerative colitis. *Gastroenterology* 1990; 98:A161.
4. Burman JH, Thompson H, Cooke WT, et al: The effects of diversion of intestinal contents on the progress of Crohn's disease of the large bowel. *Gut* 1971; 12:11–15.
5. Drenick EJ, Ament ME, Finegold SM, et al: Bypass enteropathy: An inflammatory process in the excluded segment with systemic complications. *Am J Nutr* 1977; 30:76.
6. Glotzer DJ, Glick ME, Goldman H: Proctitis and colitis following diversion of the fecal stream. *Gastroenterology* 1981; 80:438–441.
7. Goodacre RL, et al: Persistence of proctitis in 2 cases of clindamycin associated colitis. *Gastroenterology* 1977; 72:149–152.
8. Harig JM, Soergel KH, Komorowski RA, et al: Treatment of diversion colitis with short chain fatty acid irrigation. *N Engl J Med* 1989; 320:23–28.

9. Hoverstad T, Cartlstedt-Duke B, Lingaas E, et al: Influence of ampicillin, clindamycin and metronidazole on faecal excretion of short chain fatty acids in healthy subjects. *Scand J Gastroenterol* 1986; 21:621–626.

10. Korelitz BI: Clinical course, late results and pathological nature of inflammatory bowel disease of the colon initially sparing the rectum. *Gut* 1967; 8:281–290.

11. Korelitz BI, Cheskin LJ, Sohn N, et al: Proctitis after fecal diversion in Crohn's disease and its elimination with reanastomosis; implications for surgical management. *Gastroenterology* 1984; 87:710–713.

12. Korelitz BI, Cheskin LJ, Sohn N, et al: The fate of the rectal segment after diversion of the fecal stream in Crohn's disease; its implications for surgical management. *J Clin Gastroenterol* 1985; 7:37–43.

13. Korelitz BI, Dyck WP, Klion M: Fate of the rectum and distal colon after subtotal colectomy for ulcerative colitis. *Gut* 1969; 10:198–201.

14. Lee E: Split ileostomy in the treatment of Crohn's disease of colon. *Ann R Coll Surg Engl* 1975; 56:94–102.

15. Lusk LB, Reichen J, Levine JS: Aphthous ulceration in diversion colitis. *Gastroenterology* 1984; 87:1171–1173.

16. Mendonica H, Vieta J, Korelitz BI: Perforation of the colon in unsuspected amoebic colitis: report of two cases. *Dis Colon Rectum* 1977; 20:149–153.

17. Murray FE, O'Brien MJ, Birkett DH, et al: Diversion colitis: Pathologic findings in a resected sigmoid colon and rectum. *Gastroenterology* 1987; 93:1404–1408.

18. Neut C, Colombel JF, Guillemot F, et al: Impaired bacterial flora in human excluded colon. *Gut* 1989; 30:1094–1098.

19. Oberhelman HA Jr, Kohatsu S, Taylor KB, et al: Diverting ileostomy in surgical management of Crohn's disease of the colon. *Am J Surg* 1968; 115:231–240.

20. Ona FV, Boger JN: Rectal bleeding due to diversion colitis. *Am J Gastroenterol* 1985; 80:40–41.

21. Passaro E Jr, Drenick E, Wilson SE: Bypass enteritis: A new complication of jejunoileal bypass for obesity. *Am J Surg* 1976; 131:169.

22. Roediger WE: Role of anaerobic bacteria in the metabolic welfare of the colonic mucosa in man. *Gut* 1980; 21:793–798.

23. Roediger WE: The colonic epithelium in ulcerative colitis: An energy deficiency disease? *Lancet* 1980; 2:712–715.

24. Truelove SC, Ellis H, Webster CU: Place of double barreled ileostomy in ulcerative colitis and Crohn's disease of the colon. *Br Med J* 1965; 1:150–153.

25. Utlee JM, Lens J: Results of split ileostomy in Crohn's disease of colon. *Neth J Surg* 1981; 33:181–184.

26. Vernia P, Gnaedinger MS, Hauck W, et al: Organic anions and the diarrhea of inflammatory bowel disease. *Dig Dis Sci* 1988; 33:1353–1358.

PART 4

Surgery for Ulcerative Colitis

Chapter 17 _____

Selecting an Operation for Ulcerative Colitis

Norman Sohn

_____

The first ileostomy for ulcerative colitis was performed in 1913[2]; over the many years since then, the techniques have been improved. The care of the ileostomy at first was horrendous, with patients being managed with diapers and pans to collect the drainage. In 1944 the first ileostomy appliance was invented by a patient who had a background in chemistry and product development. During the next several years appliances and supplemental materials were improved, and by 1969 care had reached the level available today. Mutual self-help groups evolved, and the concept of enterostomal therapy had been introduced. All that was left for the surgeon to do was to convince the patient that life with an ileostomy was possible, and the patient was persuaded to learn to love the ileostomy.

This state of affairs was abruptly altered in 1969 when Kock introduced the continent ileostomy. In this operation the patient no longer had to wear an ileostomy appliance. In effect, the appliance was internal and concealed within the abdominal cavity. The patient no longer had to be content with an ileostomy, but had a new goal to strive for. Several years later, in the mid to late 1970s, the ileoanal pouch was developed, and it presented still new problems, hopes, and desires.

Another option is the ileorectal anastomosis, which was popularized by Aylett. The basic four operations available to a patient with ulcerative colitis are ileostomy, continent ileostomy, ileorectal anastomosis, and ileoanal pouch.

The ileoanal pouch would appear to be the ideal operation for ulcerative colitis. The colon and most of the rectum are removed. The mucosa is stripped from the distal area of the rectum, thereby totally excising all of the diseased tissue, yet preserving the important sphincter mechanism. A pouch is constructed from the ileum and anastomosed to the anus, with the sphincter muscles functioning, thereby curing the disease and allowing the patient to defecate normally.

There are limitations in this operation, however, and the decision as to which operation to provide to the patient is difficult. I will try to provide some information on which to base that decision. I have reviewed several recent papers on the ileoanal pouch, covering about 1,700 patients.[3, 4, 6, 8, 9-13] The number of deaths from this operation is low; many of the series had none, and the highest mortality rate was 1%. This is remarkable for an operation that is difficult and prone to complications.

The patient who has a successful ileoanal pouch usually has five to six bowel movements during the day and none to one at night. Continence is usually somewhat compromised, often requiring protective pads, especially at night. While this may seem to be a poor result and unacceptable to a surgeon, most patients, despite compromised continence, prefer the pouch to an ileostomy. The main risks and hazards of this operation are due to the potential for intra-abdominal sepsis; intestinal obstruction also occurs too frequently in both the early and late postoperative period. Intra-abdominal sepsis exposes the patient to additional risks, including (1) risk of adhesive obstruction; (2) risk of reoperation with intestinal trauma, perhaps leading to another intestinal resection and resulting short bowel syndrome; (3) risk of prolonged central venous therapy; (4) risk of prolonged antibiotic therapy; (5) risk of hospital-acquired infection; and (6) risk of transfusions. All of these have to be considered before advising a patient to undergo this operation. Patients have been seen who have had several of these complications, and then developed acquired immunodeficiency syndrome or chronic hepatitis as a consequence of blood transfusions that were required either during their several reoperations or as a result of their septic complications. Are these potential complications worth saving the rectum? At least in New York City, where a serious complication often results in a malpractice suit, how can the surgeon perform these operations without being involved with these inevitable legal machinations consequent to the complications? Of greater concern is the price, in the form of serious complications, ruined lives, ruined careers, and ruined marriages. Is it worth the salvage of a rectum?

The continent ileostomy (Kock pouch) was introduced in 1969 and had a flare of popularity in the 1970s. It was recognized that there were many complications associated with the Kock pouch, including sepsis, incontinence, and the need for multiple reoperations. The development of the ileoanal pouch occurred around that time. Both of these factors resulted in disappearance of the Kock pouch, except for a few medical centers. A MEDLINE search for papers on the continent ileostomy during the last 20 years shows that the annual number of papers peaked around 1980, and the interest in this operation appears to have waned subsequently. A recent report from the Cleveland Clinic shows what the potential complications are with the continent ileostomy.[5] Of 168 patients, there was one postoperative death. Late deaths, including one suicide, occurred in 3.6%. Intestinal obstruction, sepsis, and pouch excision are also reported. Reoperations appear to be an integral part of this procedure, and many of these reoperations are complex, difficult operations.

Ileorectal anastomosis for ulcerative colitis was never popular in this country. In a series published in 1988, of 59 patients 22% had to have the rectum excised and 5% developed carcinoma.[1] Most physicians consider this too high a risk for preservation of the rectum. In some patients, particularly a youngster, there may be a valid reason to try to delay the inevitable abdominoperineal resection. This type of patient could thereby have a chance to grow, marry, and have children before having abdominoperineal resection. There may be a place for this, but the risks are quite high.

The standard operation for ulcerative colitis, to which every innovation must be compared, is the panproctocolectomy with an ileostomy. What are its complications? Intestinal obstruction occurs more commonly than is desired, but significantly less frequently than with the sphincter-saving procedures.[7] It is my practice that in every patient who has an ileostomy, a Baker tube (a 9 foot long Foley catheter) is threaded from the ileostomy up to the ligament of Treitz and left in place for approximately 10 to 12 days. This has reduced our postoperative obstruction rate to about 2%; only half of these patients have required surgery for intestinal obstruction vs. a rate reported in the literature of at least 10% to 15%.

A perineal sinus can occur as a complication with an ileostomy operation or with a continent ileostomy. It is not present in a sphincter-saving procedure. In ulcerative colitis delayed healing occurs in about 25%, but only one-third of those need a reoperation for that problem. Most of these reoperations are minor local procedures designed to enhance wound healing in the perineum and are not a complicated intra-abdominal operation.

Stomal stenosis occurs infrequently in an ileostomy, and usually can be corrected by simple ambulatory procedures. Peristomal hernias and stomal prolapse occur very infrequently.

Of greatest importance is that sepsis, with its devastating effects, is not an expected complication of the ileostomy operation. Unless performing the procedure in a patient who has a perforated colon, one would not expect sepsis, and it is certainly not the feared complication that accompanies the sphincter-saving procedures or the continent ileostomy. Most of the stomal complications can be prevented by proper operative technique, selecting the site for the ileostomy preoperatively, and making a satisfactory stoma.

There is no doubt that if one would compare the life-styles of patients with the continent ileostomy or the ileoanal pouch with the ileostomy, that of the patient with an ileostomy would come in a far second. It would be better not having to bother with an appliance. The advantages in the social, emotional, and sexual aspects of one's life-style are obvious. However, we await a study comparing the life-style of the patient with an ileostomy with the life-style of the patient who had complications after the ileoanal pouch or the continent ileostomy. The serious complication rate with the ileoanal pouch is around 10%, even in centers where this operation has been done frequently and by very experienced surgeons.

Which patients should have the ileoanal pouch operation? It should be seriously considered in a patient who is young, not acutely or severely ill, and willing to accept the risks of failure. An important factor would be a good emotional support system. Can the patient afford to be sick for 1 to 2 years, requiring hospitalizations for septic complications and revisions of the pouch? Will the patient lose his/her job? Will the patient lose a spouse? Will the patient lose his/her business? With these considerations in mind, this operation may be more applicable to the young patient rather than to an adult. Starting at around the age of 25 to 30, the older the patient the less desirable is this operation. Many authors consider 50 the upper limit for consideration for this trauma.

REFERENCES

1. Backer O. Hjortrup A, Kjaergaard J: Evaluation of ileorectal anastomosis for the treatment of ulcerative proctocolitis. *J R Soc Med* 1988; 81:210–211.
2. Brown JY: The value of complete physiological rest of the large bowel in the treatment of certain ulcerative lesions of this organ; with description of operative technique and report of cases. *Surg Gynecol Obstet* 1913; 16:610–613.

3. Dozois RR, Kelly KA, Welling DR, et al: Ileal pouch–anal anastomosis: Comparison of results in familial adenomatous polyposis and chronic ulcerative colitis. *Ann Surg* 1989; 210:268–273.
4. Everett WG: Experience of restorative proctocolectomy with ileal reservoir. *Br J Surg* 1989; 76:77–81.
5. Fazio VW, Church JM: Complications and function of the continent ileostomy at the Cleveland Clinic. *World J Surg* 1988; 12:148–154.
6. Fleshman JW. Cohen Z, McLeod RS, et al: The ileal reservoir and ileoanal anastomosis procedure. Factors affecting technical and functional outcome. *Dis Colon Rectum* 1988; 31:10–16.
7. Francois Y, Dozois RR, Kelly KA, et al: Small intestinal obstruction complicating ileal pouch-anal anastomosis. *Ann Surg* 1989; 209:46–50.
8. Keighley MR, Winslet MC, Flinn R, et al: Multivariate analysis of factors influencing the results of restorative proctocolectomy. *Br J Surg* 1989; 76:740–774.
9. Nicholls RJ, Holt SD, Lubowski DZ: Restorative proctocolectomy with ileal reservoir. Comparison of two stage vs. three stage procedures and analysis of factors that might affect outcome. *Dis Colon Rectum* 1989; 32:323–332.
10. Oresland T, Fasth S, Nordgren S, et al: The clinical and functional outcome after restorative proctocolectomy. A prospective study in 100 patients. *Int J Color Dis* 1989; 4:50–56.
11. Pescatori M, Mattana C, Castagneto M: Clinical and functional results after restorative proctocolectomy. *Br J Surg* 1988; 75:321–324.
12. Skarsgard ED, Atkinson KG, Bell GA, et al: Function and quality of life results after ileal pouch surgery for chronic ulcerative colitis and familial polyposis. *Am J Surg* 1989; 157:467–471.
13. Wexner SD, Wong WD, Rothenberger DA, et al: The ileoanal reservoir. *Am J Surg* 1990; 159:178–185.

Chapter 18 _____

Results of Ileo Pouch Anal Anastomosis

Zane Cohen

The pelvic pouch procedure has gained remarkable enthusiasm during the past decade.[1] It is an operation that can potentially cure a patient of ulcerative colitis while maintaining normal gastrointestinal continuity. This will avoid an ileostomy, with its resultant potential psychosocial difficulties. At the outset one must remember that total proctocolectomy and ileostomy is still considered the standard operation for patients requiring surgery for ulcerative colitis. Any other operation for ulcerative colitis will be compared with it regarding risks, complications, and results. Although problems such as skin irritation, effluent odor, and psychologic problems related to a stoma are documented, most patients adapt extremely well to an end ileostomy, and function satisfactorily. Although it would seem obvious that restoration of gastrointestinal continuity would provide a better quality of life, we have not been able to demonstrate this with use of scientific methods.[10] Despite this, in my own practice 95% of patients who require surgery for ulcerative colitis will wish to have a pelvic pouch procedure.

From the inception of the Kock pouch to the development and modifications of the pelvic pouch, it has been shown that an ileal reservoir can be constructed out of the terminal ileum without any serious long-term metabolic side effects.[9] The Kock pouch has never been a particularly popular operation, mainly because of the very high complication rate related to sliding of the nipple valve and resultant incontinence. Despite this, once established, patients are quite happy with this operation, which allows them to avoid a permanent ileostomy. However, it was not unexpected that both Parks et al.[11] and Utsunomiya et al.[14] simultaneously but independently developed the pelvic pouch procedure, using an S and a J pouch, respectively. With this operation there are significant complications, and it remains for us to justify its use compared with total proctocolectomy and ileostomy. One must not look at the pelvic pouch procedure in isolation, however. One must also consider the complications that can occur after a total proctocolectomy and ileostomy. Intestinal obstruction, an unhealed perineal wound, as well as numerous stomal problems can result from total proctocolectomy and ileostomy (see Chapter 17).

At issue at the present time are, in particular, the modifications being used to construct the pelvic pouch and related maneuvers. The current most popular technical modifications leave a short segment of diseased anorectal mucosa that is potentially at risk for developing carcinoma. This may or may not be justified based on improved functional results, and is discussed in more detail later in this chapter.

PREOPERATIVE CONSIDERATIONS

Indications and Contraindications

The preoperative assessment is worthy of discussion. Patients deserve a thorough explanation of the benefits and potential complications of all the options of surgery for ulcerative colitis. This must be presented to the patient in an honest and unbiased way, and the patient must participate in the final decision making. Documentation of the nature of the disease by radiologic, endoscopic, and pathologic methodology is extremely important. We do not perform this operation knowingly in patients who have Crohn's disease. The high recurrence rate as well as the higher known complication rate in patients who do have Crohn's disease would advise one to avoid this operation in this particular group of patients.[2]

The patient's anal sphincter function is of critical importance to the outcome of the procedure. The patient's age is of relative importance. We are hesitant performing this operation in patients older than 50 years, but we will assess them on an individual basis rather than by a chronologic cutoff. It is my own belief that contact with other patients and an assessment of the literature by the patient are important considerations.

In my experience patients tend to help in the decision making process. They can do this only by being knowledgeable about the operation. Therefore, I do provide them with literature to read regarding not only the pelvic pouch procedure but also other options of surgical management, and they are given an opportunity to speak with other patients who have done well in addition to those who have done poorly after each of the procedures. The majority of the patients will take this opportunity to speak with other patients. It must be added here that none of the surgical operations is perfect. When a patient inquires regarding an operation and believes this will be a panacea for all of his or her emotional problems in life, I will not perform an operation. This type of patient often has deep-rooted emotional difficulties, and should be assessed for these problems before any surgical intervention.

It is important to talk further about the contraindications to the operation. An absolute contraindication for me is Crohn's disease. I have done several operations in patients with Crohn's disease known to us only after completion of the pelvic pouch operation. Their results have been poor. Perianal sepsis, severe debility, and nutritional depletion are also contraindications to initially performing a pelvic pouch procedure. In addition, cancer of the lower part of the rectum should be removed by performing a proper cancer operation with use of oncologic principles rather than trying at all costs to save the sphincter mechanism.

The relative contraindications to the pelvic pouch procedure are emergency surgery for either toxic megacolon or acute hemorrhage, patients who have already had part of their small intestine removed, and patients who have severe incontinence. Although emergency surgery should be considered lifesaving, there may be occasions when a pelvic pouch procedure can be performed. This may apply to those patients requiring surgery for hemorrhage. This has been reported both by us and by the Mayo Clinic series patients.[3] Patients who have already had part of their small intestine removed are another group on whom I hesitate to operate because they may develop complications requiring pouch removal, resulting in a relatively short bowel with metabolic difficulties. Severe incontinence is not a definite contraindication. Patients may be incontinent because of the severity of the disease, and may become perfectly continent after the disease has been removed. One of the most difficult areas is what to do with the patient who has severe dysplasia in the lower part of the rectum. The question is whether the pelvic pouch procedure should be offered. This is also an issue that will be discussed later herein.

PATIENTS

We have now performed the pelvic pouch procedure in more than 300 patients. There are an almost equal number of male and female patients, and the age distribution reveals a mean of 32 years. The great majority have had ulcerative colitis, but 12 have had Crohn's disease known to us only after construction of the pouch. We initially performed a J pouch procedure, but later switched to an S pouch. We have reverted back to using a stapled J pouch merely because of the convenience and the ease with which it can be created. We do not believe that there is a better functional result with either the J pouch, the S pouch, the W pouch, or the H pouch if assessed 1 year after surgery. We do believe the surgeon should be familiar with the different types of pouch construction, however, because during the operation the surgeon will find that different pouches will fit more easily down to the anus so that a tension-free anal anastomosis can be performed. In our own comparative series of S and J pouches, there was no difference in the functional outcome 1 year after closure of the ileostomy.[1]

POUCH PROCEDURES

The most recent 14 procedures have been performed as single-stage pelvic pouch operations. The remainder have been equally divided between two-stage and three-stage procedures. The two-stage procedure involves doing the colectomy, the pouch, the ileoanal anastomosis, and creating a loop ileostomy. The second stage is closing the ileostomy. The three-stage procedure involves an initial colectomy, the pouch procedure as the second stage, and closing the ileostomy as the third stage. A number of our patients are now referred to us already having had a colectomy and an ileostomy. They will then usually complete their surgery with two subsequent operations.

Criticism of the S pouch has been that patients do not spontaneously evacuate the pouch. This can be overcome, however, by keeping the outlet very short. It is true that if a patient has a long outlet from an S pouch, that individual will develop an overflow type of diarrhea and will have excessive stool frequency. If the S pouch is constructed properly, however, that complication does not occur. We have had experience whereby patients have had lengthy outlets and we have been able to shorten the outlet with a subsequent abdominal and perineal approach and redo the anastomosis with a shortened outlet. This has provided a much improved functional result for the patient.

What is our current technique? In the past we left a long rectal cuff with an associated mucosal proctectomy. That was a tedious, somewhat bloody procedure. We now dissect the rectum down to the pelvic floor and transect the anorectum at that level, leaving approximately

1 to 2 cm of anorectal mucosa. This has shortened the procedure considerably, and the functional results of the long rectal cuff versus the short rectal cuff are approximately the same.[1] Patients will have at best four to five semiformed bowel movements per 24 hours.

COMPLICATIONS

As was mentioned, the complication rate after this procedure is high. Our own anal anastomotic complication rate is approximately 10%. In our early experience there were seven leaks from the pouch itself. The leak rate from the pouch has diminished and almost disappeared in our own practice, however. These pouch leaks occurred early in our series when we were constructing the pouches with use of an incorrect stapling technique. Although the anal anastomotic leak rates still approach 10%, we are now able to repair some of them. The methodology of repairing these leaks has led to a very adequate functional result in approximately 50% of those patients who initially developed an anal anastomotic leak.[4] On occasion a pouch will have to be removed because of the inability to correct the local anal situation.

Small bowel obstruction occurs in more than 10% of patients, but this is not unique to this particular operation. The most frequent complication, however, is excessive ileostomy output. One must be aware that temporarily with a loop ileostomy a significant amount of small bowel is being diverted. This is a complication and problem that is easily managed but one that should be recognized early on by the attending physician or surgeon.

Through the years we have performed approximately the same number of pelvic pouch procedures per year. We perform approximately 40 to 50 per year, which is about one per week. The number of anal anastomotic leaks has not changed considerably through the years. It is different from most series in which the learning curve shows anastomotic leak rates that do decline with time and experience. In our practice that has not happened because we have introduced more individuals gradually into our team. What has changed dramatically are the number of pouches we have excised. In the past 2 years we have learned to manage the problems of anal anastomotic leaks in order to salvage these pouches and still have a satisfactory result.

Complications after ileostomy closure are also significant. In approximately 20% of patients intestinal obstruction will develop if one includes the early postoperative period. Fifteen of the patients have required reoperation because of obstruction at the ileostomy closure site.

Anastomotic strictures have occurred in less than 10% of our total patient population. Late anal fistulas have occurred in several of our patients, and, interestingly, our patients with known Crohn's disease at initial presentation have had perianal problems as opposed to pouchitis. Pouchitis in our series has been relatively common, but it is difficult to document the exact prevalence. The variability of reporting the prevalence of pouchitis in different series is mainly due to the lack of definition of this particular clinical syndrome.

CONTROVERSIES

The most current controversial area in pelvic pouch surgery is the technical aspect. More surgeons are performing this particular operation mainly because it has now become easier, and can be done in a shorter period of time with use of a stapling technique. However, utilizing this technique and leaving potentially diseased anorectal mucosa in situ theoretically produces a very small potential risk of cancer developing in the residual mucosa.

I am concerned about the possible risk of developing cancer in residual anorectal mucosa left behind with the newer stapling procedure. At the moment a number of centers are performing the pelvic pouch procedure with the anastomosis at the anorectal junction as opposed to the dentate line.[5, 6] In effect, a pouch anal anastomosis is now being performed without a mucosectomy. The major reason for the procedure being done in this way is to try to improve the functional results that patients achieve. Most of these results are measured by total stool frequency, nighttime stool frequency, soiling, and wearing a perineal pad. The important question to ask is whether these outcome measures are that important to the patient. Certainly we have shown that within limits, a range of stool frequency is not that important a consideration to the patient provided that urgency is not present. Similarly, wearing a perineal pad does not seem to be an important outcome determinant for the patient.[10] Therefore it is extremely important to weigh what the outcome measures are that are being reported vs. what the patient's true outcome measures of this operation are.

I therefore remain skeptical that we are actually representing the patient's own important outcome measures when we are reporting the results of this procedure. The rationale that a small amount of intact mucosa will allow the patient to have better sensation and be able to achieve a better functional result is still controversial.[5-7] The initial report of Johnston et al.[6] in 1987 demonstrated that an end-to-end stapled anastomosis without a mucosectomy provided higher resting sphincter pressure profiles than in those patients who had a conventionally done mucosectomy and a hand-sewn anastomosis. It is likely that while doing the hand-sewn anastomosis the anus is on stretch for a considerable period of time, thus damaging the sphincter muscle. Johnston et al.'s[6] results showed that with the stapled group, where the mucosa was left intact, 11 of 12 patients had perfect continence, whereas in the group with the mucosectomy done in a standard way only 10 of 24 patients had perfect continence while 14 had minor soiling. Subsequent studies in other centers have not substantiated a better functional result with the stapled anastomosis as opposed to the standard hand-sewn anastomosis with a complete mucosectomy.[7] The difficult question to answer is, "Which is more important—minor soiling or the potential to develop cancer in residual anorectal mucosa?" This is an impossible question to answer at the moment until a more standardized approach to the measurement of outcome is defined. Although the risk of developing cancer in the residual anorectal mucosa that is left intact and under surveillance must be extremely low, it is still probably slightly higher than had a complete mucosectomy been performed.

In our initial experience with the stapled anastomosis without a complete mucosectomy, we have now performed 25 procedures. In the first 15 of these, 14 were done as a J pouch and 1 as an S pouch. There was one postoperative leak that healed spontaneously. Only three of our patients have had follow-up for more than 3 months after ileostomy closure. We have seen no soiling or incontinence in these three patients. These results are much too preliminary to make further comment or conclusion. We will develop a surveillance program for all of those patients who have residual anorectal mucosa left intact.

To date one cancer in a rectal cuff has been reported in the literature, and that was a recent report by our group in which, in 1984, a patient underwent construction of a J-shaped pelvic pouch leaving a long rectal cuff.[12] The indication for surgery at that time was severe dysplasia. The patient did develop cancer within the cuff. A palliative procedure was attempted, but the tumor was incompletely excised and the patient has subsequently died. To my knowledge this is the only report of cancer reported in a rectal cuff, and it most likely represented residual mucosa left behind after the mucosectomy that was incomplete in this long rectal cuff. To date no carcinomas have been reported in either a pelvic or a Kock pouch. Operations with use of a short rectal cuff would reduce the risk of leaving islands of mucosa behind. However, now the tendency is to do an operation again, leaving anorectal mucosa intentionally in order to try to improve the functional results. King et al.[8] recently reported 14 patients in whom they had consecutively removed biopsy specimens from the anal mucosa while doing a pelvic pouch procedure. In four patients there were dysplastic changes, and in one anal cancer was found. A review from St. Marks Hospital has also indicated severe dysplasia found in a very small percentage of patients' anal mucosal strippings in ulcerative colitis.[13] There were a greater number of patients who had severe dysplasia in the familial polyposis group.

This would indicate to me that in patients with severe dysplasia in the colon, and in particular in those with severe dysplasia in the rectum, a complete mucosectomy should be performed. During the next year there will be an opportunity to assess a number of patients who have had this modified pelvic pouch procedure performed, and it will be important to assess the functional results quite critically. Only if these results are considerably better should we perform this operation without doing a complete mucosectomy.

SUMMARY

Overall, the pelvic pouch procedure has advanced surgery for patients with ulcerative colitis. The operation is somewhat unpredictable, however, and carries with it a relatively high complication rate. The newer procedures, leaving a small amount of intact anorectal mucosa, have not to this date proved conclusively to me that the functional results are that much improved. In addition, we are still in a situation in which results of quality of life assessment are difficult to compare between the centers because of the lack of a standardized approach. Suffice it here to say that accurate assessment of outcome measures and modifications of the procedure need to be carefully analyzed for the benefit of both the medical profession and, in particular, for those patients undergoing this particular procedure.

REFERENCES

1. Cohen Z, McLeod RS: Proctocolectomy and ileo-anal anastomosis with a J-shaped and S-shaped ileal pouch. *World J Surg* 1988; 12:217–223.
2. Deutsch AA, Gregoire R, McLeod RS, et al: The results of the pelvic pouch procedure in patients with Crohn's disease. *Dis Colon Rectum* 1991; 34(6) 475–477.
3. Dozois RR, Kelly KA, Welling DR, et al: Ileal pouch-anal anastomosis: Com-

parison of results in familial adenomatous polyposis and chronic ulcerative colitis. *Ann Surg* 1989; 210:268–273.

4. Fleshman JW, McLeod RS, Cohen Z: Improved results following use of an advancement flap technique in the treatment of ileo-anal anastomotic complications. *Int J Color Dis* 1988; 3:161–165.

5. Heald RJ, Allen DR: Stapled ileoanal anastomosis: A technique to avoid mucosal proctectomy in the ileal pouch operation. *Br J Surg* 1986; 73:571–572.

6. Johnston D, Holdsworth PJ, Nasmyth DG, et al: Preservation of the entire anal canal in conservative proctocolectomy for ulcerative colitis: A pilot study comparing end to end ileoanal anastomosis without mucosal resection and endoanal anastomosis. *Br J Surg* 1987; 74:940–944.

7. Keighly MR, Wyshioka K, Kmiot W: Prospective randomized trial to compare the stapled double lumen pouch and the sutured quadruple pouch for restorative proctocolectomy. *Br J Surg* 1988; 75:1008–1011.

8. King DW, Lubowski DZ, Cook TA: Anal canal mucosa in restorative proctectomy for ulcerative colitis. *Br J Surg* 1989; 76:970–972.

9. Kock NG, Darle N, Hulten L, et al: Ileostomy. *Curr Probl Surg* 1977; 14:1–52.

10. McLeod RS: Quality of life in patients undergoing surgery for ulcerative colitis. *Gastroenterology* (in press).

11. Parks AG, Nicholls RJ, Belliveau P: Proctocolectomy with ileal reservoir and anal anastomosis. *Br J Surg* 1980; 67:533.

12. Stern H, Walfisch S, Mullen B, et al: Cancer in an ileoanal reservoir: A new late complication? *Gut* 1990; 31:473–475.

13. Tsunoda A, Talbot IC, Nicholls RJ: Incidence of dysplasia in the anorectal mucosa in patients having restorative proctocolectomy. *Br J Surg* 1990; 77:506–508.

14. Utsunomiya J, Invarna MD, Imajo M, et al: Total colectomy mucosal proctectomy and ileoanal anastomosis. *Dis Colon Rectum* 1980; 23:459.

Ileoanal Anastomosis With Proximal Pouch: A Gastroenterologist's Perspective

Daniel H. Present

_____

Few gastroenterologists have extensive experience with ileoanal anastomosis with proximal pouch (IAPP) procedures, and I hope this presentation will leave you with several new concepts when referring patients for this type of alternative surgery. First, let us review the indications for surgery in ulcerative colitis and try to reach some agreement as to when the colon should be removed.

1. When fulminant colitis occurs, the Oxford group[13] treats for only 5 days before sending patients to surgery, whereas we at Mount Sinai believe strongly that at least a 7- to 10-day trial of intravenous steroids should be allowed. With the use of cyclosporine, we will probably be able to salvage the colon in 75% of patients in whom 7 to 10 days treatment with intravenous steroids has failed (see Chapter 29). I would therefore conclude that fulminant colitis per se is not a firm indication for colectomy.

2. Regarding toxic megacolon, we have shown at Mount Sinai Hospital that one can dependably decompress almost all patients with toxic megacolon with a comprehensive medical regimen, and we conclude that this serious complication is also not a definite indication for surgery.[12]

3. Massive bleeding is a rare indication for colectomy, since most patients will stop bleeding after intravenous steroids are initiated.

4. Free perforation is a definite indication for surgery, and unfortunately most free perforations are caused by the gastroenterologist and the colonoscope.

(I hope at this point that you are beginning to understand the concept that "urgent surgery" is not often required in ulcerative colitis and that intense medical management should be used primarily in most of these patients.)

5. The finding of cancer is a definite indication for colectomy. The risk of cancer is cited as a prime indication for colectomy, and, although this risk is real, the statistical information varies, ranging from 5% to 40% after 20 to 30 years of disease. I personally believe that the risk is in the lower range of these statistics, and do not advocate prophylactic colectomy in these long-standing cases, except when the disease activity is persistent, is of moderate degree, and is affecting the quality of life. Regarding dysplasia, most gastroenterologists believe it is true that high-grade dysplasia does lead to cancer, and I agree that this finding is a good indication for colectomy. On the other hand, surgery for low-grade dysplasia is still controversial, and more data are required before this finding becomes a definite indication.

6. Although steroid intolerance and toxicity have been a frequent indication for surgery, with the advent of immunosuppressive drugs and other newer therapeutic agents this has become a less common indication.

7. Intractability as an indication for colectomy is in the eye of the beholder. Intractability should not be an indication for the treating gastroenterologist, but, rather, the physician should help the patient to decide as to the appropriate time to undergo surgery. "This is the patient's decision!" If the patient is having five to six bowel movements a day and has grown weary of being "tied to bathrooms," and if this is the main reason for opting for a new alternative procedure, it is the surgeon's responsibility to tell the patient that after the IAPP procedure he/she will still have five to six bowel movements a day (albeit with better control). The patient needs to be made aware that although surgery will improve the quality of life, life will not be at the desired 100% level.

Should patients have alternative surgery early or later in the course of their disease? Practice styles differ greatly throughout the country. For example, if a patient is referred to the Mayo Clinic for surgery, by a general practitioner or internist, surgery is likely to be performed early.

Contrariwise, if the patient is referred to Lenox Hill Hospital or Mount Sinai Hospital, we often try for several years to control the disease process with more intricate types of medications, such as immunosuppressive drugs. The argument for surgery by many advocates is the inevitability of colectomy. In my opinion I do not think surgery is inevitable; approximately 10% of patients in my practice require colectomy, whereas in other centers with less aggressive medical approaches surgery is carried out in 20% to 50% of patients with ulcerative colitis. What is the argument for later surgery? I believe that one very good argument is the newer therapeutic agents that are becoming available. Nonsystemic steroids (budesonide, tixocortol pivalate), which currently are being administered topically, will probably be delivered to specific sites in the bowel with use of coated oral preparations (see Chapters 30 and 31). Hydroxychloroquine is currently being studied in controlled trials in patients with ulcerative colitis, and the early data tend to indicate that this agent will be successful. Immunosuppressive drugs such as 6-mercaptopurine and azathioprine, are now being accepted as effective and safe and are salvaging many chronically active colons. Cyclosporine in preliminary studies has shown efficacy in severe active ulcerative colitis, and methotrexate has also shown efficacy in chronic ulcerative colitis in noncontrolled trials.[4, 6] Several new inflammatory inhibitors are also in the early stages of testing and have shown some efficacy. Physicians must consider all these new therapeutic modalities when referring a patient for surgery for the indication of chronicity.

Those gastroenterologists who refer few patients for operations are not quite sure where to send them for surgery. Although these procedures were initially limited to the major medical centers, they are now being performed in many institutions, and, in fact, several variations of IAPP procedures are now being utilized. The type of pouch is not the most important variable, but the learning curve of experience is a major factor in the success rate. A higher failure rate can be expected with the first 50 patients.

Surgery is said to be "curative," but the data presented by both Drs. Cohen and Sohn have shown this procedure not to be "curative" in terms of complications and functional outcome (see Chapters 17 and 18). It must be emphasized that the new ileoanal procedures require two operations. I agree with Dr. Sohn that taking a 40-year-old patient who is supporting a family and referring that patient for an IAPP procedure is not the same as referring an 18-year-old who has 1 to 2 years to "spare," if there is a significant complication, as occurs in 6% of patients. I think it is very important to listen to the patient as to his or her personal needs. Regarding functional results, I agree with Dr. Cohen that they are "good" now, with most patients having five to six controlled bowel movements a day 12 to 18 months after surgery.

Long-term follow-up in patients with IAPP surgery regarding pouchitis is uncertain, and it is very important that we continue to monitor these patients for this complication.[10, 11] I believe that one of the failures of almost all of the reported studies is the lack of involvement by the initial managing gastroenterologist in postoperative care. This occurred because it was a new operation performed at only a few centers. I believe that if these patients had been in the hands of gastroenterologists we would have discovered the increased incidence of pouchitis much sooner. I think our surgeons are very good scientists, but gastroenterologists can add to clinical management.

If you question, as I have done, a large group of patients who have undergone the operation as to their major complaints, they report that they wish they had had good data about all the functional results, the severity of complications, and the possible time missed from work. Many patients did not realize that there still would be significant dietary restrictions, as well as some athletic and exercise restrictions. I do not think there is one paper in the literature on the effect of diet in patients with the new IAPP procedure. The effect of medications is also uncertain, and 50% of the patients at the Mayo Clinic are still taking antidiarrheal agents.[10] Patients also requested, before surgery, the answer to the question, "Would you please tell me the worst possible scenario?" These patients also would have preferred more organized mutual support groups.

Recently most surgeons discount the Kock pouch as a possible alternative procedure for patients with ulcerative colitis. This interests me and is strange, since we had an excellent experience at Mount Sinai Hospital with Kock pouches.[3] A literature review shows that the overall mortality with this procedure was less than 2%. The reoperation rate is 36%, but, as in the IAPP procedure, the learning curve was steep, and in the hands of more experienced surgeons and in later series, the reoperation rate was only about 10% (similar to the Brooke ileostomy). Very few pouches have to be removed, and continence is in the 90% range. At my institution, Mount Sinai Hospital, the reoperation rate is 10%, and continence is 94%. I personally believe that the Kock pouch is a very good operation, and with years of observation has held up with very few long-term complications and no risk of cancer.

An infrequently discussed option for ulcerative colitis is the ileorectal anastomosis. A review of the Cleveland Clinic series reveals a surgical mortality of 1%, and if one compares it with the IAPP procedure, anastomotic leak occurs less frequently. Functional results are also equal to the IAPP procedure, and quality of life improves in 80% of patients.[9] What is important about the functional results is appropriate patient selection. If one selects patients with distensible rectums, this will be a much more successful operation. One can evaluate the rectal distensibility with either barium enema or with balloons. Colonoscopy tells little about rectal distensibility. In favor of this operation is that we will soon have available topical agents, such as budesonide and tixocortol pivalate, that will provide better treatment of the retained rectal segment and probably will provide improved functional results. The high long-term failure rate and subsequent resection are related to the long-term cancer risk. The risk is 10% to 20% in 25 years on literature review. With the use of surveillance biopsy for dysplasia and with flow cytometry, we may be able to pick up "precancers" earlier in those patients at greatest risk. If dysplasia is found the patient will then have the option of standard ileostomy or IAPP.

In summary, an ileorectal anastomosis is a safe procedure with a complication rate lower than or equal to the IAPP, has good functional results, and whether the long-term cancer risk is too great is primarily the patient's decision.

1. Are there age limitations to these procedures? Patients do well even if more than 50 years of age, and so there may be no age limit. I have heard of one patient in whom the procedure was performed at the age of 73.

2. What is the role of diet after surgery? I am intrigued to find that in France patients have an average of three to four bowel movements daily after the IAPP procedure compared with five to six daily in the United States. The French say that it is probably the fast food that we eat in the United States compared with a healthier diet in France. The role of diet is still not clarified.

3. Can patients with indeterminate colitis undergo this procedure? In patients with indeterminate colitis results are good in the majority of patients in most series, so that one can comfortably recommend the IAPP procedure in this subgroup.

4. Is pregnancy feasible after the IAPP procedure? Regarding pregnancy, reports from the Mayo Clinic show that pregnancy is really not a problem after alternate surgery and that most of these patients can conceive and deliver normally.[8]

5. Will the long-term functional results deteriorate? With a greater than 10-year follow-up, the long-term functional results appear to be maintained.

6. Can this alternative be performed as a one-stage procedure? It has recently been reported that a number of patients have done well with a one-stage technique with a low incidence of complications. The functional results in this series were excellent.[7]

7. Can the operation be performed in patients with Crohn's disease? I have reviewed the literature as to whether the Kock pouch is effective in patients with Crohn's disease. The complication rate reported in Kock pouches in Bloom et al.'s[1] series of patients with Crohn's disease is exactly the same as that seen in patients with ulcerative colitis. Likewise, data from several series indicate that if one performs an IAPP procedure on a patient thought to have ulcerative colitis who subsequently is found to have Crohn's disease, only 15% will lose their pouches. Therefore I suggest that the issue of whether some patients with Crohn's disease are really candidates for these alternative procedures should be rethought, especially with improved medical therapy that would be available for treatment of recurrence.

The two most important new controversies regarding the IAPP procedure are concerned with cancer risk* and recurrent pouchitis. As Cohen[2] has pointed out, the site of ileoanal anastomosis is important for future potential cancer risk. Some surgeons are performing this procedure and leaving about 4 to 5 cm of the mucosa to improve functional results. If we recall, in patients who have had ileorectal anastomosis with approximately 15 to 20 cm of the mucosa left, the risk of cancer is about 10% to 20% in 25 years. Therefore leaving any segment of rectum is potentially risky and controversial.

Pouchitis may be mild in some patients but severe and recurrent in others. The prevalence ranges from 6% to 27%, and, if one reviews the Mayo Clinic data, the prevalence is increasing with more years of observation.[10] The diagnosis is made on the basis of watery stools, passage of blood, increased frequency, and abdominal cramps. Diagnosis requires endoscopic confirmation. We are not routinely performing endoscopy in patients "without" symptoms, however, and if one looks at some series in which this is done there is almost always some pouch inflammation.

What is the cause of pouchitis? Various associations have been made by surgical investigators, such as noting that it is more common in patients with extensive colitis, or in those who have had backwash

---

*Editor's Note: This would be controversial. There is still a question as to whether an ileoanal pouch anastomosis is appropriate when dysplasia has been demonstrated in the intact colon, before any resection.

ileitis, or in those who have had extraintestinal manifestations. It has also been attributed to bacterial overgrowth, the type of reservoir, and ischemia. It is conceivable that this is a brand new disease, "ulcerative colitis of the ileum," since the entity is rarely seen in patients with familial polyposis who have had an IAPP procedure.

I would therefore like to pose a simple question. Since long-standing inflammation is associated with cancer in patients with ulcerative colitis, will recurrent pouchitis with chronic inflammation lead to cancer of the pouch in these patients? Thus far this has not occurred in Kock pouches, but if surgeons do leave 3 to 4 cm of rectal mucosa, will this technique plus pouchitis produce a high prevalence of cancer with long-term follow-up[5]? Thus far, cancer has developed in one patient with an IAPP procedure and in several patients dysplasia has been found in biopsy specimens.[2]

We must therefore not conclude that we have "cured" patients with ulcerative colitis by performing an IAPP procedure, and, despite significantly improving the quality of their lives, we must still continue to observe these patients closely for potential long-term complications.

REFERENCES

1. Bloom RJ, Larsen CP, Watt R, et al: A reappraisal of the Kock continent ileostomy in patients with Crohn's disease. *Surg Gynecol Obstet* 1986; 162:105–108.
2. Cohen Z: Surgery in inflammatory bowel disease. *Curr Opin Gastroenterol* 1989; 5:514–519.
3. Gelernt IM, Bauer JJ, Krell I: The continent ilostomy. *Pract Gastroenterol* 1977; 1:47–51.
4. Kozarek RA, Patterson DJ, Gelfand MD, et al: Methotrexate induces clinical and histologic remission in patients with refractory inflammatory bowel disease. *Ann Intern Med* 1989; 110:353–356.
5. Lavery IC, Tuckson WB, Easley KA: Internal anal sphincter function after total abdominal colectomy and stapled ileal pouch-anal anastomosis without mucosal proctectomy. *Dis Colon Rectum* 1989; 32:950–953.
6. Lichtiger S, Present DH: Preliminary report: Cyclosporine in treatment of severe active ulcerative colitis. *Lancet* 1990; 336:16–19.
7. Matikainen M, Santavirta J, Hituner KM: Ileoanal anastomosis without covering ileostomy. *Dis Colon Rectum* 1990; 33:384–388.
8. Nelson H, Dozois RR, Kelly KA: The effect of pregnancy and delivery on the ileal pouch-anal anastomosis functions. *Dis Colon Rectum* 1989; 31:384–388.
9. Oakley JR, Jagelman DG, Fazio VW: Complications and quality of life after ileorectal anastomosis for ulcerative colitis. *Am J Surg* 1985; 149:23–29.

10. Pemberton JH, Kelly KA, Beart RW: Ileal pouch anal anastomosis for chronic ulcerative colitis—long term results. *Ann Surg* 1987; 206:504–513.
11. Phillips RKS, Ritchie JK, Hawley PR: Proctocolectomy and ileostomy for ulcerative colitis. A long term study. *J R Soc Med* 1989; 82:386–387.
12. Present DH, Wolfson D, Gelernt IM, et al: Medical decompression of toxic megacolon by "rolling." *J Clin Gastroenterol* 1988; 10:485–490.
13. Truelove SC, Jewell DP: Intensive intravenous regimen for severe attacks of ulcerative colitis. *Lancet* 1974; 1:1067–1070.

Discussion

Dr. Sohn: A comment on Dr. Heller's paper*—he spoke here a few months ago and he is able to get the rectum calmed down with the new topical agents. Most of the patients with colitis that we operate on, except if it is for dysplasia or cancer, have severe rectal disease. I doubt it would ever be calmed down with anything. I am not sure this population Dr. Heller operates on is the same population that we operate on. They still have a high risk of cancer. We did not have any cancer, but everyone else reports it.

Dr. Cohen: I think it depends on when you start treating these patients and how aggressively, and he feels the budesonide is much more effective. Most of my patients have active rectal disease, but it is not that terribly severe. You can control the disease if you use continuous 5-ASA agents. I frankly use 5-ASA in combination with hydrocortisone enemas. I use them together, and it may be with the new agents it will be better. The issue is distensibility of the rectum, whether you can ever use it again.

Dr. Sohn: If the rectum is well controlled by any means, I doubt that patient will be referred to me for a colectomy.

Q: (1) Why is the cancer risk so much higher in the small bit of mucosa retained in the pouch operation? (2) Did you determine, in the patients who underwent pouch operations and were subsequently found to have Crohn's disease, they did in fact have Crohn's disease on the basis of review of collective symptoms, or did you determine they had Crohn's disease by self-definition rather than nature of problems as they develop?

Dr. Cohen: Question 2 first. Of the 12 patients, 6 of them had the procedures done in 3 stages—at colectomy, and at review of the colectomy specimen the ulcerative colitis was found. At the time of creation of the pouch when we did the proctectomy on the rectal segment, it was

*Dr. Göran Heller from Stockholm.

called Crohn's disease. That may go along with what we were talking about, getting a better and more accurate diagnosis from rectal biopsy than from colonic biopsy. I do not really know, but that is the way it occurred in over half of them. The others were the manifestations of severe perianal disease later on, after the pouch had been present for up to 2 years. Some of them require pouch removal, and we are finding granulomas.

Q: What did a review of the colectomy specimens reveal?

A: Exactly the same—the colectomy specimens on review were all called ulcerative colitis.

Dr. Sohn: Do you think it could be any other entity or a Crohn's-like disease?

Dr. Cohen: I would think we are creating a new situation here, perhaps creating some stasis in terms of emptying with these procedures. We do have pouchitis now at the site of inflammation. I think it is a different entity than just having the rectum intact. We did not answer the first question regarding the cancer risk in retained rectal mucosa. I do not think we can answer it yet. I do not mean to overplay the risk of cancer in the small segment. I am not saying it is excessive; we do not know about it, but it certainly is more than exists when leaving nothing at all.

Dr. Korelitz: What we are ignoring is the fact that dysplasia tends to be multifocal. Therefore, when it is found in the rectal segment should we really consider doing an ileoanal pouch at all?

Dr. Cohen: I thought I had put that into perspective by saying that is a relative contraindication to me, dysplasia in the rectum, of doing the pouch procedure. What I said later on was that we have to look not necessarily at this operation where we are leaving mucosa to see if the functional result is not only better but also if what is being measured is what is actually important to the patient. I agree if there is a patient with dysplasia in the lower rectum that I do not think that patient should have a pelvic pouch procedure.

Dr. Korelitz: It should be noted that today with many of the former indications for colectomy falling by the wayside, dysplasia is a frequent indication for colectomy.

Dr. Cohen: I agree with you, but then if a patient has severe dysplasia in the lower rectum, I would say that patient should not have a pelvic pouch procedure. If the patient has dysplasia in the colon, I would say he should not have an operation whereby you leave him at potentially increased risk of developing cancer in the remaining mucosa. Therefore that patient should have a conventional mucosectomy—what we would consider a curative procedure. Now in the only case reported—I know there are others of cancer in the pelvic pouch procedure but ours is the only case that had been reported—that was for the indication of severe dysplasia. It was in a patient with a long rectal cuff where it was difficult to do the mucosectomy. So that patient did develop cancer, and what I am saying is that in that situation in 1990 that particular patient should not have that operation.

PART 5

Surveillance in Ulcerative Colitis and Crohn's Colitis

Mucosal Dysplasia in Inflammatory Bowel Disease

Gregory Lauwers

An increased risk of colorectal cancer is unequivocal in ulcerative colitis and has also been reported in Crohn's colitis[11, 18] (Table 20–1). Dysplasia, a premalignant neoplastic change, has been demonstrated in the colonic epithelium in both ulcerative colitis[29, 36] and Crohn's colitis[8, 22] (see Chapters 22 and 23).

Screening programs of selected patients have been based on the recognition of premalignant changes in the colonic epithelium.[25] The diagnostic features and significance of dysplasia in biopsy material have been the subject of much debate. Nonetheless, clinical guidelines have been developed according to the degree of mucosal dysplasia.[31]

HISTORICAL BACKGROUND

In 1925 Crohn and Rosenberg[7] reported the first case of rectal adenocarcinoma complicating a case of ulcerative colitis. In 1948 Warren and Sommers[34] described the first case of colonic adenocarcinoma arising in association with Crohn's colitis.[34] Since that time several reports have confirmed that inflammatory bowel disease (IBD) exposes the patient to a higher risk of developing colonic adenocarcinomas.[19, 23, 24] In extensive colitis, cumulative risks of 7.2% and 16.5% at 20 and 30 years, respectively, have been reported.[20] Two factors influence the development of colonic adenocarcinoma[23, 24]: (1) the duration of the disease with low risk for less than 10 years and progressively increased risk thereafter; (2) extensive disease with higher risk for pancoliltis than for

TABLE 20–1.
Features of Colorectal Cancer in IBD*

	Ulcerative Colitis	Crohn's Colitis
Age at cancer (mean	49	56
cancer incidence O/E)†	7–29×	4–20×
Multiple cancers (%)	8–43	11
High risk after disease	8–10	15–20
duration (yr)		
Occurrence at site of	Yes (95%)	Usually (66%)
overt disease		
Excluded bowel at risk‡	Yes	Yes
Dysplasia-associated	Yes	Yes

*Modified from Rosenstock E, Farmer RG, Petras R, et al: *Gastroenterology* 1985; 89:1342–1346.
†Observed/expected ratio.
‡Excluded rectal stump in ulcerative colitis; excluded colon in Crohn's colitis.

left-sided colitis.[23, 24] In the past prophylactic colectomy and procto-colectomy were advised, based on these two assertions.[9] This radical attitude was altered by two observations. First, most of the patients with IBD (more than 80%) do not develop colorectal cancer.[16] Second, in 1967 Morson and Pang[29] showed that precancerous epithelial lesions were associated with colonic adenocarcinoma in patients with IBD. They were the first to indicate that these mucosal alterations could be used as a marker of patients entering a precancerous phase. Since then retrospective analysis of colons of patients with ulcerative colitis resected for adenocarcinoma were shown to reveal dysplastic changes in the mucosa adjacent to or distant from the tumor.[36]

Conversely, colons removed for dysplasia have been shown to harbor adenocarcinomas.[32] It has also been demonstrated that dysplasia is often widespread in flat mucosa and detectable on rectal biopsy.[29] Thereafter sigmoidoscopy and rectal biopsy were recommended in the follow-up of patients at risk, and the finding of dysplasia was an indication for prophylactic surgery.[16] This schema was later modified by several studies, suggesting that in about 30% of cancer cases in ulcerative colitis no associated dysplasia was present. In addition, in 27% of colectomies performed for dysplasia, no cancer was present.[30]

It thus appeared that because dysplasia is not always associated with carcinoma, its diagnosis should be used as an aid to the management of patients with IBD, but not as an indication for radical surgical intervention. Although these results show some contraindications, it is presently widely accepted that epithelial dysplasia is the earliest morphologic evidence of neoplastic transformation and the precursor of malignancy in the colonic mucosa.[31]

DIAGNOSIS OF MUCOSAL DYSPLASIA

Mucosal dysplasia has been accepted as an unequivocal neoplastic alteration of the colonic epithelium.[31] Early studies failed to present a standardized classification of dysplasia. This was achieved in 1983, by Riddell and other pathologists,[31] forming the IBD-Dysplasia Study Group under the auspices of the National Foundation for Ileitis and Colitis (NFIC).

As a result of their effort, dysplasia is now recognized by well-defined cytologic and architectural criteria.

Histopathologic Diagnosis

The cytologic abnormalities recognized are cellular and nuclear pleomorphism, nuclear hyperchromasia, loss of nuclear polarity, and marked stratification of nuclei. Architectural alterations, exceeding those resulting from repair, are also considered to represent dysplastic changes. The classification presented by Riddel et al., and still widely in use, shows three diagnostic categories[31]:

1. Negative for dysplasia
2. Indefinite for dysplasia
   a. Probably negative
   b. Unknown
   c. Probably positive
3. Positive for dysplasia
   a. Low grade
   b. High grade

Negative for Dysplasia

Biopsies of the colon do not show preneoplastic epithelial lesions. Instead they may show either inactive colonic epithelium or active colitis with crypt abscesses, cryptitis, and inflamed lamina propria (Fig 20–1).

All epithelial changes seen within the crypts involved by acute active inflammation are identified as reactive changes.

Indefinite for Dysplasia

There is probably no rationale to establish such a subgroup, but it is rather the expression of the inherent difficulty the pathologist may encounter in determining which changes are reactive as opposed to neoplastic (Fig 20–2). The subcategorization into probably negative, unknown, and probably positive appears extremely subjective and

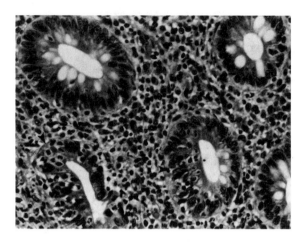

FIG 20–1.
Active colitis. There is an increased amount of acute and chronic inflammatory cells within the lamina propria. Cryptitis is also present, with acute inflammatory cells within the glandular epithelium *(arrowheads)*. (Hematoxylin-phloxin-saffron stain; original magnification ×250.)

unreproducible, with wide variations in the diagnosis by different pathologists.[27]

Positive for Dysplasia

The diagnosis made according to the criteria described is relatively easy, once the changes due to repair and reaction have been discounted.

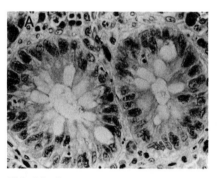
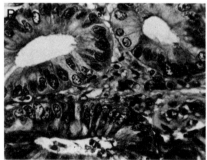

FIG 20–2.
Low-grade dysplasia **(A)** vs. repair **(B)**. In **(A)**, the nuclei have irregular contours and are somewhat hyperchromatic nuclei with chromatin clumping. In **(B)**, the oval-shaped, vesicular nuclei with conspicuous small nucleoli are typical of regenerative changes. (Hematoxylin-phloxin-saffron stain; original magnification ×400.)

In low-grade dysplasia the cytologic and architectural criteria may not all be present. Crypts are lined by columnar cells with moderately enlarged and hyperchromatic nuclei. Nuclear crowding is present. Minimal stratification is seen, but the nuclei are confined to the basal half of the cells. Some mucus differentiation can be seen (Fig 20–3).

In high-grade dysplasia, all the criteria are met. Nuclear changes with prominent hyperchromasia, pleomorphism, and loss of polarity are more pronounced. Nuclear crowding is obvious, and nuclear stratification is marked with atypical nuclei extending into the upper half of the cells. Mucus differentiation may be absent (Fig 20–4).

Architectural alterations may also be the reflection of dysplasia. This is true when the changes exceeding repair exhibit villous or tubuloadenomatous patterns[31] (Fig 20–5).

Dysplasia Associated With a Lesion or Mass

Most frequently dysplasia arises in flat mucosa. Nonetheless, dysplasia has been found associated with a macroscopic lesion detected during colonoscopic examination. Different types of lesions have been

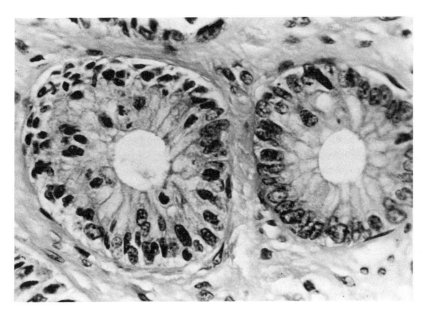

FIG 20–3.
Mucosa positive for low-grade dysplasia. The enlarged nuclei still remain in the lower half of the cells (minimal stratification). Nuclear hyperchromasia is present, as well as chromatin clumping. (Hematoxylin-phloxin-saffron stain; original magnification ×400.)

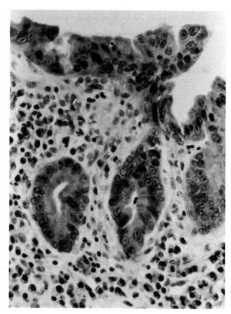

FIG 20–4.
Mucosa positive for high-grade dysplasia. The nuclei are enlarged, with prominent nucleoli. Stratification, overlapping, and loss of polarity of the nuclei are present. Note that the changes are more striking on the surface epithelium. (Hematoxylin-eosin stain; original magnification ×250.)

described: either a simple polypoid mass, or plaquelike lesions, or multiple polyps.[3] Biopsies of these lesions display low- or high-grade dysplasia or no dysplasia at all (Fig 20–6).

Several publications[3, 32] demonstrated that patients with dysplasia associated with a lesion or mass (DALM) are likely to have a colon cancer already present but still undetected. Blackstone et al.[3] saw 7 carcinomas in 12 patients with DALM but only one among 27 patients with flat dysplasia. Although the association was more frequent with a single polypoid mass, adenocarcinoma was also found in a patient whose presenting symptom was a plaquelike lesion or multiple polyps. It is also important to mention that low-grade and high-grade DALM are seen in association with colonic cancer.[3, 32] Therefore the indication for surgery is widely accepted even with low-grade dysplasia revealed at biopsy when a macroscopic lesion is present.[3, 32]

Reliability of the Diagnosis of Mucosal Dysplasia

This classification has the merit of offering a uniform terminology for colonic mucosal dysplasia. As such it has been possible to compare

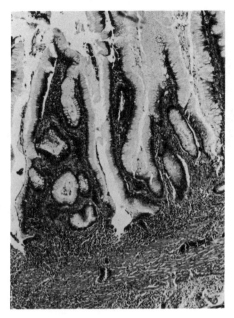

FIG 20–5.
Mucosa positive for low-grade dysplasia, showing a prominent villous pattern. The architectural features, exceeding those of repair, are more convincing than the bland cytology. (Hematoxylin-eosin stain; original magnification ×100.)

series and to facilitate communication between pathologists and gastroenterologists. Based on the clinical value of the classification, Riddell et al.[31] issued guidelines for the management of patients (Table 20–2). Still, practicing pathologists may have some difficulties using this classification.

It must be emphasized that the recognition of dysplasia is somewhat subjective. It is relatively easy to recognize high-grade dysplasia, but it may be extremely difficult to separate reactive or regenerative cytologic atypia (due to inflammation) from indefinite and low-grade dysplasia. Nevertheless, the IBD Dysplasia Study Group concluded that the classification is consistent and reproducible, and accordingly they presented a high percentage of agreement between observers. This applied mostly to the diagnosis of high-grade dysplasia and to that of no dysplasia.[31]

Other retrospective studies acknowledged the high degree of reproducibility of the classification, with agreement ranging from 66% to 83%[12] and even reaching as much as 96%.[32] More recent works claim much poorer agreement between pathologists. However, Dixon et al.[10]

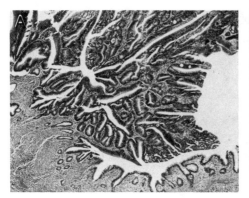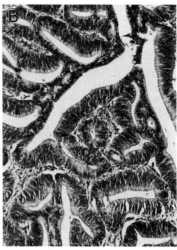

FIG 20–6.
DALM, low grade; colonoscopic surveillance detected a polypoid mass. This sessile, ade-nomatous-like lesion was found in the resected colon. Cytologic features are consistent with low-grade dysplasia. (Hematoxylin-eosin stain; original magnification ×100–×250.) **A,** low power; **B,** high power.

found an agreement rate of 49% to 72%, obtaining more acceptable rates of 68% to 84% when only the diagnosis of either "dysplasia" or "no dysplasia" was offered. More recently Melville et al.[27] showed compara-ble results, with poor agreement between pairs of pathologists ranging from 42% to 65%, but again better reproducibility when only the diag-nosis of "no dysplasia" was considered.

TABLE 20–2.
Clinical Guidelines for Classification of Dysplasia*

Biopsy Findings	Management

Negative
  Indefinite
  Probably negative
Indefinite, unknown and probably
  positive
	Usual surveillance

Positive	
Low grade	{ Short follow-up (3–6 mo), followed by repeat biopsy { Short-term follow-up (3 mo)
High grade	{ Consider resection if macroscopic lesion { Consider colectomy after confirmation of dysplasia

*From Riddell RH, et al: *Hum Pathol* 1983; 14:931–966. Used by permission.

Such variations may bring some concern as to the ability of the pathologists to diagnose dysplasia accurately in patients with IBD. Nonetheless, it should be remembered that all these results are from retrospective studies. In actual practice the pathologists can review the previous material and the clinical information (i.e., the presence of a grossly identifiable lesion would increase the suspicion). Finally, we think that a second opinion by a pathologist familiar with these problems should be recommended when the diagnosis has radical therapeutic implications.

Alternative Methods

Epithelial Mucus Alterations

Biochemical alteration in cell membrane glycoconjugate and epithelial mucin in colonic pathology has been long recognized. In 1969 Filipe[15] showed that the colonic mucosa adjacent to an adenocarcinoma has a reduction or even absence of sulfomucin and a predominance of sialomucin. Later Ehsanullah et al.[13] showed similar modifications in ulcerative colitis, with significant alteration of sialomucin associated with cancer and dysplasia in ulcerative colitis. They also suggested that staining of mucosa may increase the accuracy in the interpretation of epithelial atypia or dysplasia.

Some authors contested this conclusion, arguing that similar alterations were seen in active and inactive chronic ulcerative colitis.[2] Nonetheless, others[14] suggest that patients with sialomucin-predominant mucus in active or inactive ulcerative colitis and without dysplasia were still at higher risks of developing later dysplasia and carcinoma. Allen et al.[1] advocated the use of different staining techniques to enhance the specificity of mucus-secreting alteration.

More recently the use of lectin, a natural glycoprotein binding to specific carbohydrates, has been developed. According to some authors alterations of lectin binding may precede histologic dysplasia, allowing earlier detection of patients at risk.[4] Yet others disagree, demonstrating a strong correlation between lectin binding and severe inflammation.[2] Therefore it appears that the biochemical alteration of mucus can be used only as an adjunct to the histologic and flow cytometric assessment of colonic epithelium.

Flow Cytometry

In 1984 Hammarberg et al.[21] performed DNA analysis in ulcerative colitis with use of flow cytometry. They advocated this technique as a possible adjunct in the surveillance of patients with ulcerative colitis.

Nonetheless, if an additional study[28] indicated aneuploidy to be a specific marker of neoplastic change, others showed that the occurrence of DNA aneuploidy is related to the duration of disease.[17]

Surprisingly, although DNA aneuploidy was shown to correlate with dysplasia and carcinoma, it was seen in only 48% of the dysplasias and in 78% of the carcinomas.[26] Conversely, a high rate of DNA aneuploidy was observed in histologic sections of mucosa showing negative findings with or without inflammation and reactive hyperplasia.[28] Interestingly, Fozard et al.[17] found that less than one-third of carcinomas in ulcerative colitis are aneuploid, compared with about 60% in sporadic colon cancer in the general population. Although these contradictory results limit the practical value of flow cytometry, it is nonetheless widely accepted that the determination of the DNA status of the colonic mucosa is a useful adjunct in the assessment of dysplasia and in the surveillance of precancerous conditions in IBD.[28]

Cytogenetics

Well-documented studies have shown the constant existence of genetic alterations that play a role in the development of colonic adenocarcinoma.[33] These changes consist mostly of alterations of chromosomes 5, 17, and 18 and of mutations of the *ras* and *c-myc* genes. In 1974 Xavier et al.[35] pointed out cytogenetic alterations in inflamed and dysplastic mucosa of patients with chronic ulcerative colitis.

More recently investigators have attempted to detect oncogenic alterations in ulcerative colitis with dysplasia. Ciclitira et al.,[6] with use of monoclonal antibodies, showed that the *c-myc* protein product, although it may be expressed in the nuclei of dysplastic cells in ulcerative colitis, was also present in cases of severe inflammation without dysplasia, failing therefore to segregate dysplastic changes and regenerative atypia. In addition, the *ras* mutation found in the usual colonic adenocarcinoma was not recognized in the ulcerative colitis–associated colonic adenocarcinoma.[5] As it appears, most of the information gathered on the genetic alterations found in sporadic colonic adenocarcinoma does not apply to carcinoma in patients with ulcerative colitis, suggesting that the development of cancer in IBD may involve some unexplored pathway.

CONCLUSION

The search for an ideal marker of the patients with IBD entering a precancerous phase is still in progress. The recognition and histopathologic characterization of mucosal dysplasia have been the first step.

Nonetheless, epithelial dysplasia is far from being the ideal marker, essentially because of the subjectivity involved in its diagnosis. New techniques (i.e., lectin binding, flow cytometry, and cytogenetics), although not yet perfected, will undoubtedly be major tools for the assessment of patients with IBD in the future. For the present, regular colonoscopic surveillance, with biopsies and their histopathologic interpretation, is the safest way to follow patients with IBD at risk of developing colonic cancer.

REFERENCES

1. Allen DC, Connolly NS, Biggart JD: Mucin profiles in ulcerative colitis with dysplasia and carcinoma. *Histopathology* 1988; 13:413–424.
2. Ahnen DJ, et al: Search for a specific marker of mucosal dysplasia in chronic ulcerative colitis. *Gastroenterology* 1987; 93:1346–1355.
3. Blackstone MO, et al: Dysplasia-associated lesion or mass (DALM) detected by colonoscopy in long-standing ulcerative colitis: An indication for colectomy. *Gastroenterology* 1981; 80:366–374.
4. Boland CR, et al: Abnormal goblet cell glycoconjugates in rectal biopsies associated with an increased risk of neoplasia in patients with ulcerative colitis: Early results of a prospective study. *Gut* 1984; 25:1364–1371.
5. Burmer GC, et al: C-Ki-ras mutations in chronic ulcerative and sporadic colon carcinoma. *Gastroenterology* 1990; 99:416–420.
6. Ciclitira PJ, Macartney JC, Evan G: Expression of C-Myc in nonmalignant and premalignant gastrointestinal disorders. *J Pathol* 1987; 151:293–296.
7. Crohn BB, Rosenberg H: The sigmoidoscopic picture of chronic ulcerative colitis (nonspecific). *Am J Med Sci* 1925; 170:220–227.
8. Craft CF, et al: Colonic "precancer" in Crohn's disease. *Gastroenterology* 1981; 80:578–584.
9. deDombal FT, et al: Local complications of ulcerative colitis: Stricture, pseudopolyposis, and carcinoma of colon and rectum. *Br Med J* 1966; 2:1442–1447.
10. Dixon MF, et al: Observer variation in the assessment of dysplasia in ulcerative colitis. *Histopathology* 1988; 13:385–397.
11. Dobbins WO: Dysplasia and malignancy in inflammatory bowel disease. *Annu Rev Med* 1984; 35:33–48.
12. Dundas SAC, et al: Can histopathologists reliably assess dysplasia in chronic inflammatory bowel disease? *J Clin Pathol* 1987; 40:1282–1286.
13. Ehsanullah M, Filipe MI, Gazzard B: Mucin secretion in inflammatory bowel disease: Correlation with disease activity and dysplasia. *Gut* 1982; 23:485–489.
14. Ehsanullah M, et al: Sialomucins in the assessment of dysplasia and cancer-risk patients with ulcerative colitis treated with colectomy and ileo-rectal anastomosis. *Histopathology* 1985; 9:223–235.
15. Filipe MI: Value of histochemical reactions for mucosubstances in the diag-

nosis of certain pathological conditions of the colon and rectum. *Gut* 1969; 10:577–586.

16. Fozard JBJ, Dixon MF: Colonoscopic surveillance in ulcerative colitis dysplasia through the looking glass. *Gut* 1989; 30:285–292.
17. Fozard JBJ, et al: DNA aneuploidy in ulcerative colitis. *Gut* 1986; 27:1414–1418.
18. Greenstein AJ, Sachar DD: Inflammatory bowel disease and colorectal cancer, in Seitz HK, Simanowski UA, Wright NA (eds): *Colorectal Cancer: From Pathogenesis to Prevention.* Berlin, Springer, 1989.
19. Gyde SN, et al: Malignancy in Crohn's disease. *Gut* 1980; 21:1024–1029.
20. Gyde SN, et al: Colorectal cancers in ulcerative colitis: A cohort study of primary referrals from three centers. *Gut* 1988; 29:206–217.
21. Hammarberg C, Slezak P, Tribukait B: Early detection of malignancy in ulcerative colitis. *Cancer* 1984; 9:291–295.
22. Korelitz BI, Lauwers GY, Sommers SC: Rectal mucosal dysplasia in Crohn's disease. *Gut* 1990; 31:1382–1386.
23. Lennard-Jones JE, et al: Cancer in colitis: Assessment of the individual risk by clinical and histological criteria. *Gastroenterology* 1977; 73:1280–1289.
24. Lennard-Jones JE, et al: Cancer surveillance in ulcerative colitis. *Lancet* 1983; 2:149–152.
25. Lennard-Jones JE, et al: Precancer and cancer in extensive ulcerative colitis: Findings among 401 patients over 22 years. *Gut* 1990; 31:800–806.
26. Melville DM, et al: Dysplasia and deoxyribonucleic acid aneuploidy in the assessment of precancerous changes in chronic ulcerative colitis. Observer variation and correlation. *Gastroenterology* 1988; 95:668–675.
27. Melville DM, et al: Observer study of the grading of dysplasia in ulcerative colitis: Comparison with clinical outcome. *Hum Pathol* 1989; 20:1009–1014.
28. Melville DM, et al: DNA aneuploidy in ulcerative colitis. *Gut* 1987; 28:643.
29. Morson BC, Pang LS: Rectal biopsy as an aid to cancer control in ulcerative colitis. *Gut* 1967; 8:423–434.
30. Ransohoff DF, Riddell RH, Levin B: Ulcerative colitis and colonic cancer. Problems in assessing the diagnostic usefulness of mucosal dysplasia. *Dis Colon Rectum* 1985; 26:383–388.
31. Riddell RH, et al: Dysplasia in inflammatory bowel disease: Standardized classification with provisional clinical applications. *Hum Pathol* 1983; 14:931–966.
32. Rosenstock E, Farmer RG, Petras R, et al: Surveillance for colonic carcinoma in ulcerative colitis. *Gastroenterology* 1985; 89:1342–1346.
33. Vogelstein B, et al: Genetic alterations during colorectal tumor development. *N Engl J Med* 1988; 319:525–532.
34. Warren S, Sommers SC: Cicatrizing enteritis (regional enteritis) as a pathologic entity: Analysis of one hundred twenty cases. *Am J Pathol* 1948; 24:475–501.
35. Xavier RG, et al: Tissue cytogenetics studies in chronic ulcerative colitis and carcinoma of the colon. *Cancer* 1974; 34:684–695.
36. Yardley JH, Keren DF: "Precancer" lesions in ulcerative colitis. *Cancer* 1974; 34:835–844.

Chapter 21 _____

Experience With Surveillance in Ulcerative Colitis

Audrey Woolrich

In patients with long-standing ulcerative colitis, the risk of developing carcinoma of the colon or rectum is greater than in the general population. As with any surveillance program, the ideal purpose is to identify those individuals who are at the greatest risk of developing carcinoma or to discover those with a malignancy at its earliest stage, so as to favorably influence the prognosis.[3] Dysplasia is a premalignant marker for carcinoma. When present it can be classified as low or high grade as outlined by the Dysplasia Study Group[5] (see Chapter 20).

Finding high-grade dysplasia has been accepted as predictive of carcinoma, but until recently the significance of low-grade dysplasia has generally remained unclear.[6] The prevalence of dysplasia and carcinoma increases with disease duration, starting approximately 7 years after the onset of ulcerative colitis. Extent of involvement is also a factor, being greater in patients with universal disease than in those with left-sided colitis or proctitis.

Colonoscopy allows the clinician to visualize the mucosal surface of the colon grossly. Some macroscopic lesions can be removed, and biopsy specimens can be taken of others. Biopsy specimens can be taken from areas suspicious for dysplasia or neoplasia, such as elevations, erythematous, indurated sites or pseudopolyps containing variants in hue and texture. Not all clinicians and pathologists examining patients for inflammatory bowel disease agree on the ideal surveillance program for ulcerative colitis, but the consensus appears to be that patients with left-sided or universal involvement should have an annual colonoscopy with screening biopsies beginning 7 years from the onset of disease (see

Chapters 13 and 20). Two to four surveillance biopsy specimens are generally taken from each 10 to 15 cm area of colon from cecum to rectum as the colonoscope is withdrawn. If there is no evidence of disease activity, the biopsy specimens are taken randomly from flat mucosa.

Ideally the surveillance examination should be performed during a period of disease inactivity. Dysplasia can be identified in the presence of ulcerative colitis activity, however, even though inflammation presents an obstacle to its interpretation.[1] In practice, a patient may undergo a surveillance colonoscopy at a time when there are no bowel symptoms but endoscopically there is disease activity; nevertheless, surveillance biopsy specimens should be obtained.

If there is no dysplasia or neoplasia discovered on a surveillance colonoscopy, the patient is told to return in 1 year. This will vary with extent, duration, and clinical activity of disease. Compliance can be a problem, especially if the patient is in a period of disease remission. The cost and inconvenience of yearly colonoscopy can be a deterrent to a successful surveillance program, but it must be emphasized to the patient that the possible alternative of developing colorectal cancer is more costly.

If dysplasia is found, the patient should return for repeat examination. When the dysplasia is low grade it has been our practice to repeat the examination with additional biopsies in 3 months; but when it is high grade, low grade in multiple sites, or associated with a mass lesion, the reexamination should be immediate. Only when the subsequent biopsy findings are normal at least twice can the interval be extended to 6 months, and thereafter to 1 year, with interim sigmoidoscopy and biopsies.

Unfortunately the process of obtaining surveillance biopsy specimens is not a scientific or even reproducible practice. Because of the large surface area of the colon there is a large degree of sampling error. What appears grossly normal to the endoscopist at a site where tissue is removed during a surveillance colonoscopy may indeed be adjacent to an area of dysplasia. The endoscopist is sampling only a fraction of mucosal surface at risk. This situation must be addressed when one is interpreting subsequent biopsy material that may or may not be from the site of previous dysplasia. It has been proposed that both low-grade and high-grade dysplasia may regress. This phenomenon may be explained in part by sampling error, however.[4] Another disconcerting aspect of surveillance colonoscopy is that, despite annual examinations, carcinoma can be encountered without finding previous dysplasia. If the carcinoma occurs without previous dysplasia, however, more often than not, when the surgical specimen is reviewed, there are sites of dysplasia in the resected colon. These are just a few problems with the present method of surveillance.

A recent review of the experience of Dr. Burton I. Korelitz in his large inflammatory bowel disease practice in New York City (Woolrich et al.[8]) supports the importance of a surveillance program. During a 10-year period from 1977 to 1987, colonoscopic biopsy specimens were obtained from 121 patients who had ulcerative colitis for 7 or more years and who had at least one prior colonoscopy. Four hundred fifty-eight colonoscopies were performed. In 50% the purpose of the colonoscopy was surveillance alone. If the primary goal of the examination was for determination of extent or severity of disease, biopsy specimens were still obtained for surveillance; this accounts for the other 50%. Of the 121 patients, 27 (22.3%) were found to have dysplasia or neoplasia. Low-grade dysplasia was encountered in 22 patients (18%). Twenty of the patients with dysplasia, along with two patients in whom colonoscopy revealed a true polyp, went on to have a total of 99 subsequent surveillance colonoscopies, with a mean of four, at varying intervals. Three of the 121 patients had carcinoma without previously reported dysplasia. These patients underwent surgery, and their resected specimens all contained dysplasia as well as the carcinoma. The dysplasia or neoplasia was found during the first reviewed colonoscopy after 7 years of colitis in 12 of the 27 patients, with the mean duration of disease being 16 years. Dysplasia in this study served as an indicator of future carcinoma in 18%.

Patients in this study were requested to return for repeat examination when the dysplasia was encountered, but they did not necessarily comply. Usually they returned within 3 months, but some did not return until they needed to be seen for active disease or were motivated by educational programs such as those of the National Foundation for Ileitis and Colitis.*

Of the 22 patients undergoing subsequent examinations, in only 7 was dysplasia or neoplasia revealed in the second set of biopsies. During the next 1 to 66 months they underwent one to four examinations, and the presence and degree of dysplasia changed in most cases. An example of sampling error vs. dysplasia regression was demonstrated in one patient, who initially had low-grade dysplasia and then high-grade dysplasia followed by a biopsy of low grade, and then two sets of biopsies showing negative findings; slides of the resected colon, removed because of resistant disease and the previous finding of dysplasia, con-

*Editor's Note: This Foundation is now known as the Crohn's and Colitis Foundation of America (CCFA).

tained multiple sites of low-grade dysplasia. Another patient in whom low-grade dysplasia was found initially returned after 2 years, not for surveillance, but with an obstructing rectosigmoid carcinoma, and the colectomy specimen also contained low-grade dysplasia.

In 15 patients with surveillance biopsies showing dysplasia, the subsequent biopsies did not reveal dysplasia or neoplasia, but after two to ten examinations in four patients, low-grade dysplasia was found once again. Two of these patients were later found to have adenocarcinomas, at 105 and 112 months from the time the initial dysplasia was reported. The biopsy results immediately before the discovery of the carcinoma were negative for dysplasia, as were many of the previous biopsies, with an occasional interval report of low-grade dysplasia. After the conclusion of the study, one patient was found to have metastatic adenocarcinoma 6 months after the last of four serial sets of colonoscopic biopsies failed to reconfirm the low-grade dysplasia found 3 years earlier.[2]

Overall, surveillance during this study led to the discovery of 7 cases of carcinoma in 121 patients (6%). Carcinoma was preceded by dysplasia in 4 of these 22 patients (18%). This is similar to the findings in 877 patients summarized by Waye[7] in a review of colonoscopic surveillance in ulcerative colitis. In another study, Rosenstock et al.[6] found that the predictive rate for carcinoma was 40%, but the classification of dysplasia was limited to high grade. Other studies have not made a distinction between high- and low-grade dysplasia.

In consideration of the problem of sampling error, even if dysplasia is reported as low grade, it should not be ignored. Even if multiple series of subsequent biopsy reports show the findings to be negative and the interval between colonoscopies is extended, the patient should not be omitted from the surveillance routine. Furthermore, the presence of active disease should not diminish the recognition of true dysplasia and its significance as a premalignant lesion.

REFERENCES

1. Korelitz BI: Response to review of selected summary. *Gastroenterology* 1986; 92:2044.
2. Korelitz BI: Considerations of surveillance, dysplasia, and carcinoma of the colon in the management of ulcerative colitis and Crohn's disease. *Med Clin North Am* 1990; 74:189–199.
3. Lofberg R, et al: Colonoscopic surveillance in long-standing total ulcerative colitis—a 15 year follow up study. *Gastroenterology* 1990; 99:1021–1031.
4. Ransohoff DF, Riddell RH, Levin B: Ulcerative colitis and colonic cancer,

problems in assessing the diagnostic usefulness of mucosal dysplasia. *Dis Colon Rectum* 1985; 28:383–388.

5. Riddell RH, et al: Dysplasia in IBD: Standardized classification with provisional clinical applications. *Hum Pathol* 1983; 14:931–968.

6. Rosenstock E, et al: Colonoscopic surveillance for dysplasia and cancer in chronic ulcerative colitis. *Gastrointest Endosc* 1984; 30:145.

7. Waye J: Endoscopy in idiopathic IBD, in Kirsner JB, Shorter RG (eds): *Inflammatory Bowel Disease*, Philadelphia, Lea & Febiger, 1988.

8. Woolrich AJ, Sommers SC, Korelitz BI: Dysplasia and neoplasia at colonoscopy in the routine management of ulcerative colitis. *Gastroenterology* 1989; 96:A552.

Chapter 22

Management of Dysplasia in Ulcerative Colitis and Crohn's Disease

Burton I. Korelitz

By way of review, the following is what we do and do not know about cancer in ulcerative colitis:

1. With duration of disease the risk increases.

2. With extent of disease the risk increases. The location of the colitis is important in the sense that if it is universal, the risk is greater; if it is left sided the risk is not as great.

3. We do not know anything about the influence of the initial severity of the disease.

4. We do not know anything about the contribution of diagnostic radiation years before.

5. We do not know anything about the influence of drug therapy on the risk of cancer.

6. Dysplasia and cancer are both hard to find in most cases. With strictures, in ulcerative colitis particularly, the risk of a carcinoma being masked is fairly high.

7. Whereas in the general population most colon cancers are distal, in ulcerative colitis they are distributed throughout the entire colon.

8. Some cancers are synchronous in different areas, and some are extensive in their distribution.

Dysplasia can be patchy in distribution, alone or in multiple areas at the same time, may have a slightly elevated underlying mucosal pattern or not, usually has no underlying mass lesion such as a polyp, and the entire mucosal surface is at risk. The following classification was established by the dysplasia work group of pathologists[17]:

Negative
  Normal mucosa
  Inactive (quiescent) colitis
  Active colitis
Indefinite
  Probably negative
  (Probably inflammatory)
Unknown
  Probably positive
  (Probably dysplastic)
Positive
  Low-grade dysplasia
  High-grade dysplasia

Most studies on the outcome of dysplasia are based on finding either low-grade or high-grade dysplasia; there are no reported studies on the follow-up of "indefinite for dysplasia," either "probably negative" or "probably positive."

Many practical issues about surveillance should be considered:

1. *Is dysplasia reversible?* Barring the missing of dysplasia in biopsy specimens taken at subsequent colonoscopies, dysplasia does seem to come and go in most experiences. This in turn raises (2)

2. *The question of sampling.* How many biopsy specimens should be taken and how close to each other should they be? Dr. Waye takes a biopsy specimen every 10 cm. I personally believe that taking two to three biopsy specimens in the general field every 10 cm will at least increase the yield somewhat.

3. *Colonoscopy* might be *incomplete* for technical reasons. Therefore biopsy of the right side of the colon can be omitted, and dysplasia from this region can be missed.

4. *Time constraints of the pathologists.* Naturally if they spend more time looking at the slides for dysplasia the yield will increase, but in a busy general hospital this introduces all kinds of difficulties.

5. *Carcinoma can occur without dysplasia.*

6. *Patient compliance.* Patients really do not want to come back for surveillance if they are otherwise feeling well.

7. Downgrading of the degree of dysplasia because of inflammation.

The word *downgrading* has appeared in the literature for a long time, and implies that active disease seen on colonoscopy, even though the dysplasia might otherwise be considered high grade, should be reduced to low grade. If it otherwise might be considered low grade it should be reduced to "indefinite" or "no dysplasia at all." Sommers* never agreed with this; he believes that dysplasia could be recognized independently of the presence of inflammation.[10a] In our own experience in the Lenox Hill Hospital study, there can be activity as seen endoscopically even when the patient is asymptomatic (see Chapter 21). Furthermore, we have learned that there is better compliance for surveillance when the patient is symptomatic. Therefore, if there really is no need to consider downgrading, we should recognize that most of our surveillance is going to be accomplished during periods when the patient is symptomatic.

What data have been accumulated on the outcome of studies of dysplasia in regard to cancer? In the 1977 report of Dobbins of 453 colectomies for ulcerative colitis, 108 patients had cancer of the colon when the operative specimen was carefully examined; 88% of these had dysplasia.[4a] This is a very convincing association. In surveillance studies dysplasia has occurred in about 15%. Dysplasia has proved to be predictive of carcinoma in about 15% of these. If specifically high-grade dysplasia is found, it is predictive of carcinoma in 40% (i.e., from the study of Rosenstock and Farmer at the Cleveland Clinic).[18a] In our study we found carcinoma without dysplasia in 6%, and we found dysplasia in 22 patients (18%) on examination after 7 years (Chapter 21). We then found it on the next examination in 7 of 22 patients, but it was not found on the next examination in 15 of 22 patients. After many examinations that showed negative findings, low-grade dysplasia showed up again in 4 instances. Carcinoma was ultimately shown in those 4 patients where there had been previous dysplasia and then long intervals without dysplasia. So carcinoma was found by surveillance, whether with or without dysplasia, in 7 of 121 patients (or 6%).

These are my recommendations for colonoscopic surveillance based on my experience:

1. Colonoscopy should be initiated after 7 years of disease. You might ask whether a carcinoma complicating ulcerative colitis has ever been found in less than 7 years? Yes, but fortunately they are rare, and for all practical purposes 7 years is a reasonable time to consider starting.

*Dr. Sommers was the former Director, Department of Pathology, Lenox Hill Hospital.

2. Take three biopsy specimens every 10 cm; that is my experience, that is what I started doing, and that is what I still do. Dr. Waye, as I have mentioned, takes one biopsy specimen every 10 cm. When I asked him why he did not take three, he said he did not have time. That is a reality. Why every 10 cm as opposed to 20 cm? Maybe it should be every 5 cm. This is a very time-consuming process without really knowing whether it provides a proportionate yield.

3. Biopsy of suspicious lesions should always be done in addition to biopsy of the flat mucosa. Biopsy of any lesion not apparently belonging to the general contour or coloring should be done. These include lumps, bumps, and plaques, as well as masses, polyps, and pseudopolyps that vary in contour or hue.

4. When an interim sigmoidoscopy is performed in the routine management of ulcerative colitis, take a couple of extra biopsy specimens at that time. It is just such biopsies that have given a high yield of dysplasia. This does not, however, in any way substitute for the surveillance colonoscopy.

The usual areas where the biopsy specimens are taken include the cecum, ascending colon, proximal transverse colon, distal transverse colon, descending colon, sigmoid colon, and rectum. Extra biopsy specimens should be taken when the colon is very long, particularly on the left side. The total numbers are somewhere between seven and eight sets of biopsy specimens.

The following are my recommendations on the management of dysplasia:

1. If high-grade dysplasia is found in conjunction with a "mass lesion," colectomy is indicated.

2. If low-grade dysplasia is consistently found in conjunction with a mass lesion, colectomy is indicated.

3. If high-grade dysplasia is found on more than one occasion, without a mass lesion, and there are no extenuating circumstances such as "proctitis only," associated severe illness, or old age, colectomy is indicated.

4. The same pertains to low-grade dysplasia after it has been found on three or more consecutive examinations, but a special physician-patient relationship might modify this.

5. If dysplasia does not lead to immediate surgery, the frequency of subsequent colonoscopy should not extend beyond 3 months, whether high grade or low grade.

Even high-grade dysplasia can disappear even though it is less likely to do so than low-grade dysplasia. Low-grade dysplasia may become high grade, or it may become carcinoma, and a long hiatus in time between examinations that reveal the dysplasia does not guarantee any safety. If we find high-grade dysplasia and the next time there is no dysplasia, the colonoscopy should still be repeated within 3 months. If we find low-grade dysplasia and the next time it is low grade again the colonoscopy should also be repeated within 3 months. If we find low-grade dysplasia and the next time there is no dysplasia at all, perhaps we could wait for 6 months. If we find high-grade dysplasia in two consecutive sets of biopsies, or if the high-grade dysplasia accompanies a mass of any kind, that patient should be operated on. Even if the dysplasia is low grade, if it is persistent it warrants surgery. The only exception to that might be the elimination of the dysplasia with a trial of steroids. I am not really sure that I have seen the dysplasia disappear with steroids, but I agree it is worth a try.

6. If we find dysplasia in multiple sites, the prognosis worsens and the patient warrants surgery.

7. When the classification of dysplasia is not absolute and the degree of severity would influence the decision, a second experienced pathologist should also render an opinion. If the classification of dysplasia is not the problem, there is no value to having a review by the second pathologist.

8. The issue of cost benefit arises quite often, and I must state that I am not influenced by this.[16] If I think colonoscopic surveillance is the right thing to do, my relationship with my patient on a 1:1 basis is the priority, and I will worry about the cost benefit later. I do think if one finds no dysplasia on the second round, and it was low grade before, the interval between colonoscopies can be increased, and that perhaps improves the cost-benefit relationship.

CANCER IN CROHN'S DISEASE

We have learned from the studies at Mount Sinai Hospital that the risk of some extraintestinal cancers is increased in Crohn's disease.[6, 7] The increase in lymphomas in Crohn's disease has been emphasized. We know that cancer of the ileum occurs in ileitis and is statistically very significant even though rare. We know about bypassed loops where the risk of cancer is high, but we are seeing less of this because less bypassed loops are being created. The real problem comes with cancer of the colon and rectum complicating long-standing Crohn's disease.[9] Those segments of the bowel that are most at risk are those with the longest duration of disease. We think that sites of stricture and fistulas are more prone to the development of cancer than other sites in Crohn's disease, and particularly when the two occur together. There are cases of Crohn's disease with multifocal carcinomas and metachronous carcinomas. We have also learned that the bowel in Crohn's disease is prone to the development of dysplasia just as in ulcerative colitis.

In my study with Sommers and Lauwers,[11] 812 rectal biopsy specimens were taken from 356 patients with Crohn's disease; we found dysplasia in 22 specimens (5.1%, or 18 patients). The dysplasia was mild in 13 specimens, and moderate in 9. Tissue was taken from the rectal mucosa, which showed either active disease or appeared normal. The specimens were taken for a variety of reasons, including research. These patients were observed for many years to determine the ultimate outcome, and we found three instances of neoplasm. One was merely an adenomatous polyp at the site of an ileorectal fistula that must have been close to the biopsy site, but there were two carcinomas of the colon. One occurred in a 34-year-old man 13 years after the dysplasia was found, 26 years after onset of Crohn's disease, and he died of metastases. The other was a 36-year-old woman with dysplasia found on rectal biopsy; a year later carcinoma of the sigmoid was found. This was determined at follow-up, and that patient had died of metastases.

Obviously these observations should influence us toward a surveillance program knowing that dysplasia occurs in Crohn's disease just like it does in ulcerative colitis. Theoretically this should be more difficult in Crohn's disease because of the many limiting factors. Often the colonoscope cannot be introduced as far into the colon as in ulcerative colitis because of narrowed lumina, strictures, and abscesses. In most of the patients who require surveillance, however, Crohn's disease has responded to medical therapy, and a full colonoscopy is feasible. In my experience to date colonoscopic surveillance in Crohn's disease has yielded low-grade dysplasia in 5%, and the dysplasia was predictive of cancer in 11%.

Carcinoma in Crohn's disease with or without dysplasia is being reported more often. I have had four cases just within the last few years. Even if the lumen is stenosed and does not permit proximal passage of the colonoscope, lumen within the stricture is accessible to biopsy and cytology.

My overall conviction about surveillance in Crohn's disease, just as in ulcerative colitis, is that it should be pursued. It has been shown for ulcerative colitis that when dysplasia is found the clinical outcome has improved because of compliance by way of surveillance. Because of the fear of cancer, the patient is more likely to come for follow-up examination and get better care.

It is also my conviction that as long as dysplasia remains the best indicator, more intensive surveillance will be necessary.

REFERENCES

1. Blackstone MP, Riddell RH, Rogers BHG, et al: Dysplasia associated lesion or mass (DALM) detected by colonoscopy in long standing ulcerative colitis: An indication for colectomy. *Gastroenterology* 1981;80:366–374.
2. Collins RH Jr, Feldman M, Fordtran JS: Dysplasia and colon cancer surveillance in patients with ulcerative colitis. *N Engl J Med* 1987;316:1654–1658.
3. Cooper DJ, Weinstein MA, Korelitz BI: Complications of Crohn's disease predisposing to dysplasia and cancer of the intestinal tract: Considerations of a surveillance program. *J Clin Gastroenterol* 1984;6:217–224.
4. Craft CF, Mendelsohn G, Cooper HS, et al: Colonic "precancer" in Crohn's disease. *Gastroenterology* 1981;80:578–584.
4a. Dobbins WO III: Current status of the precancer lesion in ulcerative colitis. *Gastroenterology* 1977;73:1431–1433.
5. Fochios SE, Sommers SC, Korelitz BI: Sigmoidoscopy and biopsy in surveillance for cancer in ulcerative colitis. *J Clin Gasteroenterol* 1986;8:249–254.
6. Greenstein AJ, Sachar DB, Smith H, et al: Cancer in universal and left sided ulcerative colitis: Factors determining risk. *Gastroenterology* 1979;77:290–294.
7. Greenstein AJ, Sachar DB, Smith H, et al: A comparison of cancer risk in Crohn's disease and ulcerative colitis. *Cancer* 1981;48:2742–2745.
8. Hamilton SR: Colorectal carcinoma in patients with Crohn's disease. *Gastroenterology* 1985;89:398–407.
9. Korelitz BI: Carcinoma of the intestinal tract in Crohn's disease: Results of a survey conducted by the NFIC. *Am J Gastroenterol* 1983;78:44–46.
10. Korelitz BI: IBD and cancer, in Berk JE (ed): *Bockus Gastroenterology*, ed 4, Philadelphia, 1985; WB Saunders, pp 2346–2361.
10a. Korelitz BI: Response to review of selected summary. *Gastroenterology* 1986; 92:2044.
11. Korelitz BI, Lauwers GY, Sommers SE: Rectal mucosal dysplasia in Crohn's disease. *Gut* 1990;31:1382–1386.
12. Korelitz BI: Considerations of surveillance, dysplasia, carcinoma of the

colon in the management of ulcerative colitis and Crohn's disease. *Med Clin North Am* 1990;103–133.

13. Lennard-Jones JE: Surveillance for dysplasia: London experience, in Bayless TM (ed): *Current Management of IBD*, Toronto, BC Decker, 1989, pp 153–157.

14. Lennard-Jones JE, Morson BC, Ritchie JK, et al: Cancer surveillance in ulcerative colitis. *Lancet* 1983;2:149–152.

15. Petras RE: Dysplasia and cancer in Crohn's disease, in Bayless TM (ed): *Current Management of IBD*. Toronto, BC Decker, 1989, pp 360–363.

16. Ransohoff DF, Ridell RH, Levin B: Ulcerative colitis and colonic cancer; problems in assessing the diagnostic usefulness of mucosal dysplasia. *Dis Colon Rectum* 1985; 28:383–388.

17. Riddel RH, Goldman H, Ransohoff DF, et al: Dysplasia in IBD. Standard classification with provisional applications. *Hum Pathol* 1983; 14:931–968.

18. Riddell RH: Colonic dysplasia: Pathological identification. *Dis Colon Rectum* 1985;28:383–388.

18a. Rosenstock E, Farmer RG, Petras R, et al: Surveillance for colonic carcinoma in ulcerative colitis. *Gastroenterology* 1985;89:1342–1346.

19. Waye JD: Endoscopy in idiopathic IBD, in Kirsner JB, Shorter RG (eds): *Inflammatory Bowel Disease*, ed 3. Philadelphia, Lea & Febiger, 1988, pp 353–376.

Chapter 23 _____

Management of Cancer in Inflammatory Bowel Disease

Raul N. Lugo

Chronic inflammatory bowel disease (IBD) is considered a precancerous condition.[10, 19, 32, 48, 62] It is generally agreed that both Crohn's disease and ulcerative colitis predispose to the development of malignancies. Malignant tumors of all types have been reported and studied in association with IBD. These have been seen to occur in both the intestinal and the extraintestinal systems.[25] Some of these associations have been observed repeatedly, and some have occurred seemingly by coincidence.

Malignant tumors arising from the epithelial tissues, such as adenocarcinoma of the colon, rectum, and small bowel, have been extensively documented and frequently observed. Cases of all common types of malignancies of the gastrointestinal tract in general have been reported in the literature. Tumors arising from lymphoreticular tissues, such as lymphomas of the colon, rectum, and small intestine, and tumors of the mesenchymal tissues, such as Kaposi's sarcoma, osteosarcoma, and others, have been reported as well.

Carcinomas, lymphomas, and sarcomas have all been seen in the presence of both Crohn's disease and ulcerative colitis. There is a well-established relationship between IBD and neoplasms of epithelial and lymphoreticular origin. There are much fewer reports associating IBD with tumors of mesenchymal origin.

Although it could still be considered rare, by some, to find cancer in patients with IBD, it should not be surprising that adenocarcinoma, lymphoma, and squamous cell carcinoma are associated with ulcerative colitis, Crohn's disease, or chronic fistulous disease of the rectum.

If this is so, are all patients at risk?[9] Which patients are at risk, and what can be done to determine who is at risk? How can precancerous conditions be detected, evaluated, and treated? When should routine surveillance begin, and in whom should surveillance be performed? Should prophylactic surgery be recommended for all patients with long-standing extensive disease, or only in patients with dysplasia? In patients with carcinomas, lymphomas, and sarcomas of the colon, rectum, and small bowel, what is the best surgical and medical therapy? Is there a role for chemotherapy or radiotherapy in the management of malignant diseases in IBD?

ADENOCARCINOMA AND ULCERATIVE COLITIS

It has been thought that only patients with ulcerative colitis carried a higher risk for development of colorectal cancer than the average population. There is convincing evidence that patients with Crohn's disease also carry a higher risk. The risk of developing colorectal cancer in the presence of IBD has been estimated to be as high as 19-fold that in the general population.[27] Others have estimated the risk in patients with ulcerative colitis to be 5 to 11 times higher. When chronic ulcerative colitis has been present for more than 10 years, the prevalence of cancer approaches 15 to 30 times the risk in the general population. In a study reported from Denmark, the risk of intestinal cancer is 1.4% in ulcerative colitis after 18 years, twice the risk of the general population.[7] Although the risk of cancer in IBD is increased, it still remains low. The prophylactic treatment of patients with chronic ulcerative colitis with panproctocolectomy, or the sphincter-saving total abdominal colectomy with mucosal proctectomy and ileoanal pouch anastomosis, can prevent the development of malignancy in the colon and cure a patient with an early or incidental carcinoma, in the presence of high-grade dysplasia.*

In ulcerative colitis, the increased risk of developing an intestinal malignancy is limited to the colon and rectum. The tumors are often multifocal. Adenocarcinoma of the colon and rectum in ulcerative colitis has been reported in the age range from 19 to 89 years. The duration of the colitis has ranged from 5 to 26 years in these patients. A clinical subgroup of patients with extensive or total ulcerative colitis and a his-

---

*Editor's Note: Whether a pouch should be created in the presence of dysplasia remains controversial. (See Chapter 18 and Discussion that follows.)

tory of symptoms for more than 10 years is at greatest risk. This group can be advised to have prophylactic colectomy.*

Epithelial dysplasia has been found to be a marker for cancer; thus patients with biopsy evidence of epithelial dysplasia are at increased risk of development of cancer.[34] Although the cause of the inflammation-dysplasia-carcinoma sequence is not known, the temporal relationship between ulcerative colitis and adenocarcinoma of the colon and rectum is well charted. The cumulative risk of colon cancer developing in patients with ulcerative colitis has been said to increase 10% to 20% for every decade of duration of disease after the first 10 years.[31] In a prospective study of patients with long-standing colitis, those found to have high-grade dysplasia were found to have carcinomas resected at surgery.[39]

Environmental factors may have an independent role, or a role in the deregulation of genetic factors and oncogenes that may have been suppressed by nonenvironmental factors. Research into molecular biology, genetics, and the regulation of oncogenes may reveal etiologic factors not previously suspected.[8, 15]

PREVALENCE

The reported prevalence of colorectal adenocarcinoma developing in patients with IBD is varied in the literature. Dennis and Karlson[14] found four cancers per 100 patient years occurring after 10 years of colitis. They suggested that this figure (4% per year) is higher than the risk of proctocolectomy (2%), so that after 10 years proctocolectomy is indicated. Other investigators agree with proctocolectomy after the first 10 years of the development of ulcerative colitis because of the risk of developing carcinoma. Some emphasize that total involvement of the colon is an important additional criterion before the recommendation of colectomy.*[16, 42] Others suggest waiting until the development of high-grade dysplasia as a prerequisite to the recommendation of prophylactic total proctocolectomy. For patients electing to have prophylactic surgery because of a variety of risk factors that make the patient and the doctor concerned about the high risk of developing colorectal carcinoma, a sphincter-saving total colectomy with mucosal proctectomy

---

*Editor's note: In practice, prophylactic colectomy rarely is recommended, and still more rarely accepted unless the quality of life also is compromised by disease activity.

and ileoanal pouch is an alternative surgical procedure to panprocto-colectomy and permanent ileostomy.[47]

In 1985, Turunen and Jarvinen,[61] from the Helsinki University Central Hospital, reported a 16-year series of 235 patients operated on for ulcerative colitis. Sixteen patients developed 21 colorectal malignancies, including adenocarcinoma and lymphoma. In 44% of their patients cancer developed within 10 years of the onset of the colitis.* Those advocates of early, periodic, long-term surveillance endoscopy are supported by the clear demonstration of the risk of developing malignant tumors of the colon or rectum, soon after the onset of the ulcerative colitis rather than after a delay of decades.

In patients with ulcerative colitis, the risk of malignant transformation is greater when ulcerative colitis begins in childhood.† The prevalence of cancer is twice as high if the colitis began before the age of 25. Three percent of children with ulcerative colitis will develop cancer of the colon by the age of 10, and 20% will develop cancer during each ensuing decade. In patients with ulcerative colitis the risk of malignant conversion is greater when ulcerative colitis has been present for more than 10 years, involves the entire colon, has continuous symptoms rather than intermittent ones, and was of severe onset. Approximately 40% of patients with total colonic involvement with ulcerative colitis will die of colon cancer if they survive the ulcerative colitis.

Changes in the natural history of IBD have been reported in Norway.[43, 58] The current mortality from ulcerative colitis of 4% in 10 years is similar to that from Crohn's disease, and is quite different than that from earlier series (>20% in 10 years). The proportion of patients getting severe attacks has fallen from 14.6% in the 1960s to less than 10% in the presently reported series. Since patients with severe attacks are now better controlled with modern nonsurgical therapy, the acute mortality has declined. There is an increased number of patients receiving chronic sulfasalazine maintenance therapy as well as therapy with other medications. These patients are now living longer. The forces that have influenced the development of the disease are in these patients now controlled, but still present, and the carcinogenic influences continue to act on the colonic mucosal cells. Now cancer is equally common in patients with Crohn's disease as in patients with ulcerative colitis.

*Editor's Note: This experience has been exceptional. Reports on carcinoma before 10 years of ulcerative colitis can be found, but are rare.

†Editor's Note: Until recently all studies emphasized duration of disease rather than onset in childhood, but a recent report from Sweden (Ekbom et al, *N Engl J Med*) suggests that the pendulum is swinging in the other direction.

PATHOGENESIS

Researchers in Israel have proposed that the depletion of stem cells of the colonic mucosa may result in the development of neoplasia.[64] They suggest that, by the action of any one of the multiple environmental factors or processes, such as viruses, chemotherapy, or inflammation, on the stem cells of the mucosa, there will be mucosal stem cell depletion and, in turn, the development of malignant tumors. Thus chronic inflammatory disease of the bowel, under the added influence of drug therapy or nutritional carcinogens such as the nitrites, may potentially be responsible for the depletion of the stem cells in this disease and thus explain the increased risk of cancer seen in ulcerative colitis.

Research has been done in the laboratory with Crohn's disease tissue filtrates in nude mice and their possible role in the development of malignancies on an immunologic basis.[12] Multiple defects in cellular and humoral immunity have been well demonstrated in these two diseases.[17, 24] Aparicio-Pages et al.,[4] in the Netherlands, demonstrated that natural immunity, as expressed by natural killer cell cytotoxicity in the peripheral blood of patients with Crohn's disease and ulcerative colitis, is depressed compared with natural immunity in control subjects. Improvement in cytotoxicity was accomplished in vitro with phytohemagglutinin stimulation to levels similar to control subjects. The intestinal mononuclear cells in patients with active Crohn's disease and ulcerative colitis have also been found to produce decreased amounts of interferon-γ.[20, 37] Because of the importance of inteferon-γ in the integrity of cellular immunity, its impaired availability may be relevant in the pathogenesis of cancer in IBD. If immune deficiency has any role in the pathogenesis of malignancies in the IBDs, this work may provide an insight into immunorestoration as a treatment for the prevention of the development of cancer in these diseases.

The presence of misplaced mucosal epithelium in ulcerative colitis and Crohn's disease has been observed. This fact may help understand the observation of the unusual histologic growth pattern of submucosal adenocarcinoma underlying a flat, nondysplastic mucosa in ulcerative colitis. There are many cases in which cancer has been identified in the colon or rectum of patients with ulcerative colitis in which there were no signs of dysplasia. The effects of mucosal inflammation and repair may be related to the pathogenic mechanisms involved in the evolution of misplaced mucosal epithelium. In a report from Belfast, Northern Ireland, there was a high incidence of misplaced mucosal epithelium seen in association with Crohn's disease, ulcerative colitis, and ulcerative colitis complicated by carcinoma.[2] There were no foci of misplaced mucosal epithelium in specimens with noncolitic colorectal carcinoma. These observations would justify the recommendation of prophylactic proctocolectomy in patients with chronic inflammatory colitis and in patients with dysplasia without evidence of carcinoma.

It is suggested that patients with colitis have a genetic predisposition for the development of colorectal carcinoma[3, 13, 27, 38] and that long-standing inflammation is not of primary importance in the initiation or promotion of cancer in this disease. This belief is supported by the fact that, although the median period of time in which patients with ulcerative colitis take to develop colorectal carcinoma is 14 years, the duration of the presence of the disease has been as short as 4 years and as long as 44 years.[7]

Since the development of flexible fiberoptic colonoscopy, the association between epithelial dysplasia and carcinoma in IBD has been recognized. Riddell[46] presented the concept of dysplasia in which the polyp-cancer sequence in the noncolitic colon was compared with the dysplasia-cancer sequence in ulcerative colitis. This association has also been observed in the small bowel of patients with Crohn's disease.

It is therefore unclear whether immunodeficiency, inflammation, genetics, dietary factors, or other environmental factors are responsible for the pathogenesis of malignancies in IBD independently, or associated in a multifactorial way.

TISSUE MARKERS

Various different cell surface antigens have been studied on the mucosal cells of the small bowel and colon of patients with IBD in an attempt to develop techniques of early detection of the transformation of benign mucosal cells to malignant cells. Tissue concentrations of carcinoembryonic antigen (CEA) have been found to be significantly higher on the mucosal cells of patients with chronic IBD than on normal colonic mucosal cells.[21] Immunohistochemical staining for CEA has revealed that the intensity of CEA staining parallels the histologic degrees of dysplasia and neoplasia.[11] The expression of CEA has been seen to be more pronounced in areas of high-grade dysplasia and invasive carcinoma. Radioactively labeled anti-CEA monoclonal antibody has been found though to cross-react with the benign tissues of patients with IBD.[6] This situation may give false-positive findings when screening patients with IBD for the presence of colorectal adenocarcinoma. It is thus unclear at this time whether the presence of CEA on the mucosal cells of patients with IBD precedes or predicts the development of dysplasia or neoplasia.

Tumor-associated glycoprotein antigen (TAG-72) has been found to be expressed on dysplastic mucosal cells and in the nondysplastic mucosal cells of patients with IBD.[59, 63] It has rarely been detected in normal colonic mucosal epithelium.

Carcinoma-associated antigens (CA-19-9 and CA-50) are frequently expressed in the tissues of patients with ulcerative colitis and Crohn's disease, as well as in the tissues of patients with numerous benign conditions such as diverticular disease and sigmoid volvulus.[22]

It is clear that despite the identification of new cell surface antigens and their potential relationship to the development of neoplasia, new insights into the cellular changes that precede the development of malignancy must be obtained. This form of tissue typing is therefore of limited value in predicting the risk of developing either dysplasia or neoplasia. Furthermore, there are still no absolutely reliable methods for detecting precancerous changes in the colon of patients with IBD except by the detection of dysplasia with biopsy. It is therefore not justified at this time to recommend surgery based on the observation of abnormal cell surface antigens on the mucosal cells of patients with IBD. Hopefully research into flow cytometry may provide insight into the chromosomal and genetic changes that may precede the cellular changes seen in dysplasia.[8] We are awaiting reports in this area of investigation.

SIGNS AND SYMPTOMS, DETECTION AND TREATMENT

Early cancer can be symptomless. If symptoms are present they are frequently indistinguishable from colitis symptoms. Only in patients undergoing regular surveillance can colorectal carcinoma be detected at an early stage. In patients who do not undergo routine surveillance, cancers are frequently found at a more advanced stage (see Chapter 21). In a prospective study of patients with long-standing colitis, those found to have high-grade dysplasia were frequently found to have carcinoma at the time of resection.[39]

In a recent report from the University of Chicago, Lashner et al.[35] described a very strong association between dysplasia, neoplasia, and colonic strictures in patients with ulcerative colitis. Previous studies have reported similar findings, but with a variable prevalence of the dysplasia and cancer associated with the strictures. In Lashner et al.'s study, at resection, the patients with strictures were found to have neoplastic disease ranging from dysplasia to Dukes' stage D carcinoma. All of the cancers were located at the site of a stricture. These findings suggest that a true colonic stricture in ulcerative colitis is frequently associated with either dysplasia or carcinoma. Thus a stricture should be considered a strong risk factor for carcinoma in the presence of ulcerative colitis. These strictures require intensive colonoscopic surveillance, and surgical resection if adequate biopsy of the stricture is not possible.*

Because of the risk of cancer in ulcerative colitis, some authors advocate prophylactic colectomy after 10 to 15 years.[18, 42, 60] This can be clearly justified on the basis of the evidence presented. The most common recommendation though seems to be a policy of close observation and frequent surveillance. Surgery can be reserved only for patients with biopsy-proved severe dysplasia, dysplasia associated with a lesion or a mass, or in dysplasia associated with a stricture in ulcerative colitis. But, as already presented, carcinoma can develop without any evidence of dysplasia or stricture formation.

The procedure of choice in the emergency surgical management of ulcerative colitis or Crohn's colitis is subtotal colectomy and ileostomy with preservation of the rectum.[28, 36] Once the emergent nature of the disease is controlled, the following are the choices for the management of the retained rectum. They consist of removing the rectum totally and creating a permanent ileostomy, leaving the rectum in situ without resection, or creating an ileoanal anastomosis with a pouch (see Chapters 17 and 18). In the cases in which the rectum is spared either as a mucous fistula, a Hartmann's pouch, or is saved in the form of an ileorectal anastomosis, there is an increased risk of development of rectal adenocarcinoma in the general population.[30] When cancer occurs in the retained rectum, it is more commonly found at a more advanced stage and of a higher malignant grade. These findings should alert us to the danger of carcinomatous transformation in the retained rectum and should accentuate the need for regular long-term follow-up, the need for precancerous markers, and the liberal use of prophylactic proctectomy.

There are a number of reports of patients who have undergone colonic resection with ileostomy for ulcerative colitis in whom carcinoma has developed at the site of the ileostomy.[55, 57] These tumors on the average occur 24 years after colectomy and ileostomy. These stoma-related malignancies have been found in association with dysplasia and

---

*Editor's Note: This is a clinical decision. The vast majority of strictures in ulcerative colitis do not contain a carcinoma (see Chapter 12).

metaplasia in the surrounding mucosa of this mucinous adenocarcinoma. Gadacz et al.[23] have suggested that there is a transition from ileal mucosa to colonic mucosa to colonic dysplasia to adenocarcinoma. On the basis of their observation of metaplasia, dysplasia, and carcinoma, they suggest annual evaluation of the ileostomy for colonic metaplasia and dysplasia. In the presence of dysplasia they recommend ileal resection with stomal revision; and, for carcinoma, wide local excision.

A recent report presented two cases of adenocarcinoma developing in ileostomies of patients with Crohn's disease. In both of them mucosal dysplasia was identified.[55]

PREVENTION AND SURVEILLANCE

The cause and cure of IBD remain evasive, and treatment remains empiric. The major goals of therapy remain control of inflammation and relief of symptoms.

In view of the fact that cancers in ulcerative colitis may be present without symptoms, and that many cases have been reported within 10 years of the onset of the disease, it is necessary to establish periodic surveillance programs in these patients as soon as the diagnosis of colitis is made. Since the etiologic factors that result in carcinogenic transformation in these patients are unknown, and treatment rarely results in a complete remission of the IBD, cancer surveillance is critical. A definite improvement in 5-year survival should be obtained if prophylactic surgery is performed when the patients develop an identifiable high risk. For patients at high risk who decline prophylactic colectomy, an aggressive surveillance program involving regularly performed colonoscopy and biopsies is a reasonable alternative. Until a better screening strategy is developed, total periodic colonoscopy with biopsy of the colonic mucosa will still be the surveillance procedure of choice and the mainstay of follow-up.[1] This approach would reduce the number of tumors found in advanced stages for which the mortality would be higher, for which the recurrence rate would be higher, and for which only palliative surgery would be possible.

Patients frequently refuse to cooperate with a surveillance program if there is a lack of symptoms or a lack of information; or they are not screened if there is an inadequate follow-up system. Better education of the medical profession as well as the patients is necessary.[40] In a study from West Germany regarding the needs and fears of patients with IBD, the most commonly asked questions were regarding the possibilities of remission of the disease and the possibility of developing cancer.[49] Cancer was the fear factor selected most often. Because of this fear, the well-informed patient should be more willing to undertake a program of periodic surveillance endoscopy and should be more willing to report symptoms at an earlier stage. The patient should be more willing to co-operate with diagnostic testing and undergo surgical procedures if the risk of malignant disease can be well documented and justified. The prognosis and long-term survival of these patients should improve.

CROHN'S DISEASE

It is now generally accepted that Crohn's disease also carries a higher risk of malignancy. Some authors believe that cancer is now equally common in patients with Crohn's disease and ulcerative colitis.[58] In Crohn's disease the increased rate of cancer is higher in the large bowel and the small bowel both in areas of apparently normal bowel and in areas involved with inflammation.[48] The tumors have been found to develop frequently in areas of dysplasia within areas of Crohn's disease in both large and small intestine.[34] The dysplastic changes seen in the bowel adjacent to the tumors are identical to the characteristic precancerous dysplastic changes well described in ulcerative colitis. Diffuse signet ring adenocarcinoma and mucinous adenocarcinoma have both been described, although mucinous adenocarcinoma seems to be more common, and is associated more often with the areas of dysplasia. This association between the dysplasia and cancer seen in the colon in ulcerative colitis is similar to the pattern seen in the small bowel. The same pattern is seen in the small bowel where cancers develop in or near areas of dysplasia and in or near areas of active Crohn's inflammation.[44] When the tumors are located in the small bowel they tend to be discovered at a more advanced stage, and therefore tend to have a poor prognosis.

The cancers in Crohn's disease appear to occur at an earlier age than in the average population. The earlier the onset of the disease the higher the risk of developing cancer. In the patients with onset before the age of 21, the risk of developing colorectal carcinoma has been estimated to be up to 20 times higher than in the general population. Typically, regardless of age, the diagnosis is difficult to make because the signs and symptoms are frequently misinterpreted as representing a recurrence of Crohn's disease. Skepticism or ignorance as to the possibility of the development of cancer in young people with Crohn's disease tends to lead to a delay in diagnosis. Misinterpretation of the symptoms of the cancer as being those of active inflammation may lead to a delay as well. Although one is reluctant to operate on patients with Crohn's disease without an absolute indication, surgery is justified if the radiographic imaging studies suggest the presence of malignancy in the small bowel. It is well known that the differential diagnosis between inflammatory and neoplastic disease is often difficult to make in patients with Crohn's disease.

A case of intramucosal adenocarcinoma has been observed in the ileum of a 54-year-old woman with a 21-year history of Crohn's disease; resection was done for the treatment of recurrent low-grade intestinal obstruction.[39] Adjacent to the area of carcinoma, the mucosa showed various degrees of dysplasia consistent with the precancerous changes that have been described in IBD.

Small bowel adenocarcinoma has been reported in many patients who have undergone bypass rather than resection of segments of Crohn's disease. Adenocarcinoma in segments of ileitis that have undergone in continuity bypass has been reported to develop in 22 patients.[52] These patients' presenting symptoms have been typical of recurrent IBD. They have also had clinical pictures consisting of intestinal obstruction, abdominal mass, intra-abdominal abscess, and fistula. In many of these patients dysplasia has been seen at areas of inflammation next to or near the sites of malignancy, and in general the prognosis is very poor because of the frequently advanced stage of the local disease at the time of the diagnosis.

Chronic long-standing perineal inflammation, as is seen in chronic fistulous disease of the rectum in Crohn's disease, may be etiologically related to the development of carcinomas in this area. Cases of early and advanced rectal adenocarcinoma, as well as cloacogenic and squamous cell carcinoma, and Bowen's disease have been seen in these patients with significant perianal disease.[26, 56] The confusing clinical picture of rectal carcinoma with that of benign perianal disease also leads to delays in diagnosis.

Squamous cell carcinoma of the rectum is managed in patients with IBD in the same manner as in patients without IBD. A combination of radiation therapy along with concomitant 5-fluorouracil and mitomycin-C is well established as the therapy of choice for the treatment of squamous cell carcinoma of the rectum, as well as cloacogenic carcinoma and basaloid carcinoma. Many variations of this program have emerged, but all still consist of radiation therapy along with some form of chemotherapy. For patients in whom this program has failed, and who have either persistent or recurrent tumor, surgical resection of the rectum is indicated. More radical excision of the perineal tissues may be necessary to accomplish a curative resection. This is justified, because second-line chemotherapy for the treatment of these tumors is rarely curative.

Thus an increased awareness of the association of Crohn's disease and cancer and an awareness that the malignancies may develop in areas of apparently normal bowel should encourage the development of surveillance programs for patients with Crohn's disease, since the patients do have a similar risk of developing carcinoma that has been recognized for ulcerative colitis.[10] Careful evaluation of all new symptoms and routine surveillance endoscopy should detect dysplasia with biopsy and should arouse the suspicion of malignancy in the vicinity of the dysplasia. Early treatment of these patients should improve the prognosis of those with IBD.

SCLEROSING CHOLANGITIS AND CHOLANGIOCARCINOMA

Primary sclerosing cholangitis is seen in association with IBD (see chapter 5). Sclerosing cholangitis is most commonly seen in younger patients with extensive ulcerative colitis. It is also seen in patients with Crohn's disease.[51] Patients with ulcerative colitis and sclerosing cholangitis have an increased risk of development of colorectal cancer and also a risk of development of cholangiocarcinoma in either the intrahepatic or extrahepatic biliary tree. Patients with ulcerative colitis who have abnormal liver function test results are likely to have sclerosing cholangitis. The disease may be clinically silent, with nonspecific symptoms or biliary sepsis at initial presentation. When suspected, it is easily identifiable by endoscopic retrograde cholangiopancreatography. Percutaneous transhepatic cholangiography is also useful in the diagnosis and management of the disease.

Cholangiocarcinoma in patients with sclerosing cholangitis is more common in patients with ulcerative colitis than in patients of similar age without ulcerative colitis. The incidence of biliary tract carcinoma in patients with ulcerative colitis has been estimated to be 0.4%. In a series of 103 cases of proximal biliary tract cancer, 8% of the patients had coexisting ulcerative colitis. Eight cases of gallbladder carcinoma associated with ulcerative colitis have been reported in a separate series. Cholangiocarcinoma and gallbladder carcinoma are surgically curable in the early stages. Few cures are in fact accomplished because of the usually advanced nature of the tumors at the time of initial discovery. Cures are difficult to obtain because the radical nature of the resections needed to expect a cure. Liver transplantation has been performed for the treatment of sclerosing cholangitis and in selected cases of cholangiocarcinoma. Radiation therapy, delivered either by external beam or by a variety of brachytherapy techniques, has failed to obtain reproducible cures.

Colorectal cancers have been seen to develop after liver transplantation for sclerosing cholangitis and ulcerative colitis. It is therefore necessary to observe patients with ulcerative colitis and sclerosing cholangitis for the two neoplastic diseases that are particularly likely to develop, namely, colorectal carcinoma and cholangiocarcinoma.

Immunoblastic sarcoma, now known and classified as high-grade, large-cell, immunoblastic lymphoma, has also been reported in a patient with ulcerative colitis who had undergone liver transplantation for sclerosing cholangitis.

INTESTINAL LYMPHOMA

Intestinal lymphoma has been reported in patients with Crohn's disease and ulcerative colitis.[5, 29, 33] Colorectal lymphoma has been seen in patients with ulcerative colitis and in patients with Crohn's colitis. In 1989 primary malignant lymphoma of the large intestine was reported as a complication of chronic IBD in the colon and rectum of ten patients in Gloucestershire, United Kingdom.[53] Three of the patients had Crohn's disease of the sigmoid colon or rectum, and seven had chronic ulcerative colitis. The patients with ulcerative colitis had a history of colitis ranging from 6 to 20 years. The history of Crohn's disease ranged from 30 months to 20 years. Colorectal lymphoma has presenting symptoms with features indistinguishable from those of colorectal adenocarcinoma. In a report from St. Mark's Hospital in London, Shepherd et al.[54] observed that 7 of 45 patients with primary colorectal lymphoma had chronic ulcerative colitis, with a history of colitis ranging from 6 to 20 years. Primary intestinal lymphoma has been seen in patients with only left-sided colitis, in patients with extensive colitis, in patients with fissuring, fistulas, and extensive anal involvement. In the St. Mark's report there was a predominance of patients with extensive colitis at a ratio of 7:1.

Although there is a heterogeneity of histologic variations of primary intestinal lymphomas found in Crohn's disease and ulcerative colitis, there is an overwhelming predominance of B cell type lymphomas, with a predominance of high-grade tumors. Granulomatous T cell type lymphoma has been reported, as well as lymphomas of polymorphic and of equivocal phenotypes.[50] These neoplasms are thought to arise from the mucosa-associated lymphoid tissue. The cellular and humoral immuno-logic defects already discussed in this chapter are thought to be of etiologic significance in the development of malignancies in these diseases.

The prognosis of primary intestinal lymphoma in IBD appears to be dependent on factors already known to be of prognostic significance for primary intestinal lymphoma not associated with IBD. The prognosis is found to be related to grade. A predominance of high-grade tumors suggest that the outlook is generally worse. When a modified Dukes' staging system was applied in one study, there was a trend for early stage to give a prognostic advantage.[54] This concept supports the view that surgery should be the primary treatment of choice for localized intestinal lymphomas associated with Crohn's disease or ulcerative colitis, with radiotherapy or chemotherapy being reserved for advanced-stage or high-grade tumors. It is difficult to recommend a specific chemotherapeutic program for lymphoma in this situation, since the chemotherapeutic combinations are so often changing in this modern era. But, with the cure rates reported today for many varieties of lymphoma, it is advisable in most instances to treat intestinal lymphoma with chemotherapy as well as surgery. This is especially true in view of the predominance of high-grade lymphomas and the usually systemic nature of non-Hodgkin's lymphoma.

INTESTINAL SARCOMAS

Colonic Kaposi's sarcoma has been reported in human immunode-ficiency virus (HIV)–negative and HIV-positive patients with ulcerative colitis. A case was reported at Mayo Clinic of Kaposi's sarcoma in the colon of a young heterosexual man with chronic ulcerative colitis whose tests were negative for HIV. Similarly, a case of non–acquired im-munodeficiency syndrome (AIDS)–related Kaposi's sarcoma of the colon was seen in a patient with ulcerative colitis by Meltzer et al.[41] in New York. AIDS and later colonic Kaposi's sarcoma have been observed to develop in a male patient with a 14-year history of ulcerative colitis.

Gastrointestinal Kaposi's sarcoma is usually asymptomatic in AIDS patients. A case of AIDS-related colonic Kaposi's sarcoma has been reported by a group in Australia. The patient had an ulcerative colitis–type illness that ultimately required emergency total colectomy for toxic megacolon. In another report, in a 37-year-old HIV-positive male homosexual, persistent diarrhea with mucus production developed. After barium enema and rectal biopsy a diagnosis of ulcerative colitis was made. Cutaneous and colonic Kaposi's sarcoma later developed in this patient.

EXTRAINTESTINAL MALIGNANCIES

Extraintestinal malignancies have been recorded in many different organ sites, most without any apparent association. There are no statistically significant increases in the overall observed-to-expected ratios of extraintestinal malignancies in either Crohn's disease or ulcerative colitis, except reticuloendothelial tumors, such as leukemias in ulcerative colitis and lymphomas in both ulcerative colitis and Crohn's disease. Other tumors found in higher than expected rates include perianal squamous cell carcinoma and squamous cell carcinoma of the vagina.

Extraintestinal sites of malignancies that have been observed in patients with IBD include skin, breast, lung, genitourinary, cervix, and pancreatic islet cell. Soft tissue sarcomas, extraosseous osteogenic sarcoma, and desmoid tumors have been observed as well.

Treatment of IBD with certain medications, particularly the immunosuppressive drugs, is thought possibly to be responsible for the development of some of the extraintestinal malignancies. In a large series reported on the management of IBD with the use of 6-mercaptopurine, of 396 patients, 12 neoplasms were observed.[45] Only one case of diffuse histiocytic lymphoma of the brain was believed probably to be associated with the use of 6-mercaptopurine.

REFERENCES

1. Albert MB, Nochomovitz LE: Dysplasia and cancer surveillance in inflammatory bowel disease. *Gastroenterol Clin North Am* 1989; 18:83–97.
2. Allen DC, Biggart JD: Misplaced epithelium in ulcerative colitis and Crohn's disease of the colon and its relationship to malignant mucosal changes. *Histopathology* 1986; 10:37–52.
3. Alstead EM, McConnell RB: Genetic aspects of inflammatory bowel disease and gastrointestinal cancer. *Acta Gastroenterol Belg* 1984; 47:139–148.
4. Aparicio-Pages MN, Verspaget HW, Pena AS, et al: Natural, lectin- and phorbol ester–induced cellular cytotoxicity in Crohn's disease and ulcerative colitis. *J Clin Lab Immunol* 1988;27:109–113.
5. Baker D, Chiprut RO, Rimer D, et al: Colonic lymphoma in ulcerative colitis. *J Clin Gastroenterol* 1985; 7:379–386.
6. Bares R, Fass J, Truong S, et al: Radioimmunoscintigraphy with ^{111}In labelled monoclonal antibody fragments (F(ab')2 BW 431/31) against CEA: Ra-

diolabelling, antibody kinetics and distribution, findings in tumour and non-tumour patients. *Nucl Med Commun* 1989; 10:627–641.

7. Binder V: Epidemiology, course and socio-economic influence of inflammatory bowel disease. *Schweiz Med Wochenschr* 1988; 118:738–742.

8. Bleiberg H, Buyse M, Galand P: Cell kinetic indicators of premalignant stages of colorectal cancer. *Cancer* 1985; 56:124–129.

9. Brandt LJ, Dickstein G: Inflammatory bowel disease: Specific concerns in the elderly. *Geriatrics* 1989; 44:107–111.

10. Clamp SE, Wenham JS, Softley A, et al: Sampling gastroenterologists' opinions and attitudes at two world congresses. *Scand J Gastroenterol (Suppl)* 1984; 95:59–69.

11. Cuvelier C, Bekaert E, De Potter C, et al: Crohn's disease with adenocarcinoma and dysplasia. Macroscopical, histological, and immunohistochemical aspects of two cases. *Am J Surg Pathol* 1989; 13:187–196.

12. Das KM. Simon MR, Valenzuela I, et al: Serum antibodies from patients with Crohn's disease and from their household members react with murine lymphomas induced by Crohn's disease tissue filtrates. *J Lab Clin Med* 1986; 107:95–100.

13. Delpre G, Kadish U: A genetic predisposition for colorectal cancer in inflammatory bowel disease (letter). *Gut* 1988;29:1618.

14. Dennis C, Karlson KE: Cancer risk in ulcerative colitis: Formidability per patient year of late disease. *Surgery* 1961; 50:568.

15. Deschner EE, Winawer SJ, Katz S, et al: Proliferative defects in ulcerative colitis patients. *Cancer Invest* 1983; 1:41–47.

16. Dobbins WO III: Dysplasia and malignancy in inflammatory bowel disease. *Annu Rev Med* 1984;35:33–48.

17. Doldi K, Manger B, Koch B, et al: Spontaneous suppressor cell activity in the peripheral blood of patients with malignant and chronic inflammatory bowel diseases. *Clin Exp Immunol* 1984; 55:655–663

18. Ekelund G, Lindhagen T, Lindstrom C, et al: Surgical treatment of inflammatory bowel disease—a review of some current opinions and controversies. *Jpn J Surg* 1987; 17:413–424.

19. Feczko PJ: Malignancy complicating inflammatory bowel disease. *Radiol Clin North Am* 1987; 25:157–174.

20. Fiocchi C, Youngman KR, Yen-Lieberman B, et al: Modulation of intestinal immune reactivity by interleukin 2. Phenotypic and functional analysis of lymphokine activated killer cells from human intestinal mucosa. *Dig Dis Sci* 1988; 33:1305–1315.

21. Fischbach W, Mossner J, Seyschab H, et al: Tissue carcinoembryonic antigen and DNA aneuploidy in precancerous and cancerous colorectal lesions. *Cancer* 1990; 65:1820–1824.

22. Frykholm G, Enblad P, Pahlman L, et al: Expression of the carcinoma associated antigens CA 19 9 and CA 50 in inflammatory bowel disease. *Dis Colon Rectum* 1987; 30:545–548.

23. Gadacz T, McFadden DW, Gabrielson EW, et al: Adenocarcinoma of the il-

eostomy: The latent risk of cancer after colectomy for ulcerative colitis and familial polyposis. *Surgery* 1990; 107:698–703.

24. Gibson PR, Jewell DP: Local immune mechanisms in inflammatory bowel disease and colorectal carcinoma: Natural killer cells and their activity. *Gastroenterology* 1986; 90:12–19.

25. Greenstein AJ, Gennuso R, Sachar DB, et al: Extraintestinal cancers in inflammatory bowel disease. *Cancer* 1985; 56:2914–2921.

26. Greenstein AJ, Meyers S, Szporn A, et al: Colorectal cancer in regional ileitis. *Q J Med* 1987; 62:33–40.

27. Gyde SN: Cancer in inflammatory bowel disease. *Scand J Gastroenterol* 1989; 170(suppl):79–80.

28. Haas PA, Haas GP: A critical evaluation of the Hartmann's procedure. *Am Surg* 1988; 54:380–385.

29. Hope-Ross M, Magee DJ, O'Donoghue DP, et al: Ulcerative colitis complicated by lymphoma and adenocarcinoma. *Br J Surg* 1985; 72:22.

30. Johnson W, McDermott FT, Hughes ES, et al: The risk of rectal carcinoma following colectomy in ulcerative colitis. *Dis Colon Rectum* 1983; 26:44–46.

31. Katzka I, Brody RS, Morris E, et al: assessment of colorectal cancer risk in patients with ulcerative colitis: Experience from a private practice. *Gastroenterology* 1983; 85:22–29.

32. Kimura K, Koyanagi Y, Aoki T, et al: High-risk group: Colorectal cancer. *Gan To Kagaku Ryoho* 1987; 14:2650–2657.

33. Kirkeby HJ, Jakobsen J: Ulcerative colitis and malignant lymphoma of the intestine: Causal relation or differential diagnostic problem? *Ugeskr Laeger* 1983; 145:2224–2225.

34. Korelitz BI, Lauwers GY, Sommers SC: Rectal mucosal dysplasia in Crohn's disease. *Gut* 1990; 31:1382–1386.

35. Lashner BA, Turner C, Bostwick DG, et al: Dysplasia and cancer complicating strictures in ulcerative colitis. *Dig Dis Sci* 1990; 35:349–352.

36. Lavery IC, Jagelman DG: Cancer in the excluded rectum following surgery for inflammatory bowel disease. *Dis Colon Rectum* 1982; 25:522–524.

37. Lieberman BY, Fiocchi C, Youngman KR, et al: Inferferon gamma production by human intestinal mucosal mononuclear cells: Decreased levels in inflammatory bowel disease. *Dig Dis Sci* 1988; 33:1297–1304.

38. Lynch HT, Schuelke GS, Lynch JF: Genetics of rectal cancer. *Bull Cancer (Paris)* 1984; 71:1–15.

39. Manning A: Screening by colonoscopy for colonic epithelial dysplasia in inflammatory bowel disease. *Gut* 1987; 28:1489–1494.

40. Mayberry JF: Information booklets for patients with inflammatory bowel disease. *Int Disabil Stud* 1988; 10:179–180.

41. Meltzer SJ, Rotterdam HZ, Korelitz BI: Kaposi's sarcoma occurring in association with ulcerative colitis. *Am J Gastroenterol* 1987; 82:378–381.

42. Morson BC: Precancer and cancer in inflammatory bowel disease. *Pathology* 1985; 17:173–180.

43. Myren J, Bouchier IA, Watkinson G, et al: The O.M.G.E. Multinational In-

flammatory Bowel Disease Survey 1976–1982. A further report on 2,657 cases. *Scand J Gastroenterol* 1984; 95(suppl):1–27.

44. Perzin KH, Peterson M, Castiglione CL, et al: Intramucosal carcinoma of the small intestine arising in regional enteritis (Crohn's disease): Report of a case studied for carcinoembryonic antigen and review of the literature. *Cancer* 1984; 54:151–162.

45. Present DH, Meltzer SJ, Krumholz MP, et al: 6-Mercaptopurine in the management of inflammatory bowel disease: Short and long term toxicity. *Ann Intern Med* 1989; 111:641–649.

46. Riddell RH: Inflammatory bowel disease. Differential diagnosis and cancer of the small and large bowel. *Dig Dis Sci* 1985; 30:11S–13S.

47. Sackier JM, Wood CB: Ulcerative colitis and polyposis coli: Surgical options. *Surg Clin North Am* 1988; 68:1319–1338.

48. Sales DJ, Kirsner JB: The prognosis of inflammatory bowel disease. *Arch Intern Med* 1983; 143:294–299.

49. Scholmerich J, Sedlak P, Hoppe Seyler P, et al: The information needs and fears of patients with inflammatory bowel disease. *Hepatogastroenterology* 1987; 34:182–185.

50. Schrock TR: Conceptual developments through colonoscopy. *Surg Endosc* 1988; 2:240–244.

51. Schrumpf E, Fausa O, Aadland E, et al: Primary sclerosing cholangitis and inflammatory bowel disease. *Tidsskr Nor Laegeforen* 1990; 10:1212–1216.

52. Senay E, Sachar DB, Keohane M, et al: Small bowel carcinoma in Crohn's disease. Distinguishing features and risk factors. *Cancer* 1989; 63:360–363.

53. Shepherd NA, Hall PA, Williams GT, et al: Primary malignant lymphoma of the large intestine complicating chronic inflammatory bowel disease. *Histopathology* 1989; 15:325–337.

54. Shepherd NA, Hall PA, Coates PJ, et al: Primary malignant lymphoma of the colon and rectum. A histopathological and immunohistochemical analysis of 45 cases with clinicopathological correlations. *Histopathology* 1988; 12:235–252.

55. Sherlock DJ, Suarez V, Gray JG: Case reports: Stomal adenocarcinoma in Crohn's disease. *Gut* 1990; 31:1329–1332.

56. Slater G, Greenstein A, Aufses AH Jr: Anal carcinoma in patients with Crohn's disease. *Ann Surg* 1984; 199:348–350.

57. Smart PJ, Sastry S, Wells S: Case report: Primary mucinous adenocarcinoma developing in an ileostomy stoma. *Gut* 1988; 29:1607–1612.

58. Softley A, Clamp SE, Watkinson G, et al: The natural history of inflammatory bowel disease: Has there been a change in the last 20 years? *Scand J Gastroenterol (Suppl)* 1988; 144:20–23.

59. Thor A, Itzkowitz SH, Schlom J, et al: Tumor-associated glycoprotein (TAG-72) expression in ulcerative colitis. *Int J Cancer* 1989; 43:810–815.

60. Turunen MJ, Peltokallio P: Surgical results in 657 patients with colorectal cancer. *Dis Colon Rectum* 1983; 26:606–612.

61. Turunen MJ, Jarvinen HJ: Cancer in ulcerative colitis: What failed in follow up? *Acta Chir Scand* 1985; 151:669–673.
62. Walker AR, Segal I: Colorectal cancer: Some aspects of epidemiology, risk factors, treatment, screening and survival. *S Afr Med J* 1988; 73:653–657.
63. Wolf BC, Demillia JC, Salem RR, et al: Detection of the tumor associated glycoprotein antigen (TAG 72) in premalignant lesions of the colon. *J Natl Cancer Inst* 1989; 81:1913–1917.
64. Zajicek G: Inflammation initiates cancer by depleting stem cells. *Med Hypotheses* 1985; 18:207–219.

Discussion

DR. SACHAR: If you look at most studies of cancer risk ever published from anywhere around the world, whether they are prospective studies, population-based studies, or surveillance studies, the figures are nearly identical. After the first 10 years of disease, the cancer risk is ½% to 1% per year. There are some higher figures from Chicago that point out that the "hazard rate" may increase a little above the ½% to 1% level as more and more years go by. The Chicago study suggested that at about 20 years the annual risk may go as high as 3% and that at 30 years it could be as high as 5%. There are some lower figures published from Copenhagen, but that series comprised many patients who had already had colectomies. I must say that after a total proctocolectomy the risk for developing colorectal cancer is substantially lower. In brief, you can rely on the figures of ½% to 1% annual cancer risk after the first 10 years of colitis. In fact, these are precisely the figures we saw from Dr. Korelitz' presentation: a 6% prospective risk from a group of 120 patients with a mean follow-up of 16 years. That means in 6 years after the first 10 there was a 6% risk, which is 1% per year. You will always get the same figures if you calculate them correctly.

The question I would ask you, Dr. Korelitz, given what you have said about sampling error, what is the rationale for making the recommendation not to do anything about finding dysplasia until you have done it over again. You said you had to find high-grade dysplasia twice before acting on it. You said you would have to find low-grade dysplasia multiple times (three times). Now I grant you how important it is to have the slide reviewed and to make sure that two to three pathologists agree it is high-grade dysplasia, but if it is high-grade dysplasia, why do you have to wait to find it again?

DR. KORELITZ: I agree with you if it is clearly high-grade dysplasia, and if there are no extenuating circumstances, it is enough. Once you have had the experience of seeing a carcinoma develop overnight in someone who had previous dysplasia, you never forget it. I don't feel that the one-time finding of low-grade dysplasia, even if confirmed by another pathologist, is sufficiently conclusive to warrant colectomy for its own sake. It should, however, warrant very careful surveillance.

Dr. Sachar: Having gotten Dr. Korelitz to agree with me, at least in part, I will quit.

Q: Can folic acid supplements reduce the risk of colon cancer in ulcerative colitis?

Dr. Sachar: *That is a very interesting observation that just came out of Lashner and Hanauer's report in which they suggested from their surveillance group of 99 patients that those who were not on folate supplementation, whether or not they were taking Azulfidine, had a higher risk of dysplasia and cancer than those who were taking folate supplements. The problem is that they never give the data. They tell us there is an increased relative risk in the group not taking folate, but they never tell us exactly how many cancers or dysplasias arose in the patients taking folate vs. those not taking folate. Not only do we have to take their word for it that the relative risk now increased, but also the increase was not in any event statistically significant, i.e., the 95% confidence levels for the relative risk overlapped unity. Nonetheless, I feel it is a provocative finding. I don't feel it is established that folate deficiency contributes to cancer nor that giving folate to patients will prevent cancer. But two facts emerge. First, the hypothesis is testable. You can, as was pointed out by Rosenberg in a recent editorial in* Gastroenterology, *go back to the data and show the actual calculations or, even better, you can test the hypothesis prospectively. Second, it is cheap and harmless to give folate supplementation, so why not do it anyhow, especially for patients who are on sulfasalazine?*

Q: What was the Dukes classification of the tumors in Dr. Woolrich's series?

Dr. Woolrich: Of the seven tumors found, four were Dukes A, two were Dukes C, and one was Dukes D.

Dr. Sachar: The general experience is that those cancers detected purely by surveillance programs have always tended to have better prognostic Dukes classifications than those found in the course of ordinary clinical follow-up. The hypothesis therefore is that it is a good thing to do surveillance because when you find a cancer it will be earlier and therefore curable. From that concept the hypothesis emerges that if you do surveillance you will save lives. The bottom line conclusion, however, has never been established by any study.

In other words, it has never been shown that a surveillance program for dysplasia saves any lives that would otherwise have been lost if the patients were followed up with equal clinical intensity but not surveyed routinely for dysplasia. One recent study on the subject from the University of Chicago, for example, was unable to show that their surveillance program of 99 people over a period of years reduced cancer mortality. Maybe we need to look for better markers like DNA aneuploidy, altered mucin histochemistry, or oncogenes, since dysplasia may not be the best way to do it.

Q: Can colonic dysplasia spontaneously regress?

DR. SACHAR: No one really knows the answer to that question. It is almost impossible to know whether dysplasia actually waxes and wanes or if it is simply the sampling that varies. What do our pathologists say about it?

DR. LAUWERS: Part of the issue is whether all cases diagnosed as dysplasia really are dysplasia. For high-grade dysplasia I believe so, but whatever is low grade may fall into the range of disagreement among pathologists. Maybe those low-grade dysplasias that seem to disappear were really reactive atypia that was secondary to inflammation and activity of disease.

DR. SACHAR: My bias is that reactive atypia may regress, but that real dysplasia persists, if you can only find it again.

Q: If you see a raised lesion and biopsy shows low-grade dysplasia, has anyone thought about using some sort of endoscopic means to obliterate that area?

DR. SACHAR: That is not the issue. The concern is not that a dysplasia-associated lesion or mass is necessarily the specific site that degenerates into malignancy, so that if you obliterate that you are okay. The issue is that a lesion is a marker for a whole colon at high risk. What you need to do is not endoscopy to obliterate the dysplastic mass, but surgery to remove the entire colon.

Q: But if you follow it along every 3 months anyway, why not go on and get rid of it.

DR. SACHAR: I would not follow it every 3 months, I would do a colectomy at that point.

DR. KORELITZ: My slide included it as an indication for surgery. Even low-grade dysplasia plus mass warrants colectomy.

Q: There was a paper in *Cancer* about a year ago suggesting a correlation between CEA levels and the Dukes classification, and I was wondering if anyone uses CEA levels to follow the dysplasia.

Dr. Sachar: They are talking about tissue CEA, not serum CEA. That CEA issue has been repeatedly studied, and our own study of 112 patients many years ago showed that circulating CEA levels are absolutely useless and bear no correlation with cancer risk, dysplasia, or anything else. There have been some studies with histochemical staining, however, suggesting that tissue CEA might be a more objective marker of dysplasia. This is just one of many immunohistochemical techniques, oncogene probe techniques, and DNA aneuploid techniques that are all trying to objectify dysplasia. I feel that is where the future lies. The 1990s will see the substitution of more objective, more sensitive, and more predictive biomarkers than for the subjective morphological reading of dysplasia. We will probably start with morphometrics and go on from there to other forms of biomarkers, but we cannot rely on serum CEA.

PART 6 _____

Drug Therapy

_____

Chapter 24 _____

Efficacy of Current Drugs in Inflammatory Bowel Disease

Henry Janowitz

_____

One can predict without fear of contradiction that the 1990s will see a continuing flood of new drugs. Some will be what I ironically call "old wine" in "new bottles," but undoubtedly we will see lots of new drugs. Their place in our scheme of therapy undoubtedly will be related to how they compare with our current drugs. My colleagues, Peter Salomon, Asher Kornbluth, and Henry Sachs, and I have been trying to make an analysis of the current drugs we are using in controlled trials. My emphasis will be mostly on ulcerative colitis, for which some data exist, and there may be a few comments on Crohn's disease where there is a greater paucity of information.

We know our drugs are better than placebo or we would not use them. That was true for a long time for antacids in ulcer disease. We knew they worked but we had not proved it. How much better are our placebos than current drugs in the management of mild to moderate ulcerative colitis? There are no controlled trials of severe disease, severe ulcerative colitis, or fulminating ulcerative colitis. I think this is unethical, and we are unlikely ever to see controlled trials of these conditions.

Equally important, how much better are current drugs than placebos in maintaining remission in ulcerative colitis? Of course, the trendy word these days is meta-analysis. We tried to do a meta-analysis of placebo-controlled trials; we had to start somewhere, so we started with single drugs vs. placebo in mild to moderate ulcerative colitis. This is just the first step in such an analysis. We excluded trials in patients who were allowed to continue pretrial drugs. This is really an abstraction, but I think for the purpose of analysis we have to begin somewhere, and this is what we decided to do. For the first part, we will cover drug vs. placebo, in which we excluded for the moment drug vs. drug comparison, although I will have something to say about that. We also excluded drugs that were no longer used.

We could find only 11 trials of therapy of mild to moderate active disease and five trials of maintenance therapy that fulfill these criteria. I already pointed out that we are not talking about severe ulcerative colitis.

We are talking here about how much better than these placebos are our drugs. What is the "therapeutic advantage," or what is referred to as the "therapeutic gain," of using a drug vs. placebo. The difference, of course, between drug and placebo is the therapeutic advantage in this concept.

The agents used in these studies included steroids, sulfasalazine, 5-aminosalicylic acid, and related compounds. Excluded from analysis were drug-vs.-drug trials, studies that allowed patients to continue taking pretrial medications.

In the therapeutic trials, a total of 363 patients were treated for 15 to 42 days for single episodes of mild to moderate ulcerative colitis. Success rates were computed in three categories: complete clinical remission, complete or partial remission, and complete sigmoidoscopic remission.

It is clear that there is an advantage in using the available drugs. A complete or partial remission will be achieved in 75% of patients with single-drug therapy, compared with only 27% with placebo. Sigmoidoscopic improvement lagged behind clinical improvement, but a therapeutic gain was nevertheless evident.

In the 5 maintenance trials, 361 patients were treated for either 6 or 12 months. Among patients receiving single-drug therapy, 73% were in remission at 6 months, and 71% remained in remission at 12 months. In contrast, 51% of those receiving placebo remained in remission at 6 months, and only 24% were in remission at 12 months.

In those five trials, the difference between a drug and a placebo in maintaining remission in patients with mild to moderate ulcerative colitis is not very striking at the end of the first 6 months. At the end of 1 year, however, it becomes clear that continuation of the maintenance drug is worthwhile.

I think we have all observed that our patients doing fairly well on sulfasalazine get tired of taking it because they cannot see that they are much better off than before, since they are still in remission. It is at the end of the year that it is clear that it is worthwhile continuing with maintenance drug. Incidentally, on all of these I have not shown whether we have the appropriate statistics; the rate differences, the confidence limits, and the *P* values that we hope to publish when we finish this study.

To summarize, with placebo vs. a single drug in mild to moderate ulcerative colitis, a partial remission will be achieved in 75% of patients with single-drug therapy compared with only about 25% in patients on placebo. As far as remission, we maintained up to 12 months in approximately three-fourths of patients with single drug, while on placebo one-half of the patients remained in remission for 6 months, but only one-fourth were in remission at the end of 12 months.

DRUG COMPARISONS

Another meta-analysis was undertaken to examine data from 13 trials in which various drugs were compared. For each agent the percentage of clinical improvement in the drug-vs.-host studies was also compared with that in the drug-vs.-placebo studies.

There was no significant difference when any of these drugs was compared or tested against another. Furthermore, the magnitude of each agent's therapeutic effect in comparative trials was comparable to that in the placebo-controlled studies.

MAINTENANCE STUDIES

There were 11 trials with about 250 patients in which maintenance studies were done. Here we compared the maintenance of sulfasalazine in drug-vs.-drug and in drug-vs.-placebo trials. There was no statistical significance between them at either 6 or 12 months. This leads us to conclude at this point regarding this kind of study that it may not be necessary ethically and probably scientifically to do placebo studies anymore when we have a positive control study where the numbers are of the same magnitude.

UNRESOLVED ISSUES

Despite 30 years of trials, we do not have the requisite data to predict difference in response based on duration of attack being studied, whether it was the first or one of many attacks. We lack data on relationship to the extent of disease. I believe that the duration of the illness makes some difference in whether the patient will respond again in a new episode. So please, if you are going to do any control trials give us all that data in the original protocols. Sort out the patients and tell us how many attacks they have had, their duration, extent of disease, and duration of disease.

TREATMENT OF SEVERE ULCERATIVE COLITIS

Regarding severe ulcerative colitis, we will not have any controlled trials, so the best we can expect to have are data based on comparison of drugs. There are only a few studies of comparisons of drugs in severe or fulminant ulcerative colitis, but there are the three studies on corticotropins vs. hydrocortisone. I am not presently interested in the difference between these drugs or a comparison as such, but rather what was the overall result of treating patients with severe ulcerative colitis with steroids in a controlled setting. In the London study by Powell-Tuck et al.[4] a small group of 16 patients was studied. Fifty-six percent of patients improved, and 40% underwent surgery. In the New Haven study, which is confused by the fact that they included patients with acute Crohn's disease and acute ulcerative colitis, the overall rate of improvement was about 68%.[2] While the difference between the drugs is approached but did not have statistical significance, only about two-thirds of patients improved in the severe situation.

In our study of 66 patients, the overall remission rate of fulminant and severe ulcerative colitis with one or another of the steroids was only 42%.[3] In the subgroups the best overall remission rate was 55% or 63%. Steroids obviously have not solved the question of ulcerative colitis in these studies.

Another way of approaching the severe fulminant ulcerative colitis, since we are not going to have any controlled trials, is to consider Truelove et al. and Jarnerot's "atomic blast" therapy. Truelove: 5 days, intravenous steroid, antibiotics, 5-aminosalicylic acid or sulfasalazine, and steroid enemas[5,6]; 100 trials in 87 patients with remission in 60%, 40% going on to surgery. The advantage of the therapy was 20%. Jarnerot's study was not quite so dogmatic as to the day of surgical guillotine: 62 patients treated with a similar program; 47% did not go to the operating room, and 53% did.[1] How would you calculate the therapeutic advantage?

It is obvious the treatment of severe ulcerative colitis has not been solved by the use of intravenous steroids alone, and it is in the light of this that I look forward to hearing what the status of cyclosporine is in these fulminant cases compared with what is already available in the literature.

REFERENCES

1. Jarnerot G, Rolny P, Sandberg-Gertzen H: Intensive intravenous treatment of ulcerative colitis. *Gastroenterology* 1985; 89:1005–1013.
2. Kaplan HP, Portnoy B, Binder HJ, et al: A controlled evaluation of intravenous adrenocorticotropic hormone and hydrocortisone in the treatment of acute colitis. *Gastroenterology* 1975; 69:91–95.
3. Meyers S, Lerer PK, Feuer EJ, et al: Predicting the outcome of corticoid therapy for acute ulcerative colitis: Results of a prospective, randomized, double-blind clinical trial. *J Clin Gastroenterol* 1987; 9:50–54.
4. Powell-Tuck J, Buckell NA, Lennard-Jones JE: A controlled comparison of corticotropin and hydrocortisone in the treatment of severe proctocolitis. *Scand J Gastroenterol* 1977; 12:971–975.
5. Truelove SC, Jewell DP: Intensive intravenous regimen for severe attacks of ulcerative colitis. *Lancet* 1974; 1:1067–1070.
6. Truelove SC, Willoughby CP, Lee EG, et al: Further experience in the treatment of severe attacks of ulcerative colitis. *Lancet* 1978; 2:1086–1088.

SUGGESTED READING

Korelitz BI, Margolin ML: Clinical trials in ulcerative colitis. I: Personal observations. *Am J Gastroenterol* 1988; 83:224–226.

Margolin ML, Krumholz MP, Fochios SE, et al: Clinical trials in ulcerative colitis. II: Historical review. *Am J Gastroenterol* 1988; 83:227–243.

Chapter 25 _____

Use of Asacol in Treatment of Inflammatory Bowel Disease

Steven M. Faber
Burton I. Korelitz

Sulfasalazine, developed in the 1940s for use in patients with colitis,[11] has been the most widely prescribed agent in the therapy of inflammatory bowel disease (IBD). Its use, however, has been compromised by the adverse reactions observed in up to one third of patients.[7]

Observations on the biochemical pathways of sulfasalazine have led to the understanding that, for successful therapeutic benefit, 5-aminosalicylic acid (5-ASA; mesalamine), the effective split product of sulfasalazine, must accumulate in the colon, where it has a topical action.[1,8] While sulfasalazine has been shown to inhibit colonic leuko-triene B_4 (LTB_4) synthesis,[12] 5-ASA reportedly selectively affects the cyclooxygenase pathway of arachidonic acid metabolism, and, in a dose-dependent manner, inhibits the release of LTB_4 and sulfidopeptide-LT from normal human colonic mucosa.[8]

We report our experience in treating ulcerative colitis and Crohn's disease with Asacol, Norwich Eaton's brand of 5-ASA prepared in tablets coated with an acrylic base resin (eudragit-S). In this form release is delayed until the drug reaches the distal area of the ileum and colon, where the pH is greater than 7 and the coating is dissolved.

CLINICAL TRIALS

Patient Population

Our observations on the use of Asacol in IBD are based on the review of 66 patients treated in the private gastroenterology practice of one of us (B. I. K.) between 1985 and the present. The indications for trial of Asacol were reviewed, as well as all evidence of tolerance, adverse reactions, and therapeutic effectiveness. In all patients, whether intolerant or allergic to sulfasalazine or not, Asacol was started at 400 mg, or one tablet daily, and then increased at varying rates to larger doses, up to 12 tablets per day.

The patient population consisted of 66 patients, 31 male and 35 female. Thirty-eight had ulcerative colitis, 25 had Crohn's disease, and 3 had indeterminate colitis. The distribution of involvement of the 38 patients with ulcerative colitis and the 25 patients with Crohn's disease is shown in Table 25–1.

Design and Methods

Indications for Asacol use were organized into the following categories (Table 25–2): (1) patients who had allergic reactions to sulfasalazine, (2) patients intolerant to sulfasalazine, and (3) patients with asymptomatic, nonallergic complications of sulfasalazine therapy.

In three patients the Asacol was introduced to supplement the dose of sulfasalazine in the hope of avoiding intolerance because of a still

TABLE 25–1.
Asacol Therapy of IBD in 66 Patients

	No.	Active disease	In remission	Treatment duration (in mo) Range	Mean	Maximum dosage (in g/day) Range	Mean
Ulcerative colitis							
Universal	8	4	4	4–43	16.1	1.2–3.2	2.4
Left-sided	8	6	2	5–41	12.5	1.6–4.8	2.5
Proctosigmoiditis	18	10	8	4–25	10.1	1.6–3.2	1.9
Proctitis	4	2	2	7–35	18.5	1.6–3.6	2.8
Total	38	22/38 (58%)	16/38 (42%)	5–36	14.3	1.5–3.7	2.4
Crohn's disease							
Ileitis	15	7	8	1–48	11.5	1.6–3.25	2.05
Colitis	3	2	1	9–21	14.0	0.8–3.25	1.86
Ileocolitis	2	1	1	3–27	15.0	1.6	1.6
Proctosigmoiditis	3	2	1	3–25	12.0	1.2–3.2	2.5
Proctitis	2	2	—	13–14	13.5	1.6–3.2	2.4
Total	25	14/25 (56%)	11/25 (44%)	5.8–27	13.2	1.3–2.9	2.07
Indeterminate colitis	3	2	1	10–37	24.6	1.2–3.2	5.6
Grand total	66	38/66	28/66				

TABLE 25–2.
Indications for Trial of Asacol in Patients
With IBD

	No. of Patients
Allergic reaction	
Rash	8
Urticaria	3
Pruritus	2
Oral lesions	2
Chronic interstitial nephritis	1
	16
Dominating symptom	
Headache	15
Nausea	11
Fatigue	10
Personality change	3
Heartburn	2
Fever	1
	42
Other complications	
Hypospermia	3
Abnormal liver function	2
Macrocytic anemia	1
	6
To supplement sulfasalazine	3
Failure of sulfasalazine	2

higher dose of sulfasalazine. In only one instance was the Asacol tried despite failure of sulfasalazine.

Results

When treatment with Asacol was initiated, some patients had active disease, whereas in others the disease was in remission. Table 25–3 shows the response of patients with ulcerative colitis. "Therapeutic Response" was defined as symptomatic and endoscopic improvement with Asacol alone for greater than 6 months. The column headed "±" summarizes those patients for whom we were not able to determine therapeutic response to Asacol, given the presence of concurrent medications. The column headed "0" enumerates those patients showing no response to Asacol.

Results in Ulcerative Colitis

The results show that 32% of patients with active ulcerative colitis had a therapeutic response. In another 59% the response was favorable, but concomitant medications made Asacol's role difficult to interpret, and in 9% of patients there was no response to therapy.

There were 16 patients with ulcerative colitis in remission in whom Asacol was introduced for the purpose of maintaining the remission (see Table 25–3). Forty-four percent remained symptom free for at least 6 months. In 50% the remission continued, but Asacol's role was not clear because of the use of concomitant medications. In 6%, Asacol did not serve to maintain the remission.

Results in Crohn's Disease

In 14 patients, Asacol was used to bring active Crohn's disease into remission (Table 25–4). In 8 (57%) Asacol was successful, in 4 (29%) the role of Asacol could not be determined because of concomitant medications, and in 2 (14%) there was no response to therapy. For 11 patients with Crohn's disease in remission at the start of Asacol therapy (Table

TABLE 25–3.

Response to Asacol in 38 Patients with Ulcerative Colitis

	No. of Patients	Therapeutic Response		
		+*	±†	0‡
Active				
Universal	4	1	3	0
Left-sided	6	2	4	0
Proctosigmoiditis	10	3	6	1
Proctitis	2	1	0	1
	22	7 (32%)	13 (59%)	2 (9%)

	No. of Patients	Maintenance of Remission		
		+§	±	0
Remission				
Universal	4	2	2	0
Left-sided	2	2	1	0
Proctosigmoiditis	8	3	5	0
Proctitis	2	1	0	1
	16	7 (44%)	8 (50%)	1 (6%)
Total	38	14 (37%)	21 (55%)	3 (8%)

*More than 6 months of therapy with Asacol alone, with symptomatic and endoscopic improvement.
†Not able to determine, because of concomitant medications.
‡No response.
§More than 6 months of therapy with Asacol alone, with maintenance of remission.

TABLE 25–4.
Response to Asacol in 25 Patients With Crohn's Disease

	No. of Patients	Therapeutic Response		
		+*	±†	0‡
Active				
Ileitis	7	4	3	0
Ileocolitis	1	1	0	0
Colonic	2	1	0	1
Proctosigmoiditis	2	0	1	1
Proctitis	2	2	0	0
	14	8 (57%)	4 (29%)	2 (14%)

		Maintenance of Remission		
		+§	±	0
Remission				
Ileitis	8	5	2	1
Colitis	1	1	0	0
Proctosigmoiditis	1	1	0	0
Ileocolitis	1	0	0	1
	11	7 (64%)	2 (18%)	2 (18%)
Total	25	15 (60%)	6 (24%)	4 (16%)

*More than 6 months of Asacol therapy alone, with symptomatic and endoscopic improvement.
†Not able to determine, because of concomitant medications.
‡No response.
§More than 6 months of Asacol therapy alone, with maintenance of remission

25–4), 7 (64%) successfully maintained remission during the 6 months that followed, in 2 (18%) the response to Asacol could not be determined because of other medications, and in 2 (18%) there was no response. Two of the 3 patients with indeterminate colitis had a therapeutic response, and 1 had successful maintenance of remission.

Adverse Reactions

In Table 25–5 adverse reactions coincident with the use of Asacol and the mean Asacol doses are recorded. Twenty-two patients (33%) had some type of adverse reaction. Only 9 of the 66 patients (14%) had to discontinue the Asacol because of these adverse reactions. In most patients a reduction in dose was followed by a reduction in side effects.

Later Management

At the time of follow-up, 45 of the 66 patients remained on a regimen of Asacol therapy, with 25 having thus far responded with resulting remission of disease, 15 with continued maintenance of remission, and

TABLE 25–5.
Adverse Reactions Coincident With Use of
Asacol in 66 Patients With IBD

Reaction	No. of Patients	Mean Dose (gm/day)
Headache	7	2.5
Increased frequency of bowel movements	4	2.4
Hair loss	2	3.2
Fatigue	2	2.6
Nausea	2	1.6
Rash	1	1.6
Cerebral paresthesias	1	1.6
Memory loss and swollen tongue	1	1.6
Abdominal cramps	1	1.6
Reduced concentration	1	3.2
Total	22 (33%)	

5 with effectiveness not yet established because of coincident medications. The 21 patients no longer on a regimen of Asacol therapy had stopped because of adverse reactions, surgery, loss to follow-up, noncompliance, or no response to the drug.

DISCUSSION

This retrospective study served to assess the efficacy of Asacol as used in a private gastroenterologic practice for treatment of IBD. The 66 patients we considered appropriate for a trial included 38 with ulcerative colitis, 25 with Crohn's disease, and 3 with indeterminate colitis. Of the 38 patients with ulcerative colitis and the 25 with Crohn's disease, 22 and 16, respectively, had active disease, while in 16 and 11 the disease was in remission but the patients were allergic or intolerant to sulfasalazine. The use of Asacol alone for 6 months in patients with active ulcerative colitis at an average dosage of 2.4 g/day resulted in a complete therapeutic response in 7 of 9 patients (78%). Although the numbers are small, the results are still better than those of Schroeder et al.[10] In their series of patients with mild to moderately active ulcerative colitis, after 6 weeks of therapy 24% had complete response and 50% had partial response on a regimen of Asacol of 4 to 8 g/day. Habal and Greenberg,[4] with use of Asacol for treatment of 85 patients who had active ulcerative colitis, noted a 29% rate of remission with Asacol alone during an acute attack, but a 64% overall rate of remission for mild to moderately active ulcerative colitis. Meyers et al.,[6] with use of olsalazine (Dipentum), showed that 35% of patients with active ulcerative colitis improved clinically after 21 days of the drug vs. 16% with placebo.

In our study 44% of patients whose disease was in remission remained in remission for more than 6 months on a regimen of Asacol alone. In another 50% of patients maintenance of remission was also achieved, but Asacol's role could not be determined because of concomitant medications. Dew et al.[1a, 2] with use of Asacol vs. sulfasalazine for 16 weeks in 67 patients with ulcerative colitis in remission, found that 9 of 34 on a regimen of Asacol at 1.2 g/day and 6 of 33 on a regimen of sulfasalazine showed relapse of remission of disease during the study period. These results suggest that Asacol was as effective as sulfasalazine for maintenance of remission in ulcerative colitis.

The use of Asacol alone for 6 months in patients with active Crohn's disease at an average dose of 2.4 g/day resulted in a complete therapeutic response in 8 of 10 patients (80%). Again, the numbers are small, but the results were better than expected.

Rasmussen et al.,[9] in an open trial with use of oral 5-ASA in the form of Pentasa in 18 patients at 1.5 g/day for six weeks for short-term treatment of ileitis and ileocolitis, showed that in 72% the patients' condition improved. Hanauer et al.[5] also treating Crohn's disease with Pentasa, showed a dose-related response, with 67% success rate at 4 g/day. Pentasa contains 250 mg of 5-ASA in microgranules that are coated with a semipermeable membrane of ethylcellulose. Ethylcellulose has amphioionic properties in aqueous solutions; therefore 5-ASA should, in principle, be released from the granules at either an alkaline or an acid pH. This is in contrast to Asacol; with its use release is delayed until the drug reaches the distal areas of the ileum and colon where the pH is greater than 7. Our favorable results seen with use of Asacol in ileitis may be related to earlier activation of the drug due to narrowed, inflamed bowel, which delays its transit and provides prolonged contact at the optimum pH.

Maintenance of remission was also achieved in 64% of patients with Crohn's disease. We found that 22 of 66 patients (33%) manifested adverse reactions on a regimen of Asacol therapy, with only 9 of 66 patients (14%) discontinuing the drug because of side effects. Headache was the most common. An increased number of bowel movements could be attributed to Asacol in only 4 of 66 cases.

Habal and Greenberg[4] recorded 6 of 85 patients with side effects of Asacol. The most common was severe retrosternal chest pain in 3 of 6; 4

of 6 had an increase in stool volume and frequency; 2 of 6 had maculo-papular rash, and 2 of 6 upper extremity paresthesias.[4] In our study one patient had a maculopapular rash, and one had paresthesias. Dew et al,[2] with use of Asacol, reported 6 of 35 patients with side effects of nau-sea and abdominal discomfort. Schroeder et al.[10] reported that Asacol was discontinued in only 4 of 92 patients because of adverse reactions, which included diarrhea in 2 and 1 each with nausea and with vomit-ing. Meyers et al.[6] found that 6 of 66 patients on a regimen of olsalazine developed adverse reactions, with only 4 of 66 patients withdrawing from the study, 2 with skin rash and 2 with diarrhea.

The higher prevalence of adverse reactions noted in our study of Asacol use may be explained by the vulnerability of the trial population as evidenced by the almost total incidence of allergic or toxic reaction to previous drug therapy (sulfasalazine). We also noted that a dose re-duction often gave relief from side effects, so that only 9 of 66, or 15%, had to terminate the drug.

Some studies[6, 8] have suggested that a dose-response relationship exists when using mesalamine. Determination of whether a higher dos-age will improve the therapeutic outcome in patients with more severe disease requires further investigation. Hanauer et al.[5] showed a dose-re-lated response to Pentasa in patients with active Crohn's disease, with a 67% success rate at 4 g/day.

Asacol is clearly a safe, well-tolerated therapeutic alternative in the management of both Crohn's disease and ulcerative colitis. Future dou-ble-blind, randomized studies will be necessary to demonstrate further the effectiveness of this drug in select distributions of Crohn's disease and degrees of severity of ulcerative colitis, both alone and in conjunc-tion with other agents.

CONCLUSIONS

In the 22 patients with active ulcerative colitis, therapeutic results could be assessed in 9; there was symptomatic and endoscopic re-sponse in 7 (77%). In the 14 patients with active Crohn's disease, thera-peutic results could be assessed in 10; there was symptomatic and en-doscopic response in 8 (80%). Remission was maintained in 7 of 8 (94%) patients with ulcerative colitis and in 7 of 9 (82%) patients with Crohn's disease. Adverse reactions of varying severity occurred in 33%. While most were sufficiently modified by dose reduction, the drug had to be stopped in 14%.

Asacol is effective in the treatment and maintenance of remission of

ulcerative colitis at least to the same degree as the parent drug sulfasalazine. The favorable results in Crohn's disease were unexpected,
and show greater promise than sulfasalazine. The results in ileitis were
particularly impressive (57%), since the parent drug is effective in only
25%.[3]

The overall favorable results in active and inactive Crohn's disease
may be due to the anatomic narrowing from inflammation, edema, and
nodularity in segments of small bowel and terminal ileum, causing a
more protracted topical effect of the 5-ASA in these areas, whereas the
parent product would be inert before release of the 5-ASA by colonic
bacteria. Asacol was well tolerated in 68% of patients intolerant or allergic to sulfa drugs, with a therapeutic response rate similar to that in ulcerative colitis and better than that for Crohn's disease with sulfasalazine at equivalent doses.

REFERENCES

1. Azad Kahn AK, Piris J, Truelove SC: An experiment to determine the active
   therapeutic moiety of sulfasalazine. *Lancet* 1977; 2:892–895.
1a. Dew MJ, Hughes P, Harries AD, et al: Maintenance of remission in ulcerative colitis with oral preparation of 5-aminosalicylic acid. *Br Med J* 1985;
   285:1012.
2. Dew MJ, Harris MD, Evans BK, et al: Treatment of ulcerative colitis with
   oral 5-aminosalicylic acid in patients unable to take sulphasalazine. *Lancet*
   1983; 3:801.
3. Goldstein F, Farquahar JJ, Thornton J, et al: Favorable effects of sulfasalazine on small bowel Crohn's disease. *Am J Gastroenterol* 1987; 82:848–853.
4. Habal FM, Greenberg GR: Treatment of ulcerative colitis with oral 5-
   aminosalicylic acid including patients with adverse reactions to sulfasalazine. *Am J Gastroenterol* 1988; 83:15–91.
5. Hanauer SB, Belker ME, Gitnick G, et al: Placebo controlled dose ranging
   study of oral Pentasa (controlled release mesalamine) for active Crohn's
   disease: Preliminary results. *Gastroenterology* 1990; 98:A173.
6. Meyers S, Sachar DB, Present DH, et al: Olsalazine sodium in the treatment
   of ulcerative colitis among patients intolerant of sulfasalazine. *Gastroenterology* 1987; 93:1255–1262.
7. Peppercorn MA: Sulfasalazine: Pharmacology, clinical use, toxicity and related new drug development. *Ann Intern Med* 1984; 101:337–386.
8. Peskar BM, Dreyling B, May K, et al: Possible mode of action of 5-
   aminosalicylic acid. *Dig Dis Sci* 1987; 32(suppl):51S–56S.
9. Rasmussen SN, Binder V, Maier K, et al: Treatment of Crohn's disease with
   peroral 5-aminosalicylic acid. *Gastroenterology* 1983; 85:1350–1353.
10. Schroeder W, Tremaine MD. Ilstrup DM: Coated oral 5-aminosalicylic acid

therapy for mildly to moderately active ulcerative colitis. *N Engl J Med* 1987; 317:1625–1629.

11. Svartz N: The treatment of 124 cases of ulcerative colitis with salazopyrine and attempts of desensitization in cases of hypersensitiveness to sulpha. *Acta Med Scand* [Suppl] 1948; 206:465–472.

12. Van Hees PAM, Van Tongeren JHM, Bakker JH, et al: Active therapeutic moiety of sulphasalazine and its metabolites in patients with ulcerative colitis and Crohn's disease. *Lancet* 1978; 1:277.

Chapter 26 _____

Use of Sulfasalazine and 5-Aminosalicylic Acid in Inflammatory Bowel Disease

Mark A. Peppercorn

Sulfasalazine, first known as salazopyrin, was introduced into clinical medicine by Nana Svartz, a Scandinavian rheumatologist whose primary interest was in rheumatoid arthritis. It was theorized at that time that rheumatoid arthritis might be caused by bacteria, and it was known that it responded to salicylates. Sulfasalazine links one of the first sulfonamides, sulfapyridine, to an aspirin analog 5-aminosalicylate, joined through a nitrogen-nitrogen double bond or azo bond (Fig 26–1).

The therapeutic results in rheumatoid arthritis are good, and in Europe sulfasalazine is still the primary therapy. Fortunately Dr. Svartz and her colleagues had an interest in colitis as well, and when they applied the use of sulfasalazine to treatment for colitis the results were even more striking. Sulfasalazine has since become one of the mainstays of therapy for inflammatory bowel disease (IBD).

CLINICAL USE OF SULFASALAZINE

Data from controlled trials support the use of sulfasalazine for treatment of ulcerative colitis as a first-line agent in mild to moderate active disease regardless of extent of disease.[7, 12] Most patients take 3 to 4 g to achieve response when the disease is active. It is important to start at a low dosage of 500 mg two times a day and work up for 7 to 10 days to the so-called therapeutic dose for two reasons: (1) to minimize the tendency to side effects, and (2) there are occasional patients who have a

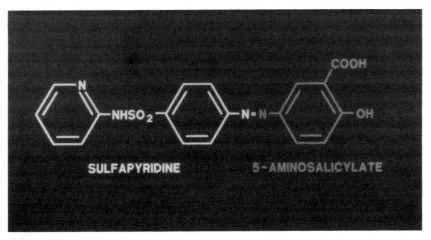

FIG 26–1.
Structural formula for sulfasalazine.

remarkable response even within days to a lower dose, which can be maintained. A liquid concentrate or pills in emulsion given in an enema also will work in distal disease. Because sulfasalazine may interfere with the absorption of dietary forms of folic, folic acid tablets (1 mg/day) are added.

Sulfasalazine has never been studied in controlled fashion in ulcerative colitis as an adjunct to other drugs such as corticosteroids, even though many of us use it in that context. It has not been studied in any fashion in severe disease where steroids are the choice of therapy, although occasionally it can be added to therapy in severe disease and may have some limited impact. One of the major roles in ulcerative colitis is in maintenance of remission.[9] Any patient who has repeated episodes of ulcerative colitis, or whose ulcerative colitis goes into remission after a moderate or severe episode of colitis, is a candidate for long-term remission therapy. One study suggested that 4 g of sulfasalazine was the optimal maintenance dose, but most patients will not take eight pills/day if they feel well. Most of us settle for 2 g daily as a maintenance dose.

In Crohn's disease the evidence of efficacy from controlled trials was a little later in coming, but certainly it has been shown convincingly that sulfasalazine is useful in mild to moderate active Crohn's disease, particularly when the colon is involved.[15] There is a debate about its utility in isolated ileal disease, although a body of anecdotal experience, including my own, suggests that there is at least a subgroup of patients with ileal disease alone who do respond.

Therefore I will use sulfasalazine generally as my first choice in mild to moderate active Crohn's disease regardless of distribution. Unfortunately and inexplicably, it has not been shown that sulfasalazine maintains remission in Crohn's disease as it does so well in ulcerative colitis. In a practice, however, many patients with Crohn's disease are maintained on sulfasalazine indefinitely, particularly if their disease has been difficult to manage. On the other hand, there is really no justification for continued use of sulfasalazine once a patient has had all obvious disease resected, since it clearly does not prevent recurrences postoperatively.

Gastroenterologists frequently are asked about the use of drugs during pregnancy and in mothers who are breast-feeding. It is clear that sulfasalazine is safe for both.[10] There are no adverse effects on pregnancy itself, there has been no evidence of fetal teratogenicity, and there are no reports of kernicterus in the nursing baby. With regard to neonatal jaundice, the competition for bilirubin binding to albumin by sulfapyridine is minimal. In general we use sulfasalazine in pregnant women just as we do in those who are not pregnant.

SULFASALAZINE TOXICITY

One of the problems with sulfasalazine, as is true with all of our treatments, is toxicity.

1. Common side effects include dyspepsia, nausea, anorexia, and headache.
2. Allergic reactions include rash, fever, and arthralgia.
3. Hematologic effects can be mild, including mild hemolysis, mild neutropenia, and folate deficiency; or severe, including severe hemolysis and agranulocytosis.
4. Male infertility can develop.
5. Severe toxic reactions can involve lung, liver, pancreas, skin, and central nervous system.

As many as 20% of patients will have side effects, sometimes limiting the use of the drug.[6] Common effects, such as nausea, anorexia, and headache, usually can be overcome by just lowering the dose. Mild allergic reactions (rash, fever, and mild arthralgia) occur in 5% to 10% of patients, and as many as three quarters of these patients can be continued on the drug through a process of desensitization in which very low doses of a tablet or liquid form gradually work up after several weeks to therapeutic doses.* The more severe adverse reactions clearly limit its use, however.

In patients with severe neutropenia or agranulocytosis, severe hemolytic anemia, or toxic reactions involving almost every organ system, the use of sulfasalazine must be stopped. Reversible male infertility may be a problem, and patients who are going to be on long-term sulfasalazine therapy should be warned. Finally, exacerbation of colitis due to sulfasalazine is an infrequent but real phenomenon.

SULFASALAZINE PHARMACOLOGY

Sulfasalazine was used clinically for many years before we understood its pharmacology. An understanding of that pharmacology and concurrently some of the issues with its toxicity have led to the development of the whole new group of agents, the aminosalicylates.[11,12] With regard to its pharmacology, after ingestion one third of the drug is absorbed in the proximal area of the small intestine (Fig 26–2). There is no hepatic metabolism of this intact drug. Whatever cycles through the liver either enters the bile and then again the small intestine or is excreted into the urine unchanged and imparts the dark yellow color to the urine that patients describe. The absorbed portion, which then returns to the intestine via the bile, joins the unabsorbed portion and traverses the small intestine until it encounters the intestinal bacterial flora, which is predominantly colonic. Intestinal bacteria of all varieties have abundant azoreductase, which breaks the azo bond. The sulfa moiety is then absorbed, achieves high levels in the blood, is metabolized by the liver, and is excreted in the urine.

The 5-aminosalicylic acid (5-ASA) moiety, in contrast, is minimally absorbed and most of it stays within the lumen of the colon in contact with active disease, if present, to be excreted in the stool. As the parent sulfasalazine traverses the colon it is virtually completely metabolized, so that there is very little if any intact sulfasalazine coming out in the stool. If sulfapyridine or the 5-ASA moiety is ingested as a single agent, each is promptly absorbed in the small bowel, metabolized by the liver, excreted in the urine, and never achieves any significant levels in the distal area of the intestine. This observation, coupled with the distribution studies, suggested that sulfasalazine might be serving as a vehicle

*Editors Note: It has been observed that not only is desensitization usually successful but also the subsequent course of IBD in patients treated with sulfasalazine is more favorable than in patients who were not allergic or intolerant to the drug. This is particularly true of ulcerative colitis.[8]

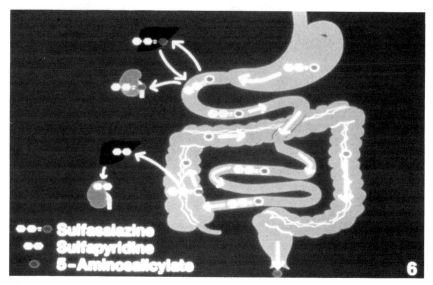

FIG 26-2.
Metabolism and distribution of sulfasalazine and its metabolites, sulfapyridine and 5-aminosalicylate.

for delivery of an active metabolite to distal disease sites. 5-ASA seemed the likely candidate since it alone remained in contact with the entire colon.

It is easy to understand, therefore, why there was interest in developing ways of delivering the presumed active metabolite of sulfasalazine, 5-ASA, alone directly to disease sites. In fact, during the past decade or more there has emerged tremendous interest in this new group of agents, the aminosalicylates.

THE AMINOSALICYLATES

Topical 5-ASA

Most of the initial attention focused on topical enema suspensions or suppositories of 5-ASA as well as 4-aminosalicylate (4-ASA), which is an isomer of 5-ASA developed because of some initial problems with the stability of 5-ASA, which may oxidize rapidly. The landmark clinical study for 5-ASA was done in 1977 by Azad-Kahn and colleagues.[1] Patients with active ulcerative colitis were randomized to enemas containing either sulfasalazine or 5-ASA or sulfapyridine. The patients were followed for 2 weeks. After 2 weeks 75% of the patients on a regimen of either sulfasalazine enemas or 5-ASA enemas achieved a clinical remission contrasted with a 40% remission in those on a regimen of sulfapyridine therapy, approximately the rate seen with placebo treatments in other controlled trials. Although sigmoidoscopic remission lagged compared with clinical improvement, two thirds of patients on 5-ASA or sulfasalazine showed endoscopic remission. This was significantly different from the 33% showing improvement on sulfapyridine therapy. There was a similar significant histologic improvement in patients treated with 5-ASA and sulfasalazine compared with sulfapyridine. Based on these results the authors concluded that 5-ASA was the active moiety of sulfasalazine, supporting the hypothesis from the basic pharmacologic data.

A further compelling study was reported by Campieri and colleagues,[5] who randomized patients with distal ulcerative colitis to either 5-ASA enemas or to hydrocortisone enemas. Within 2 weeks 93% of the 5-ASA group achieved remission clinically and sigmoidoscopically compared with 50% in the hydrocortisone group. These differences were statistically significant and quite striking.

Many of the patients studied in the early trials of 5-ASA enemas were those with distal ulcerative colitis refractory to standard therapies, including sulfasalazine, topical steroids, and even oral corticosteroids. It has been gratifying to see that in both controlled trials and in open trials there is approximately a 75% response rate in such patients with refractory distal colitis.[2] The response in such patients, however, may take up to 8 months, whereas patients with new-onset disease usually show an effect within 2 to 3 weeks.

Ideally, one would hope that any medication that will supplant or be used in place of sulfasalazine would be as effective as prophylactic therapy in ulcerative colitis. Indeed, topical 5-ASA appears to be effective at maintaining remission. In a study by Biddle and colleagues,[4] patients with ulcerative colitis of the distal area of the colon who had achieved remission on 5-ASA enemas were randomized to either 1 g 5-ASA enemas every night or to placebo enemas. During a 12 month period, 75% of patients on a regimen of 5-ASA therapy remained in clinical and sigmoidoscopic remission in contrast to an 85% relapse rate in the placebo group.

In addition to the clear efficacy of 5-ASA enemas in distal colitis (new-onset and refractory colitis), the hoped-for decrease in adverse effects compared with sulfasalazine therapy has been realized. Eighty to 90% of patients intolerant or allergic to sulfasalazine will tolerate topical 5-ASA, while 10% to 20% receiving 5-ASA therapy will experience the same adverse effect as seen with sulfasalazine.[13] Side effects have been infrequent, although anal irritation, hair loss, and cases of pancreatitis and myopericarditis have been reported.

Two problems have emerged with the routine use of 5-ASA enemas. The first pertains to the high relapse rate seen in patients who respond to treatment and then are withdrawn from therapy. It is not clear, however, whether this relapse rate is any higher than that seen with other forms of therapy, including sulfasalazine and topical steroids. There has been some concern that the relapses seen after 5-ASA withdrawal are more severe and harder to control than those after other forms of therapy. These anecdotal concerns, however, were not borne out in a recent review of a large experience with topical 5-ASA therapy.[3]

The second problem, which is not a hypothetical concern, is the cost, currently at $7 to $8 per enema. That cost may be prohibitive for certain patients, especially those with new onset of disease, in whom there are other alternatives. A number of gastroenterologists have been reluctant to use 5-ASA as first-line therapy for mild distal disease when hydrocortisone enemas and sulfasalazine are available at less expense. Since doses of 1 and 2 g appear to be just as effective as the 4 g dose currently available, cost can be contained somewhat by using half an enema nightly as initial therapy. Hopefully there will be a cost reduction in the future since, from the point of view of efficacy and safety, 5-ASA enemas can be viewed as the treatment of choice for distal ulcerative colitis.

Many questions about the use of 5-ASA enemas in distal colitis remain unanswered. I have achieved success in certain refractory patients with combinations of 5-ASA enemas and hydrocortisone enemas or 5-ASA enemas and sulfasalazine. Whether such combination treatment should be utilized initially in new-onset disease is not clear.

Moreover, the optimal maintenance schedule for patients who are going to be on long-term enema therapy is also not clear. My experience is that the majority of patients can get by with every-other-night or every-third-night treatment. I have some patients who remain well if they take one enema a week, but if they stop even this low dose they have a recurrence of symptoms. In contrast, I do have a number of patients who seem to need nightly 5-ASA enemas or the condition begins to flare. There is currently an ongoing controlled trial looking at the optimal maintenance schedule, and we should have that information soon.

The topical 5-ASA enemas are here to stay. They are a major advance; I am delighted to have them, but they are not going to be the answer for patients who have ulcerative colitis that is more proximal than the sigmoid colon. Certainly they are of no help to patients with

Crohn's disease of the ileum and right colon. In Crohn's colitis of the distal area they have not been well studied. My impression is that they are not quite as useful as in ulcerative colitis, but occasionally a patient will benefit. Because of these considerations there has been considerable interest in developing various oral preparations.

ORAL 5-AMINOSALICYLIC ACID AGENTS

There are three basic oral formulations under study.[12]

1. Slow-release or controlled-release forms. These are either coated with an acrylic resin (Asacol) or packaged in ethylcellulose microspheres (Pentasa) (see Chapter 25). These free forms of oral 5-ASA, as well as the topical forms, are known generically as mesalamine in the United States and mesalazine in Europe.

2. A form studied in England (Balsalazide), which links the 5-ASA, again through that same azo bond as sulfasalazine, to an inert vehicle. Unlike the slow-release forms, this does still require bacterial metabolism.

3. The disodium azodisalycilate, or olsalazine (Dipentum), links two 5-ASA molecules together again via an azo bond and requires bacterial metabolism. Olsalazine has recently become the only oral agent available commercially in the United States, while the other oral forms are available in Canada or Europe (or both).

Data from controlled trials have demonstrated the efficacy of various controlled-release forms and olsalazine in mild to moderate active colitis and as prophylaxis for ulcerative colitis in remission.[12] Moreover, the slow-release form, Pentasa, appears to be effective in active Crohn's disease. In contrast to the experience with sulfasalazine, oral Pentasa has shown efficacy at maintaining remission in Crohn's disease when begun within 3 months of the onset of the remission. As with sulfasalazine, there appears to be a dose-response effect when treating patients with active disease with oral 5-ASA agents. In many of the controlled trials, success was attained only at the highest dosage schedule.

As with topical 5-ASA, the majority of patients intolerant or allergic to sulfasalazine will be able to take an oral 5-ASA preparation, with serious adverse effects such as pancreatitis, pneumonitis, or pericarditis and exacerbation of colitis reported only infrequently. Watery diarrhea, which is related to dose and extent of colitis, has been reported in up to 15% of patients receiving olsalazine therapy, and may limit its use in patients with more extensive active disease. Often the diarrhea is eliminated by lowering the dose, and it tends to improve with time as the patient improves.

What will be the ultimate role of 5-ASA agents? At the very least they will be attractive alternatives in the sulfasalazine-intolerant or allergic patient. If their efficacy and more limited side effects hold up in time, one or more of the agents may replace sulfasalazine itself.

MECHANISM OF ACTION

Through work on the aminosalicylates, we may learn more about the pathogenesis of IBD itself and emerge with other new agents for treatment. The leading hypothesis regarding the mechanism of action of 5-ASA (and sulfasalazine) is that the lipoxygenase pathway of arachadonic acid metabolism is inhibited.[14] This leads to a decrease in chemotactically active substances such as leukotriene B_4, which in turn leads to a decrease in the inflammatory process. There are now studies of specific inhibitors of lipoxygenase, including fish oil, which will not only shed additional light on basic pathophysiology but also may provide us with additional forms of therapy.

REFERENCES

1. Azad-Kahn KA, Piris AJ, Truelove SC: An experiment to determine the active therapeutic moiety of sulphasalazine. *Lancet* 1977; 2:892–895.
2. Barber GB, et al: Refractory distal ulcerative colitis responsive to 5-aminosalicylate enemas. *Am J Gastroenterol* 1985; 80:612–614.
3. Biddle WL, Miner PB Jr: Long term use of mesalamine enemas to induce remission in ulcerative colitis. *Gastroenterology* 1990; 99:113–118.
4. Biddle WL, et al: 5-Aminosalicylic acid enemas: Effective agent in maintaining remission in left-sided ulcerative colitis. *Gastroenterology* 1988; 94:1075–1079.
5. Campieri M, et al: Treatment of ulcerative colitis with high dose 5-aminosalicylic acid enemas. *Lancet* 1981; 2:270–271.
6. Das KM, et al: Adverse reactions during salicylazosulfapyridine therapy and the relation to drug metabolism and acetylator phenotype. *N Engl J Med* 1973; 289:491–495.
7. Dick AP, et al: Controlled trial of sulphasalazine in the treatment of ulcerative colitis. *Gut* 1962; 5:437–442.
8. Korelitz BI, Present DH, Rubin PH, et al: Desensitization to sulfasalazine after hypersensitivity reactions in patients with IBD. *J Clin Gastroenterol* 1984; 6:27–31.

9. Misiewicz JJ, Lennard-Jones JE, Commell AM: Controlled trial of sulphasalazine in maintenance therapy for ulcerative colitis. *Lancet* 1965; 1:185–188.
10. Mogadam M, et al: Pregnancy in inflammatory bowel disease. Effect of sulfasalazine and corticosteroids in fetal outcome. *Gastroenterology* 1981; 80:72–76.
11. Peppercorn MA, Goldman P: The role of intestinal bacteria in the metabolism of salicylazosulfapyridine. *J Pharmacol Exp Ther* 1972; 181:555–562.
12. Peppercorn MA: Sulfasalazine: Pharmacology, clinical use, toxicity and related new drug development. *Ann Intern Med* 1984; 101:377–386.
13. Peppercorn MA: Advances in the drug therapy for inflammatory bowel disease. *Ann Intern Med* 1990; 112:50–60.
14. Ruo SS, Cann PA, Holdsworth CD: Crohn's disease: Clinical experience of the tolerance of mesalazine and olsalazine in patients intolerant of sulphasalazine. *Scand J Gastroenterol* 1987; 22:332–336.
15. Summers RW, et al: National Cooperative Crohn's Disease Study: Results of drug treatment. *Gastroenterology* 1979; 77:847–869.

Use of Steroids and 6-Mercaptopurine in Inflammatory Bowel Disease

Burton I. Korelitz

Two concepts based on the natural course of Crohn's disease are pertinent to the choice of drug therapy:

1. Crohn's disease is a diffuse process that involves the entire alimentary canal. Those most diseased areas we see by x-ray examination are exactly that, the major areas of involvement.
2. Historically the extent of disease remains constant unless the bowel is transected. Resection or transection of the bowel is then followed sooner or later by extension of the disease proximally.

CORTICOSTEROIDS AND ACTH

What do we know about steroids in ulcerative colitis? The following are the historical steps that summarize our knowledge:

1. Truelove and Witts, in 1955, showed that cortisone was better than placebo and then later that intravenous adrenocorticotropic hormone (ACTH) was better than cortisone in relapse of disease as opposed to the first attack.
2. Later Spencer and Kirsner showed us that there were serious side effects with prolonged use of steroids.

3. Lennard-Jones and his group showed that steroids were ineffective in preventing relapses of ulcerative colitis.

4. Later, Truelove and Jewel introduced the 5-day therapy of intravenous prednisolone in which they threw in everything (steroid enemas, antibiotics, total parenteral nutrition). Favorable results occurred in only 60% of patients. If there was no response in that 5-day period, treatment was considered a failure. Currently I believe that we know a lot more about using intravenous steroids in inflammatory bowel disease (IBD), and therefore our results are better.

5. Finally, some controversy has existed through the years about which is better as an intravenous preparation—hydrocortisone or ACTH. Meyers et al.,[5] at Mount Sinai Hospital, have shown that in the original attack ACTH is better, and in recurrent attacks when the patient is already receiving steroids, intravenous hydrocortisone is better. Based on my own experience I have believed that intravenous ACTH is better than hydrocortisone in all cases, whether the original attack, relapse, or after previous treatment with steroids.

In Crohn's disease it has been demonstrated that prednisone is better than placebo in bringing about remission, that it is most effective in small bowel disease as opposed to colonic disease, but, as in ulcerative colitis, it is not effective in preventing recurrence or extension of disease. As stated, for the sicker patients I prefer intravenous ACTH to hydrocortisone. This is administered in most cases as a slow intravenous drip with 120 units of ACTH every 24 hours. The volume of the vehicle, whether saline or water, depends on the state of hydration or depletion and existing salt and water retention. In either case, potassium should be added to the infusion.

It is important when a patient is started on oral steroids that they are at least initiated at a high dose of 60 to 80 mg. It is easier to start there, effect a remission, and then decide on the formula for the rate of reduction. If we start at a lower dose and it is not satisfactory, raising the dose in small increments might also prove not to be satisfactory. Once one starts steroids the dose should not be reduced until it is clear that the purpose is being accomplished. Otherwise the value of the steroids might be eliminated. Steroids, as has been shown in many different ways, are not maintenance drugs, and it is important to incorporate that into the thinking on management.

There are many disadvantages to use of steroid therapy in IBD (Table 27–1). Concern about these complications is particularly significant because steroids have no prophylactic value.

Steroids remain the most potent group of drugs in the treatment of

TABLE 27–1.
Complications of Steroid Therapy in IBD

Short-term Therapy	
Stimulation	Excessive appetite
Insomnia	Polyuria
Weird feelings	Hypokalemia
Steroid psychosis	Renal stones
Change in appearance	Water retention
Maintenance Therapy	
Moon facies	Fungal infections
Weight gain	Social retardation
Acne	Fractures
Depression	Osteonecrosis
Hypertension	Vascular fragility
No prophylactic value	

IBD. Because of their complications they should be considered acute-phase drugs for the sicker patients, while other drugs such as the immunosuppressives, sulfasalazine, and 5-aminosalicylic acid should be considered chronic-phase drugs. The latter are used for maintenance whether they are responsible for the remission in the first place or not.

6-MERCAPTOPURINE

If steroids cannot be eliminated or they must be reintroduced shortly after being terminated, a chronic-phase type drug should be introduced. The role of the steroids then is to "buy some time" for 6-mercaptopurine (6-MP), or another chronic-phase drug, to be given a chance to work. The steroids can be continued (and reduced) until the chronic-phase drug has become effective. Immunosuppressive drugs are not rapid-acting drugs—they have a lag period of the equivalent of 2½ months up to many months. What is the role of the steroids in buying that time? Probably it is by the lysis of established T cell clones. The response to 6-MP, however, is not dependent on the steroids except as the steroids buy time for the 6-MP to work. Then steroids should be reduced and eliminated even if it takes a few attempts to accomplish this, because steroids are not maintenance drugs.

6-MP is tolerated by most patients without any side effects. In contrast to steroids, 6-MP has prophylactic value. Table 27–2 shows the most recent computed results of 6-MP in Crohn's disease, based on data that Adler and I[1] have collected since my original double-blind, controlled study conducted with Present et al.[8] Observations show that

TABLE 27–2.
Results of 6-MP in Crohn's Disease*

1. Still better than earlier (70%)	
2. Favorable reports from other centers	
3. Indications for 6-MP in Crohn's disease with best results	
a. Eliminations of steroids	71.4%
b. Healing internal fistulas	64.1%
c. Healing perirectal abscesses	64.6%
d. Healing recurrent ileitis	80.0%
e. Healing Crohn's disease of stomach and duodenum	100%
f. Permitting elective resection	100%
g. Prophylaxis against recurrence	?

results are still better than they were earlier, an overall response rate of 70%. There have also been favorable reports from other centers, most notably by O'Brien and Bayless[7] from Johns Hopkins, whose figures match ours almost identically. There have also been reports from Sweden,[6] from Goldstein[3] in Philadelphia, from Verhave et al.[10] in Boston, and from Markowitz et al.[4] from North Shore, on the use of 6-MP and azathioprine in adults and children. They have all been favorable.

The indications for 6-MP in Crohn's disease that seem to have the best results are:

1. Elimination of steroids (more than 70%).
2. Healing internal fistulas.
3. Healing perirectal abscesses most often in conjunction with the modified Parks procedure to eradicate the perirectal fistulas and abscesses (see Chapter 15).
4. Healing recurrent ileitis after a resection (80%).
5. I have had particularly good luck with 6-MP therapy for Crohn's disease of the stomach and duodenum; it certainly is a far better modality than bypass surgery in the upper gastrointestinal tract.
6. Permitting elective resection—what does that mean? Some patients sent to us for treatment with immunosuppressive drugs have late-stage Crohn's disease with extensive disease and had not been considered surgical candidates. After a few months on a regimen of 6-MP therapy, and with clinical improvement, the borders then lend themselves to better definition and the possibility of surgical intervention with combinations of resection

and perhaps stricturoplasty. This has become an important indication for 6-MP therapy.
7. For prophylaxis. Our own latest data are not yet compiled, but again 6-MP seems to be very promising since the patients on a regimen of 6-MP therapy seem more and more to be going for years without indication of recurrent ileitis after surgery.

From this latest study of 6-MP for treatment of Crohn's disease, the mean time until elimination of steroids has been 3.4 months.[1] This is similar to the original study.[5] The duration without steroids while on a regimen of therapy with 6-MP was 2.9 years (6 months to 12 years). The duration of remission after stopping 6-MP has been 15 months, somewhere between 1 and 39 months.

The elimination of steroid dependence was a major therapeutic goal of 6-MP in ulcerative colitis also. Adler and I[2] have collected data on our 6-MP experience in ulcerative colitis. In the early studies uncontrolled data suggested that efficacy was still greater than in Crohn's disease. This has not been proved in our experience, but resistant cases of ulcerative colitis show responses that are meaningful. In 42 of 87 patients (48%) remission was accomplished successfully after a mean treatment period of 2½ months. The mean steroid-free period on a regimen of 6-MP therapy was 19 months in these patients. In addition, there were 13% (11 of 87) who had an intermediate response in which the steroids could be reduced but not eliminated. Altogether, we had 61% improvement in patients with resistant ulcerative colitis after initiating 6-MP. The mean time to eliminate steroids was even faster than in Crohn's disease, supporting the observations made many years ago when we first started using 6-MP. In other words, if it is going to work in ulcerative colitis, the mean time is usually shorter!

We have long-term follow-up data available on 29 of 42 patients with ulcerative colitis whose condition responded to 6-MP therapy, and these patients were able to maintain steroid-free remission for a mean period of 21 months (median 12½ months) after its discontinuation.[2] Therefore, 6-MP appears to have a role in treatment of ulcerative colitis as well as Crohn's disease.

The disadvantages to use of 6-MP include:

1. Fear of using it (unquestionably this has dissipated to a great extent through the years)
2. Allergic reactions
3. Interference with consideration of pregnancy
4. Inconvenience of monitoring blood counts

5. Infections
6. Neoplasms

Recently, in *Annals of Internal Medicine*, our long-term experience with toxicity to 6-MP has been published, representing Present's practice and mine.[9] We reported 400 patients observed during a 16-year period with a 90% follow-up regarding toxicity. Pancreatitis occurred in 13 patients (3%), bone marrow depression in 2%, allergic reactions in 2%, and hepatitis in less than 1%. All of these complications were reversible, and there was no mortality in this entire group of patients. After pancreatitis 6-MP cannot be used again.

We had grouped infections into those possibly related and those probably related to 6-MP. Those probably related amounted to about 1.8%. These, too, were all reversible, and there was no mortality in the entire group. Regarding neoplasm, the outstanding obstacle to use of 6-MP has been the one case of a lymphoma of the brain that developed in a man who had been receiving 6-MP therapy for a relatively short time. We presumed it was related to the 6-MP, because this is a rare type of tumor that has been reported in patients receiving transplants who have been maintained for long periods with use of high-dose immunosuppressive drugs. There was one lymphoma in our entire group of cases, and when one adds to that the experience of Kinlen in Scotland it comes out to be one case in 750 patients with IBD treated with 6-MP or azathioprine. There are other kinds of tumors found in the course of follow-up, but they did not occur more commonly in those patients treated with 6-MP than in those with IBD not treated with 6-MP.

Cancer of the colon should be a complication of particular concern because ulcerative colitis is a disease prone to the development of cancer even without immunosuppressive drugs. Present and I looked back to our experience. I counted 16 patients with cancer of the colon complicating ulcerative colitis during a 20-year period. One had taken 6-MP, and 15 had not. Present counted 18. He, too, had one patient in his entire group who had taken 6-MP. Of 34 patients, 2 had received therapy with 6-MP (6%) and 32 had not. Similarly, what about cancer of the intestinal tract complicating Crohn's disease? I could identify 7 patients in whom carcinoma of the ileum or colon developed; one had been treated with 6-MP. Present identified 10 patients, with 1 receiving 6-MP. Together, of 17 patients, 2 had received 6-MP therapy and 15 had not. While these figures are not controlled and do not include a denominator, carcinoma seems to be far more common in Crohn's disease and ulcerative colitis independent of immunosuppressive therapy than associated with it.

DURATION OF TREATMENT

How long should 6-MP be used? For the purpose of the double-blind trial, a 2-year period was established to cover 1 year on 6-MP therapy and 1 year receiving a placebo. A 2-year period of 6-MP therapy was adopted then, but remains arbitrary now. At the end of that time, if patients have done very well, some want to stop the drug, a few because of fear, but the number has decreased. A far larger number want to continue 6-MP therapy if it has been successful. A compromise seems to be to continue the drug but to reduce the dose. A fair trial once initiated requires a year. It is not clear whether the drug has been effective until a year has passed, even though the majority can tell much sooner.

Reasons for stopping 6-MP therapy have to do mostly with pregnancy, whether the patient is female or male. The issue arises frequently, since patients with IBD usually are young. If in the course of management I learn that pregnancy is the priority, I advise that the 6-MP should be stopped for 2 to 3 months before conception. On the other hand, Lennard-Jones and his associates presented data showing that azathioprine was continued throughout pregnancy with no complications.

We have patients receiving 6-MP therapy whose disease has been in remission for as long as 20 years. It seems the safety of the drug increases with time, probably with experience, and probably with better compliance of patients. In the last few years I have not seen any cases of bone marrow depression. Pancreatitis seems to be occurring less commonly. Infections also seem infrequent now. In any case, we recognize these conditions early and treat them with antibiotics so that they reverse quickly. I advise avoiding 6-MP therapy if pregnancy is the priority. If the female patient becomes pregnant while taking 6-MP, the question arises about therapeutic abortion. It has been my policy to recommend abortion if the patient is young, otherwise fertile, and has a good chance of becoming pregnant again. We do not yet know if there is any risk to the fetus in a mother receiving 6-MP therapy. Certainly it has not been demonstrated. It is still possible, however, that complications might not be realized until the child has grown and developed to finally answer that question.

When I start patients on a regimen of therapy with 6-MP, I provide them with information forms for orientation, telling why we are considering 6-MP therapy. The forms include the outcome of the trials and some information about the duration until the drug is likely to be effective. They also tell patients about all of the possible complications, so that we are partners in the venture. Then I get a permission form signed. Present does not believe this is necessary. He believes that a permission form would be more appropriate for steroids where toxicity is far greater. I usually have a second meeting with the patient and the family to discuss treatment and to answer all questions. Patients usually sign the permission form on that day, and then I give them the prescription for 6-MP.

I have a printed form for use by the clinical laboratory that the patients take with them. It instructs the laboratory to do a complete blood study with platelets and to telephone to my office the white count, platelet count, and hemoglobin level. The complete report can then be sent by mail. When the data are called into the office they are entered on this monitor form (Fig 27–1). The form is then showed to me. I write directions as to whether to continue the dose or to change it, and when the patient should have the next complete blood study. This goes smoothly and works well.

I always start at a dose of 50 mg/day, and the blood counts are done at least weekly in the first 3 weeks until the dose is established to be

Burton, I. Korelitz, MD
45 East 85 Street
New York, NY 10028
(212) 988-3800

6-MP RECORD

Name: Date of Onset: Original Dose:

DATE	WBC	HGB	HCT	PLATELET	LAST DOSE	CURRENT DIRECTIONS/DATE	NEXT CBC TO BE DONE

FIG 27–1.
Form for monitoring complete blood cell count after administration of 6-mercaptopurine.

safe. The period between blood counts can then be increased when the white count is stable. If the goal of therapy is accomplished by the initial dose, we do not have to increase the dose. On the other hand, if the therapeutic goal is not reached and if the blood count permits, we can increase the dose. If the dose is raised, the time between blood counts should be continued at, or changed to, once a week. Steroids serve to raise the white blood cell count. It has to be remembered that when steroid dosage is lowered, the white blood count can fall and the patient becomes more vulnerable. Raising steroid dosage increases the safety margin; reduction and elimination of steroids reduce the safety margin. The white blood count is more indicative of the influence of 6-MP once steroids are discontinued. Another important principle is that increasing the dose of 6-MP may lead to therapeutic success when a lower preceding dose of 6-MP had not done so. This is a move many people have not made, and it is important.

In regard to the more rapid-acting immunosuppressive drug cyclosporine, I believe it will serve as a "quick fix" when given intravenously when patients are seriously ill and refractory to steroids, thereby buying time for the safer orally administered 6-MP to take effect (see Chapter 29). I do not see that oral cyclosporine has as yet been more effective than 6-MP, but it might be tried when there are specific sensitivity reactions to 6-MP that preclude its further use.

REFERENCES

1. Adler DJ, Korelitz BI: The long term efficacy of 6-mercaptopurine in the treatment of Crohn's disease. *Gastroenterology* 1987; 92:1288.
2. Adler DJ, Korelitz BI: The therapeutic efficacy of 6-mercaptopurine in refractory ulcerative colitis. *Am J Gastroenterol* 1990; 85:717–722.
3. Goldstein F: Immunosuppressive therapy of inflammatory bowel disease. *J Clin Gastroenterol* 1987; 9:654–658.
4. Markowitz J, Rosa J, Grancher K, et al: Long-term 6-mercaptopurine treatment in adolescents with Crohn's disease. *Gastroenterology* 1990; 99:1347–1351.
5. Meyers S, Sachar DB, Goldberg JD, et al: Corticotropin versus hydrocortisone in the intravenous treatment of ulcerative colitis. A prospective randomized, double-blind clinical trial. *Gastroenterology* 1983; 85:351–357.
6. Nyman M, Hansson I, Eriksson S: Long-term immunosuppressive treatment in Crohn's disease. *Scand J Gastroenterol* 1985; 20:1197–1203.
7. O'Brien JJ, Bayless TM, Bayless JA: Use of azathioprine or 6-mercaptopurine in the treatment of Crohn's disease. *Gastroenterology* 1991; 101:39–46.
8. Present DH, Korelitz BI, Wisch N, et al: Treatment of Crohn's disease with 6-mercaptopurine. *N Engl J Med* 1980; 302:981–987.

9. Present DH, Meltzer SJ, Krumholz MP, et al: 6-Mercaptopurine in the management of inflammatory bowel disease: Short-term and long-term toxicity. *Ann Intern Med* 1989; 3:641–649.
10. Verhave M, Winter HS, Grand RJ: Azathioprine in the treatment of children with inflammatory bowel disease. *J Pediatr* 1990; 117:809–814.

Complications of Corticosteroids and Adrenocorticotropic Hormone in Treatment of Inflammatory Bowel Disease

Joseph B. Felder
Burton I. Korelitz

The number of drugs with proved efficacy for treatment of inflammatory bowel disease (IBD) is limited. Systemic steroids (adrenal corticosteroids, and adrenocorticotropic hormone [ACTH]) have long been the mainstay of treatment for acute disease and severe exacerbations. They have been shown, however, to have no role in prevention or in maintenance of remission in both ulcerative colitis and Crohn's disease.

Because of their use in many common medical disorders (allergic phenomena, collagen vascular disease, autoimmune disease, reactive airway disease, chronic obstructive pulmonary disease), most physicians have learned to use steroids with confidence early in their careers and thus have become skilled in their use. Therefore steroid therapy is often maintained, increased, reintroduced or prolonged when IBD worsens after dose reduction or cessation.

The toxicity of long-term corticosteroid therapy should not be underestimated. In our experience the sickest patients with IBD are those with severe and unremitting bowel disease and superimposed complications of long-term high-dose steroid use. The multiple of dose and time serves as an indicator or risk factor of the severity of the side effects to be expected. The following is a review of the toxicities and complications associated with steroid use in general, with special emphasis on those most commonly encountered in treating patients with

IBD. Physicians using these medications should be well familiar with these side effects.

COMPLICATIONS ASSOCIATED WITH STEROID USE IN GENERAL

Most commonly, physical "cushingoid" signs associated with steroid use include moon facies, buffalo hump, central obesity, enlargement of the supraclavicular fat pads, striae, ecchymoses, acne, hirsutism, and thinning of the skin. The most effective method in minimizing these effects is the administration of a total 48-hour dose of an intermediate-acting steroid (i.e., prednisone) in the morning, every other day, but in doing so the therapeutic value is most likely compromised.

Steroid Withdrawal

When withdrawal of corticosteroids after prolonged therapy is rapid, acute adrenal insufficiency may result. Characteristically there is a corticosteroid withdrawal syndrome consisting of hypotension, fever, arthralgias, myalgias, and malaise. Furthermore, electrolyte imbalance, with prominent hyponatremia and hypokalemia, as well as coma, can occur, and, if not recognized and corrected, can be fatal.

Fluid and Electrolyte Abnormalities

Hypokalemia and associated alkalosis are often encountered. Edema and hypertension, sometimes severe, also occur. Many steroid preparations have a sodium-retaining quality resulting from their mineralocorticoid effects that demands caution when they are being administered to those patients with preexisting cardiovascular, renal, or hypertensive disease. Patients with hypokalemia are treated with potassium supplementation, whereas hypertension and edema can usually be controlled with restriction of dietary sodium intake and the use of diuretics. Steroids can also cause increased levels of renin, which will subsequently cause hypertension and may necessitate the use of angiotensin-converting enzyme inhibitors to control it.

Abnormalities of Glucose Metabolism

Prolonged glucocorticoid therapy can cause hyperglycemia and glucosuria by increasing gluconeogenesis. This can occur independent of underlying diabetic disease or can represent the unmasking of diabetes. This complication can usually be managed with diet control and oral hypoglycemic agents, but sometimes insulin is required.

Infectious Complications

Patients treated with corticosteroids have an increased susceptibility to infection that is not specific for any particular pathogen. *Mycobacterium* tuberculosis should be ruled out in patients about to start on high-dose corticosteroids; after therapy is initiated, it will be difficult to diagnose because of a diminished immune response, with resultant decrease in skin test reactivity. In the face of infection, while the patient is receiving corticosteroid therapy, the steroids may usually be continued as long as concomitant treatment for the infection has been instituted.

Gastrointestinal Disturbances

Peptic ulcers, gastric hypersecretion, and esophagitis can complicate corticosteroid therapy. The correlation is controversial, as evidenced by the fact that we see these complications so infrequently in our patients with IBD. Messer et al.,[18] however, concluded that steroid therapy approximately doubles the risk of peptic ulceration and gastrointestinal hemorrhage. They found that even in patients treated for less than a month and in those receiving a total dose of less than 1,000 mg prednisone equivalent, the prevalence of ulcers was significantly increased. Oral and parenteral steroids seem to have the same effect, which is probably dose related. Treatment with antacids, H_2 blockers, sucralfate, or omeprazole may be indicated.

Musculoskeletal Complications

Although osteoporosis and vertebral compression can occur at any age, patients at high risk because of prolonged steroid use are elderly men, postmenopausal women, and patients whose physical activity is restricted. These patients, and young patients as well, are at an increased risk of developing osteonecrosis. Patients on prolonged therapy with corticosteroids should be followed up with radiographic examinations of the spine. Unfortunately there must be a significant amount of bone loss before it is apparent radiographically.

Steroid-induced myopathy can occur, and is characterized by weakness of the proximal limb muscles. Prolonged steroid usage is not required for this complication to develop because it can occur shortly after initiation of therapy. When any of the complications mentioned occur, termination of steroid therapy is imperative.

Behavioral Complications

Nervousness, insomnia, and increased appetite are minor side effects that are easily reversible.

Patients can experience changes in mood as well as depression and schizophrenia. Suicidal ideation has also been encountered. Previous psychiatric problems probably do not predispose the patient being treated with steroids to behavioral abnormalities anymore than occurs in other patients.

Ocular Toxity

There are reports of posterior subcapsular cataracts in patients who have received prolonged corticosteroid therapy. This is irreversible and must be corrected surgically. Ophthalmologic examinations should be performed periodically in patients when steroid therapy must be prolonged.

Growth Retardation in Children

Even small amounts of steroids used in treating children can result in inhibition or arrest of growth resulting from premature closure of the epiphyseal plates.

COMPLICATIONS FREQUENTLY OBSERVED IN COURSE OF STEROID TREATMENT OF IBD

Early Side Effects

Euphoria, agitation, depression, mania and incessant talking, and confusion may occur. We commonly see insomnia, excessive increase in appetite, and polyuria soon after steroid therapy is initiated. These symptoms often abate rapidly when the steroid dosage is decreased. It has been reported that insomnia can usually be minimized with use of a short-acting steroid preparation, or by prescribing the total daily dose as an early morning medication, but this might serve to compromise the therapeutic efficacy. As long as these side effects are controllable, we prefer continuing total dose and dosing intervals in favor of optimum therapeutic value of the steroid therapy.

Disfiguring Complications

Acne and development of a moon facies are two of the most common side effects of steroids that cause disfigurement. Acne can occur early in a course of therapy, whereas moon facies tends to appear later. The patient is constantly aware of acne and finds it most irritating. The greatest relief appears to be reassurance that the acne will resolve after termination of steroid therapy. Steroid-induced acne is usually an acne-like folliculitis in which pustules of various sizes without keratin plugs can develop in considerable profusion on the chest, back, and shoulders. Comedones and cysts are not found. These lesions can be treated with benzoyl peroxide lotion, gel, or cream (in a 5% concentration applied once a day). In most cases the liberal use of soap and water will be sufficient until full eradication of the acne occurs after steroid therapy is withdrawn. Consulting with a dermatologist is usually not necessary because this is a well-known entity, although some patients will be reassured by seeing a specialist who deals with skin when the acne has become more important to them than the underlying disease.

The "cushingoid" appearance is often disheartening to the managing physician and devastating to the patient and the family.[25] The emotional reaction can be one of severe withdrawal and depression in a young person vulnerable to the reaction and aware of his or her appearance. The only compensatory mechanism when the responsible steroids are essential for optimum therapy is the support of the managing physician with the reassurance that the disfigurement is reversible and will be gone soon.

In a study done by Spencer et al.,[26, 28] in 1962, almost all of their 288 patients with ulcerative colitis who were treated with ACTH or corticosteroids experienced acne, moon facies, striae, or a buffalo hump. The European Cooperative Crohn's Disease Study also reported moon facies and acne as the most common minor side effects encountered when treating patients with active Crohn's disease with corticosteroids.[16, 19, 29]

Infectious Complications

One of the more commonly seen infections in patients with IBD being treated with steroids is candidiasis. Oral and esophageal involvement are the most common and are usually treated successfully with clotrimazole troches (10 mg troches), one troche by mouth five times per day for 14 days; an oral nystatin suspension (100,000 units/mL), 5 mL swish and swallow four times a day; or, in worse cases, ketoconazole, 200 to 400 mg orally per day.* If esophageal symptoms are pronounced and the patient has failed to respond to the oral preparations, a 5- to 10-day course of intravenous amphotericin B may be required (0.3 mg/kg/day). Fungal vaginal infections should be treated with miconazole vaginal suppositories. Fungal infections of the bladder are best treated with amphotericin B bladder irrigations.

In the studies by Spencer et al.,[27, 28] infection appeared to be the most common serious side effect, seen in up to 28% of their studied population, but types of infections were not specified. Only one patient among thousands of patients with IBD treated with steroids by one of us (B. I. K.) had provocation of pulmonary tuberculosis.

It should be remembered that rarely a colitis is not IBD as diagnosed but really amebiasis, and an effort should be made to exclude this organism. Steroids serve to encourage the spread of amebic colitis and compromise the value of the diagnostic serologic tests. This problem has been addressed elsewhere.[12]

Fluid and Electrolyte Abnormalities

Hypernatremia leading to hypertension and edema may occur as a result of the mineralocorticoid effects of many steroid preparations. Hypertension is usually manifested as mild to moderate hypertensive episodes, and those patients with underlying hypertension are more prone to exacerbations. Treatment is the same as for steroid-induced hypertension not involving IBD, and in the more severe cases includes sodium restriction, diuretics, and sometimes angiotensin-converting enzyme inhibitors. Because we do not use steroid maintenance therapy in these patients, it is rare that this problem is encountered on an outpatient basis, and only rarely do we have to resort to low-sodium diets when steroids are being reduced.

Edema and even possible anasarca can be seen with steroid use, especially in malnourished patients with IBD who have low albumin levels.[2] This is best treated with furosemide, 20 to 40 mg/day orally. If severe enough, intravenous furosemide administration may be necessary. In some patients supplementation with intravenous salt-poor albumin is warranted.

Hypokalemia is often encountered with steroid use in the patient with IBD, especially when using intravenous steroids. For this reason it is a complication generally not encountered in the outpatient population, especially when oral steroids are purposely reduced and their use

---

*Editor's Note: Fluconazole has become available recently, and may be indicated therapy in this complication.

for maintenance therapy is avoided. When steroids are required intravenously, 20 to 40 mEq of potassium chloride/L of intravenous fluid (when the steroids are administered in 1 L of intravenous fluids over 24 hours) is usually adequate to maintain normal serum potassium levels (e.g., 120 units of ACTH in 1 L 5% dextrose in water with 20 mEq KCl/L to run by continuous intravenous infusion over 24 hours). If the patient is on a regimen of oral steroid therapy, potassium supplementation can be accomplished with oral administration of tablet or powdered forms of potassium chloride. We usually do not use the oral route of administration in this setting (especially during an acute exacerbation of IBD) because the potassium can be irritating to the gastrointestinal tract (the least irritating of these preparations appears to be potassium chloride (K-Lor) powder mixed in some water, supplied as 20 mEq packets). Instead, foods high in potassium content (bananas, celery, carrots, cantaloupe, oranges, and radishes) can be used to maintain adequate potassium levels. If patients become severely hypokalemic and the threat of muscle weakness or even paralysis is possible, potassium supplementation should be accomplished intravenously with use of runs of potassium chloride (10 mEq/hr).

Neurologic Complications

Steroid-induced myopathy and peripheral neuropathy often occur with steroid use in the patient with IBD. In some instances recovery takes many months; this is particularly true when the steroid therapy has been prolonged.

As early as 1950 Hoefer and Glaser[7] reported significant electroencephalographic changes in 13 of 15 patients receiving ACTH. Furthermore, 10 of the 15 experienced "neuropsychiatric complications." We have seen convulsions occur infrequently in patients with toxic psychosis due to steroids.

There have been multiple reports of seizures in patients with IBD who are receiving steroid therapy. The seizures have been related to steroid-induced fluid retention and hypertension in IBD. We have encountered this complication only rarely, because it appears to be related to long-term steroid therapy, which we do not use. Levine et al.[15] reported grand mal seizures occurring within 3 to 72 hours of operation in three children with Crohn's disease and two with ulcerative colitis, all of whom had been on long-term steroid therapy. In these five patients they observed an arterial hypertension peaking at 170–180/110–120 before onset of seizures, a positive cumulative fluid balance of 2 to 4 L without peripheral edema but with diminished urine output, and an elevated urine specific gravity.

Levine et al. suggest that prolonged steroid administration alters cerebral electrical activity, diminishes the threshold for seizure activity, and acts jointly with antidiuretic hormone responses to cause fluid retention and hypertension.

Mulvihill and Fonkalsrud[20] reported vasodilatation during induction of anesthesia in children who underwent surgery for IBD while on chronic high-dose prednisone. The vasodilatation caused systemic hypotension requiring treatment with intravenous fluids; this led to water retention, with resultant hypertension as well as pulmonary edema and seizures. A control group of 10 children also having operations for IBD but not on long-term steroid therapy did not experience any of these complications despite similar volumes of intravenous fluids given intraoperatively.

Shulak et al.[24] reported convulsions in 5 of 23 patients with IBD who underwent emergency colectomy; four of the five had been receiving preoperative steroid therapy. The average age of the patients was 25, in contrast to the younger age group mentioned.

Because steroids can cause a retention of fluid that can lead to hypertension as well as seizures, it is most important that fluid balance be followed closely in these patients.

Steroid Psychosis

Psychotic disorders have been described in association with ulcerative colitis and, to a lesser extent, with Crohn's disease. Steroids can also cause acute psychiatric disorders. The development of these complications in patients receiving steroids is probably dose dependent and the manifestations range from affective to schizophreniform disorders.[1] In our experience, preexisting psychiatric illness does not increase the risk for steroid-related psychiatric manifestations in the patient with IBD unless the emotional disorder was initiated by earlier steroid therapy.

The most prominent symptoms of steroid psychosis include progressive emotional lability with manic or depressive episodes, agitation, and memory impairment. Some become incomprehensible and, rarely, catatonic.

As clinical experience develops, the astute physician can recognize the changes in emotional behavior and to what extent they can be attributed to steroid usage. An effort should be made constantly to recognize the danger zone of transition between the common side actions attributable to the steroids and signs of more ominous toxic psychosis.

Accepted treatments for steroid-induced psychosis include lithium, tricyclic antidepressants, chlorpromazine hydrochloride (Thorazine) and haloperidol; electroconvulsive therapy is infrequently necessary. In earlier years chlorpromazine hydrochloride in our experience was the most effective; more recently we have favored haloperidol.

Psychologic reactions to steroids on one occasion do not invariably mean that the patient will again respond unfavorably to a second course of therapy, but drug prophylaxis may be indicated before the initiation of the second course. Most commonly, for lesser psychologic reactions, we have used clonazepam (Klonopin), 0.5 to 1 mg orally one to three times a day, and have found it to be extremely effective. It is best to involve a psychiatric consultant at this point in the case, as the psychologic effects of steroids can be multifold, and a correct diagnosis is imperative to selection of the proper treatment.

Musculoskeletal Complications

Osteonecrosis (aseptic necrosis, avascular necrosis) is one of the more serious complications of steroid therapy and is a source of concern in the patient with IBD. It is characterized by death of all the cellular elements of bone. Although it is usually seen after long-term steroid therapy, it can occasionally occur early in the treatment period. We have encountered this adverse reaction only about six times in the past 15 years. In a study done by Vakil and Sparberg[30] in 1989, osteonecrosis developed in 4.3% of a total of 161 patients with IBD who were treated with corticosteroids during a 10-year period. These patients had received steroids for a mean duration of 42 weeks at a mean daily dose of 26 mg and a mean cumulative lifetime dose of 7 g of prednisone. The mean daily dose during the month of most intensive therapy was 49 mg. The patients had complaints of joint pain in the hip or knee at initial presentation, and the osteonecrosis was frequently mistaken for the arthropathy of IBD or the arthralgia of steroid withdrawal. In 80% of patients the osteonecrosis caused by corticosteroids is bilateral.

Compared with other disease entities associated with steroid-induced osteonecrosis, the patients with IBD are younger, the dose is lower, and the duration of steroid therapy at the time of development of this problem is shorter. A study done by Kenzora and Glimcher[9] in 1985 suggested that an underlying multisystem illness impairs osteoblast function, thereby increasing susceptibility to osteonecrosis caused by other agents, which in this context are corticosteroids. This theory could very well explain the findings of Vakil and Sparberg[31] that patients with severe IBD may be more susceptible to steroid-induced osteonecrosis. A bone scan or magnetic resonance imaging should be done on patients with IBD who complain of joint pain and are, or recently were, being treated with steroids.

Growth Retardation in Children

Growth retardation is a prominent manifestation of ulcerative colitis or Crohn's disease with onset in childhood.[3] Studies of growth patterns in children have shown that low-dose steroid therapy does not retard growth, but high-dose steroids and both Crohn's disease and ulcerative colitis do. Since the pioneer studies that have demonstrated the contribution of inadequate nutrition to retarded growth, both total parenteral nutrition and oral nutritional supplementation have served to modify the problem.

Renal Complications

Renal calculi are fairly often encountered in the course of IBD. Oxalate stones have been reported in 2% to 3% resulting from increased absorption of dietary oxalate in the presence of steatorrhea and an increased permeability of the colon to oxalate.[5, 8] The prevalence of uric acid stones is increased with dehydration from chronic diarrhea, and the risk is further increased in patients with ileostomies. Renal calculi are often encountered in those patients with IBD being treated with corticosteroids, particularly when the dose is high and sustained. The stones formed are always made of calcium. Patients may pass multiple small stones without pain, but occasionally a large stone is impacted into the renal pelvis and requires nephrostomy. Temporary treatment is the same as that for ordinary calcium oxalate kidney stones, with increased hydration, low calcium and oxalate diet, and anion-binding agents. The underlying IBD still keeps the patient at an increased risk, but withdrawal of steroid therapy decreases the incidence of recurrences.

Coagulation Abnormalities

Thrombosis, as manifested by thrombophlebitis or deep vein thrombosis, occurs in patients with IBD who have been placed on a regimen of steroid therapy. It is an uncommon complication of IBD, occurring more often in ulcerative colitis than in Crohn's disease, and it has been reported in the pediatric population as well as in adults.[21] A hypercoagulable state has been recognized in association with IBD, but remains poorly defined. The risk of thrombosis is further increased by steroid therapy. Treatment with heparin is usually avoided, particularly when ulcerative colitis is active and the stools contain gross blood, but the clinical situation sometimes favors it use.

SPECIFIC COMPLICATIONS SEEN WITH INTRAVENOUS ACTH THERAPY

Allergic complications found with the use of intravenous ACTH have not been reported since 1957; at that time it was believed that these reactions were due to the animal source of the drugs administered (i.e., beef or pork pituitary). Kirsner et al.[10] reported a 5% incidence of hypersensitivity to ACTH gel or aqueous ACTH used intramuscularly or intravenously; the hypersensitivity was manifested principally by urticaria. Less often, patients experience pruritus, erythema, severe headaches, and tinnitus. These side effects are not commonly encountered today.

Kirsner et al.[10] further noted that the frequency of steroid complications with the use of ACTH was greater than with hydrocortisone, prednisone, or prednisolone. By stimulating adrenal mineralocorticoids, ACTH can produce fluid retention to a greater degree than corticosteroids.[23]

An extremely rare complication of intravenous ACTH therapy in the patient with IBD is adrenal hemorrhage.[6] ACTH causes adrenal cortical hypertrophy, hyperplasia, and hyperemia, and can lead to focal necrosis and hemorrhage. Adrenal hemorrhage can mimic an acute exacerbation of IBD or an acute condition of the abdomen, because patients may have abdominal pain, nausea and vomiting, fever, and peritoneal signs. The differential diagnosis must also include renal colic. A recent report from Mount Sinai Hospital in New York City describes four cases.[14] Only bilateral adrenal hemorrhage has caused adrenal insufficiency; unilateral hemorrhage has not. At Lenox Hill Hospital in New York City, where during the past 35 years, more than 1,000 patients with IBD have been treated with intravenous ACTH, only one case of adrenal hemorrhage resulting from intravenous ACTH has been found. The patient was a 23-year-old man being treated with 120 units of intravenous ACTH each day for a severe exacerbation of his Crohn's disease. On the 12th day of treatment, severe left flank pain with nausea, vomiting, and fever developed, and the patient was found to have a left-sided adrenal hemorrhage by computed tomographic scan. Intravenous ACTH was discontinued, and the patient's symptoms resolved within 48 hours. This complication requires termination of ACTH therapy and maintenance of corticosteroid support with intravenous hydrocortisone. Although rare, the diagnosis of adrenal hemorrhage in patients with IBD who are receiving intravenous ACTH and develop acute abdominal or flank pain in the face of apparent quiescence of their underlying illness must be considered. Obtaining a computed tomographic scan of the adrenal glands would be the next step in making the diagnosis.

PERSPECTIVES

Perioperative Complications Attributed to Steriod Use

The study in 1962 by Korelitz and Gribetz[13] found that children with ulcerative colitis who were treated with steroids had an increased prevalence of postoperative complications compared with those patients not treated with steroids. A retrospective analysis by Knudsen et al.,[11] in 1976, of 205 major operations on 95 patients with IBD previously receiving steroid therapy found that steroid therapy did not influence the overall incidence of complications and mortality rate, neither in Crohn's disease nor in ulcerative colitis. Both Korelitz and Gribetz and Knudsen et al. concluded that these risks were dependent on the clinical state of the patient at the time of surgery and whether the operation was performed electively or under adverse circumstances.

Mortality in Patients With Crohn's Disease Treated With Steroids

Prior et al., in 1970,[22] reported that the number of deaths in patients with Crohn's disease was double that expected in the general population. The disease itself was responsible for the majority of deaths, but some were attributable to prolonged corticosteroid therapy. At Lenox Hill Hospital, Mendelsohn and Korelitz[17] found that 17 of 26 deaths were attributed to Crohn's disease. One of the 17 deaths was due to steroid cardiomyopathy, but none of the others could be directly attributable to corticosteroids.

Cooke and Fielding,[4] in 1970, suggested that corticosteroid therapy in Crohn's disease can increase the overall mortality rate and need for surgery. They found that the risk of operation each year for those patients treated with steroids was twice that of those not treated, and they also found that 19% of the patients treated with steroids died, a mortality approximately two and one-half times that experienced in patients not treated with steroids. Again, these findings are probably explained by the more seriously ill patients being the ones to be put on a regimen of steroid therapy. As a generality, in recent years we have not observed any adverse effects of steroids on the postoperative course or wound healing.

CONCLUSIONS

Systemic steroids (ACTH and corticosteroids) are often used in treating patients with IBD since they represent the most potent and effective form of therapy available for acute disease and severe exacerbations. There are multiple side effects attributed to their use. These include a cushingoid appearance, electrolyte and fluid abnormalities, including hypokalemia and hypertension, infectious complications, including particularly candidiasis, gastrointestinal disturbances, musculoskeletal complications, including osteonecrosis, and psychologic and behavioral problems.

Some complications of steroids often dominate management in patients with IBD. Growth retardation can be compounded by the use of steroids. Adrenal hemorrhage can occur with the use of intravenous ACTH. Toxic psychosis, obstructing renal stones, and osteonecrosis can become the priorities in management. Most complications can be avoided by terminating or significantly reducing the steroids at the earliest feasible time that serves their purpose, before initiating maintenance therapy.

It is essential to be familiar with the complications found with steroid therapy so that they can be avoided or modified if possible. The skillful use of steroids is imperative in the treatment of some patients with IBD to reduce the need for surgery, to "buy time" for establishment of chronic-phase drugs such as 6-mercaptopurine, to improve the overall prognosis, and to save lives.

REFERENCES

1. Alcena V, Alexopoulos GS: Ulcerative colitis in association with chronic paranoid schizophrenia: A review of steroid induced psychiatric disorders. *J Clin Gastroenterol* 1985; 7:400–404.
2. Baillie J, Soltis RD: Systemic complications of IBD. *Geriatrics* 1985; 40:53–60.
3. Berger M, Gribetz D, Korelitz BI: Growth retardation in children with ulcerative colitis: The effect of medical and surgical therapy. *Pediatrics* 1975; 55:459–467.

4. Cooke WT, Fielding JF: Corticosteroids and corticotropin in the treatment of Crohn's disease. *Gut* 1970; 11:921–927.

5. Dobbins JW: Nephrolithiasis and intestinal disease. *J Clin Gastroenterol* 1985; 7:21–24.

6. Dunlap SK, et al: Bilateral adrenal hemorrhage as a complication of intravenous ACTH infusion in 2 patients with IBD. *Am J Gastroenterol* 1989; 84:1310–1312.

7. Hoefer PFA, Glaser GH: Effects of pituitary adrenocorticotropic hormone therapy: Electroencephalographic and neuropsychiatric changes in 15 patients. *JAMA* 1950; 143:620–624.

8. Hylander E, Jarnum S, Frandsen I: Urolithiasis and hyperoxaluria in chronic IBD. *Scand J Gastroenterol* 1979; 14:475–479.

9. Kenzora JE, Glimcher MD: Accumulative cell stress; the multifactorial etiology of idiopathic osteonecrosis. *Orthop Clin North Am* 1985; 16:669–679.

10. Kirsner JB, Sklar M, Palmer WL: The use of ACTH, cortisone, hydrocortisone and related compounds in the management of ulcerative colitis. *Am J Med* 1957; 22:264–274.

11. Knudsen L, Christiansen L, Jarnum S: Early complications in patients previously treated with corticosteroids. *Scand J Gastroenterol* 1976; 37:123–128.

12. Korelitz BI: When should we look for amebae in patients with IBD? *J Clin Gastroenterol* 1989; 11:373–375.

13. Korelitz BI, Gribetz D: The prognosis of ulcerative colitis with onset in childhood. II. The steroid era. *Ann Intern Med* 1962; 57:592–597.

14. Kornbluth AA, et al: ACTH-induced adrenal hemorrhage: A complication of therapy masquerading as an acute abdomen. *J Clin Gastroenterol* 1990; 12:371–377.

15. Levine AM, Pickett LK, Toubloukian RJ: Steroids, hypertension and fluid retention in the genesis of postoperative seizures with IBD in childhood. *J Pediatr Surg* 1974; 9:715–724.

16. Malchow H, et al: European Cooperative Crohn's Disease Study: Results of drug treatment. *Gastroenterology* 1984; 86:249–266.

17. Mendelsohn RA, Korelitz BI: Death in Crohn's disease (abstract 312). *Am J Gastroenterol* 1990; 85:1293.

18. Messer J, et al: Association of adrenocorticosteroid therapy and peptic ulcer disease. *N Engl J Med* 1983; 309:21–24.

19. Meyers S, Sachar DB: Medical management of Crohn's disease. *Hepatogastroenterology* 1990; 37:42–55.

20. Mulvihill SJ, Fonkalsrud EW: Complications of excessive operative fluid administration in children receiving steroids for IBD. *J Pediatr Surg* 1984; 19:274–277.

21. Paradis K, Bernstein ML, Adelson JW: Thrombosis as a complication of IBD in children: A report of four cases. *J Pediatr Gastroenterol Nutr* 1985; 4:659–662.

22. Prior P, et al: Mortality in Crohn's disease. *Lancet* 1970; 1:1135–1137.

23. Sack DM, Peppercorn MA: Drug therapy of IBD. *Pharmacotherapy* 1983; 3:158–176.
24. Shulak JA, et al: Convulsions complicating colectomy in IBD. *JAMA* 1977; 237:1456–1458.
25. Sparberg M, Kirsner JB: Long term corticosteroid therapy for regional enteritis: An analysis of 58 courses in 54 patients. *Am J Digest Dis* 1966; 11:865–880.
26. Spencer JA, Kirsner JB: Experience with short and long term courses of local adrenal steroid therapy for ulcerative colitis. *Gastroenterology* 1962; 42:669–677.
27. Spencer JA, Kirsner JB: The treatment of ulcerative colitis. *Am J Gastroenterol* 1962; 37:17–23.
28. Spencer JA, et al: Immediate and prolonged therapeutic effects of corticotropin and adrenal steroids in ulcerative colitis. *Gastroenterology* 1962; 42:113–129.
29. Summers RW, et al: National Cooperative Crohn's Disease Study: Results of drug treatment. *Gastroenterology* 1979; 77:847–869.
30. Vakil N, Sparberg M: Steroid related osteonecrosis in IBD. *Gastroenterology* 1989; 96:62–67.

Use of Cyclosporine in Treatment of Inflammatory Bowel Disease

Daniel H. Present

The use of cyclosporine in the treatment of inflammatory bowel disease (IBD) is relatively new, and there is much to be learned. I will present the current status of cyclosporine, and I must give credit to Dr. Simon Lichtiger, who has performed the major amount of work in terms of organizing the clinical trials that are about to be carried out in the United States.

There are several rationales for using cyclosporine in the management of IBD, in that there are few available therapeutic agents, and other immunosuppressive agents such as 6-mercaptopurine (6-MP), azathioprine, and methotrexate, have shown efficacy in IBD.[15] Likewise, steroids, metronidazole, and sulfasalazine also have immunosuppressive actions. Whereas 6-MP is a slow-acting drug, what is intriguing about cyclosporine is its rapid onset of action. Finally, there have been multiple case reports of efficacy in patients with IBD, and the drug is effective in other autoimmune processes, with responses seen in uveitis, Behçet's disease, psoriasis, rheumatoid arthritis, and pyoderma gangrenosum.[6]

The difference between our studies at Mount Sinai Hospital and those of other investigators relates to our use of intravenous cyclosporine as initial therapy, whereas almost every other study used oral cyclosporine. It has been shown that there is erratic absorption of cyclosporine in patients with radiation enteritis, anemia, diarrhea, and, especially, malabsorption.[3] Since these situations often apply to patients with IBD, as contrasted with other autoimmune disorders, intravenous cyclosporine may be essential in the therapy of IBD. Pharmacokinetic studies indicate that if one administers cyclosporine by bolus infusion, there is a rapid rise, often to toxic levels, with a rapid falloff. If one administers continuous infusion of cyclosporine, however, this results in steady blood levels. This is important in maintaining adequate therapeutic levels in acutely ill patients with ulcerative colitis.

Another unique factor is the mechanism of cyclosporine action. The drug has selective action on T lymphocytes rather than B lymphocytes, and predominantly inhibits T lymphocyte proliferation as well as the activation of primary helper T cells and the subsequent release of many lymphokines.[11] It inhibits the secretion of interleukin 2, with a rapid onset of action.

A review of the literature on cyclosporine for treatment of patients with IBD indicates that there are reports of only 170 treated patients with Crohn's disease and 40 with ulcerative colitis. In Crohn's disease the uncontrolled rate of response is 60% to 70%, with a 61% response rate in the one controlled trial. At the present time there are no controlled trials on treatment of patients with ulcerative colitis.

The initial case report on treatment of a patient with Crohn's disease was by Allison and Pounder.[2] The patient had extensive ileitis and steroid psychosis, and did respond to cyclosporine therapy. The side effects of hirsutism and tremor were noted. This report was quickly followed by another one in *Lancet* by Bianchi et al.[5] on two patients, one with active colitis and one with a stricture. The patient with active colitis improved, and the one with a stricture did not. No significant side effects were noted in this study.

The next development was the performance of pilot studies by multiple groups in Europe and Canada. Brynskov et al.[7] put together the data from 11 pilot studies, which included acutely ill patients as well as patients with resistant disease. Some of the patients were treated concomitantly with steroids or azathioprine, with varying doses and different durations of cyclosporine. Because of these variations the data in these 74 patients were confusing, but resulted in some guidelines. The first observation was that the drug seemed to work rapidly (within 1–3 weeks), and it seemed more effective in chronically ill patients. In responders, however, there was a rapid relapse after stopping cyclosporine. What was most exciting in this small group was that short-term toxicity appeared to be quite limited.

An interesting paper then appeared in *Gut*,[1] reporting a patient with multiple resections for ileocolitis and a short bowel syndrome. The patient was refractory to steroids and azathioprine and responded to total parenteral nutrition, but then showed relapse of disease. In this patient intravenous cyclosporine produced an excellent response, with relapse when the patient was switched to oral therapy. The patient was then restarted on intravenous cyclosporine and again improved, demonstrating that malabsorption with lowered blood cyclosporine levels was an important factor in the relapse. Another study on acute ulcerative colitis and Crohn's disease was done by Baker et al. at Oxford.[4] They believed that there was no advantage to adding cyclosporine to steroids in patients acutely ill either with ulcerative colitis or with Crohn's disease.

A critical review of the uncontrolled literature demonstrates that these were a heterogenous group of patients, that malabsorption was prominent in many pilot studies, and that there was no clear correlation of efficacy with cyclosporine levels (data on levels were not provided in almost all studies). Finally, there was no standardization of concomitant or prior medical therapy.

The paper by Brynskov et al.[8] was the first controlled trial in 71 patients with Crohn's disease. Cyclosporine, at a dose of 5 to 7 mg/kg/day, was given for 3 months, stratifying for steroids, with a response rate of 61%. Somewhat disconcerting was the 33% placebo response in patients who were said to be chronically ill. This is a frequent problem encountered with multicenter trials in that one cannot always enter a homogenous group of patients. As with the prior uncontrolled studies, the response was rapid (2 weeks), and there was good correlation of the Crohn's Disease Activity Index with the therapeutic index that was used in our 6-MP study.[16] Brynskov et al.[7] also found good correlation with serum orosomucoid levels as well as with the Van Hees Index.[17] Once again, there were few side effects requiring withdrawal.

Dr. Simon Lichtiger and I have been using cyclosporine in patients with Crohn's disease who have intractable nonobstructive disease. Standard medical therapy, including steroids, metronidazole, sulfasalazine, and often 6-MP, has been ineffective. We have also included patients with fistulous disease and steroid dependency. The criteria for efficacy were the same as used by Korelitz and me, together with our colleagues,[16] in our 6-MP trial, including individual goal improvements with criteria such as well-being, healing of fistulas, and steroid reduction and withdrawal. In the study with 6-MP and subsequently with cyclosporine, 3+ was given for total remission for every goal, 2+ for good response in which one does not have complete response for every goal, and 1+ for mild improvement. We have treated 12 patients, 10 of whom were quite ill or had fistulous disease, with cyclosporine in a dosage of 4 mg/kg/day for 14 days. A therapy regimen of oral cyclosporine was then used for at least another 28 days. In two patients we did not use intravenous cyclosporine, and the patients were started directly on the oral agent. If the patients did not improve in 2 months we considered the treatment a failure.

The following are the results in the 12 patients. In some of them we looked for steroid sparing, some for fistula healing, and some for improvement in clinical criteria. As noted, some of the patients have been on cyclosporine for almost 2 years. Four showed 3+ response, and another four showed 2+ response. We have excluded mild improvement in chronically ill patients and have labeled this as not significant. Therefore, in this group of chronically ill patients with Crohn's disease, we had a 66% response rate, which correlates well with the Brynskov data. Some perianal fistulas showed dramatic improvement in as quickly as 6 days. A patient with pyoderma gangrenosum had total healing of the lesion on the leg in 2 months. We treated another patient with an abdominal wall fistula that totally closed in 5 days. We have also treated a patient with a rectovaginal fistula with bilateral fistulas on the labia. She was unable to have intercourse for 1 year, and had to wear cotton pads continuously. Six days after intravenous cyclosporine, all fistulas had closed.

We now turn to ulcerative colitis, on which there are minimal data relating to therapeutic response in the literature. The first patient, who was treated by Gupta et al.,[10] was an older patient who did improve, but had relapse of disease on lower cyclosporine doses. Kirschner and Whitington[12] have treated children with intravenous cyclosporine, with rapid response in three of five patients. Because of their concern about maintenance of the drug in children, they have lowered the dose quickly, with frequent and prompt relapse of disease.

As was noted, the Oxford group[4] treated acutely ill patients with cyclosporine, and surgical intervention had to be carried out in 3 of 12, which is similar to their experience with steroid therapy alone, indicating no advantage to adding oral cyclosporine.

Our most exciting data have been seen in treatment of patients with ulcerative colitis with intravenous cyclosporine.[13] We have studied acutely ill patients in whom treatment with parenteral steroids for 7 to 10 days has been unsuccessful, and we have employed the standard Truelove and Witts criteria for severe ulcerative colitis. With use of the data from most centers, colons in all of these patients should have been removed if treatment for 7 to 10 days with parenteral steroids was not successful.

Our protocol for this pilot study was the administration of intravenous cyclosporine (4 mg/kg/day for 14 days). We closely monitored cyclosporine and creatinine levels, and the single goal in 14 days was to avoid colectomy. If the colon was saved and the patient was able to return home on oral medications, we considered this a phase 1 success. The patient then went on to phase 2, in which oral cyclosporine was started at 6 to 8 mg/kg/day and maintained for 6 months. The goal was total discontinuation of steroids, endoscopic healing, and clinical remission. If one does not achieve all goals, treatment of the patient is not considered a complete success in this trial. In our trial 20 patients were entered, 16 with universal disease and 4 with left-sided disease. Of the 20 patients, treatment failed immediately in 2, and colectomy was necessary during the hospitalization. Two, after having shown no improvement by our criteria, were advised to undergo colectomy, refused, and remained on high-dose steroids. Another patient had an anaphylactic reaction to the intravenous cyclosporine related to the carrier agent (cremaphor), and treatment was considered a failure. The other 15 responded, with the drug showing rapid efficacy (mean response time of 6.4 days). We avoided colectomy in 75% of patients who otherwise would have required it.

The next logical question is, What is the long-term outlook in these responders? A review of our data shows, in the two who refused colectomy, that both did have their colons removed at 3 and 9 months, respectively, despite continuation of high-dose steroids. Of the 15 responders, 12 have completed the trial, have discontinued steroids, are maintained on sulfasalazine, and are totally well. Three patients had relapse of disease, two of whom underwent colectomy; one patient who was not acutely ill after relapse was placed on a therapy regimen of 6-MP. She has had a subsequent complete remission. Therefore, 75% of the patients who initially improved have maintained their response, have had their colons salvaged, have discontinued cyclosporine, and are in clinical and endoscopic remission.

What are the major fears regarding cyclosporine administration to patients with IBD?

1. Nephrotoxicity: There are several types of renal toxicity, including an acute reaction that is dose related and is rapidly reversible with lowering of the dose of cyclosporine.[14] Chronic renal toxicity has been noted, but predominantly in patients taking high doses of cyclosporine for prolonged periods of time. There are also medications that may potentiate cyclosporine nephrotoxicity, and require caution if concurrently administered. Much of the nephrotoxicity data in the literature have occurred in patients with rheumatoid disease who are also treated with nonsteroidal anti-inflammatory agents, which may be a potentiating factor. To prevent nephrotoxicity we perform frequent tests of creatinine levels and creatinine clearances, and try to avoid concomitant

nephrotoxic agents. We attempt to maintain cyclosporine blood levels in the therapeutic range, and if the serum creatinine level rises by 30% or more we lower the dose of cyclosporine.

2. Another major fear is that of neoplasia. The overall risk of neoplasia in patients with autoimmune disease treated with cyclosporine is 1.3%. There is a high prevalence of skin cancer, central nervous system lymphomas,[9] and Kaposi's sarcoma. It is interesting, however, to note that some of the lymphomas have been monoclonal, and reverse and disappear if the cyclosporine is stopped.

There is a high percentage of annoying side effects, among which is hirsutism, which is very troublesome in women. Tremors are common, as are gingival hyperplasia, hypertension (dose related), paresthesias, and headaches.[18] The toxicity data on Crohn's disease and ulcerative colitis in 30 patients reported by Lichtiger and me[13] include a high number of these mild side effects. Serious side effects are uncommon; they include one patient with nephrotoxicity, which rapidly reversed on lowering the dose, and a patient mentioned previously with anaphylaxis to intravenous cyclosporine.

In conclusion, cyclosporine in Crohn's disease is effective in treatment of fistulas. We had moderate improvement in four of five patients, and two fistulas closed completely (one was an enterocutaneous fistula). Cyclosporine is definitely steroid sparing in Crohn's disease. Unfortunately, patients who have had a significant resection and those with diffuse small bowel disease may malabsorb when being treated with oral cyclosporine. I therefore predict that cyclosporine will be of limited value in the majority of patients with Crohn's disease because of the difficulty in maintaining therapeutic cyclosporine levels.

On the other hand, I believe the true indication for cyclosporine in patients with IBD will be in those who have acute and fulminant ulcerative colitis. It is rapidly effective in 75% of patients who are steroid nonresponders. Also, the majority of patients maintain their response for long periods of time. Short-term side effects are mild, whereas the long-term toxicity at this time is uncertain.

REFERENCES

1. Allam BF, Tillman JE, Thomson TJ, et al: Effective intravenous cyclosporine therapy in a patient with severe Crohn's disease on parenteral nutrition. *Gut* 1987; 28:1166–1169.
2. Allison MC, Pounder RE: Cyclosporine for Crohn's disease. *Lancet* 1984; 1:902–903.

3. Atkinson E, Britton T, Paull C, et al: Detrimental effect of intestinal disease on absorption of orally administered cyclosporine. *Transplant Proc* 1983; 15:246–251.
4. Baker K, Jewell DP: Cyclosporine for the treatment of severe IBD. *Aliment Pharmacol Ther* 1989; 3:143–149.
5. Bianchi PA, Monadelli M, Quarto-DiPalo F, et al: Cyclosporine for Crohn's disease. *Lancet* 1984; 1:1242.
6. Borel JF, Gunn C: Cyclosporine-A as a new approach to therapy of autoimmune diseases. *Ann NY Acad Sci* 1986; 475:307–319.
7. Brynskov J, Binder V, Riis P, et al: Low dose cyclosporine for Crohn's disease: Implications for clinical trials. *Aliment Pharmacol Ther* 1989; 3:135–142.
8. Brynskov J, Freund L, Rasmussen SN, et al: A placebo controlled double blind randomized trial of cyclosporine therapy in active Crohn's disease. *N Engl J Med* 1989; 321:845–850.
9. Cockburn I: Assessment of the risk of malignancy and lymphomas in patients using Sandimmune. *Transplant Proc* 1987; 19:1804–1807.
10. Gupta S, Keshavarzian A, Hodgson HJF: Cyclosporine in ulcerative colitis. *Lancet* 1984; 2:1277–1278.
11. Hess AD, Colomboni DM: Cyclosporine: Mechanism of action. In vitro studies. *Prog Allergy* 1986; 38:198–221.
12. Kirschner B, Whitington PF: Experience with cyclosporine in severe nonspecific ulcerative colitis (Abstract). *Pediatr Res* 1989; 117A.
13. Lichtiger S, Present DH: Cyclosporine in treatment of severe active ulcerative colitis. Preliminary report. *Lancet* 1990; 336:16–19.
14. Mihatsh MJ, Thiel G, Ryffel B: Hazards of cyclosporine therapy and recommendations for its use. *J Autoimmunity* 1988; 1:533–543.
15. Present DH: 6-Mercaptopurine and other immunosuppressive agents in the treatment of Crohn's disease and ulcerative colitis. *Gastroenterol Clin North Am* 1989; 18:57–71.
16. Present DH, Korelitz BI, Wisch N, et al: Treatment of Crohn's disease with 6-mercaptopurine. A long term randomized double blind study. *N Engl J Med* 1980; 302:981–987.
17. Van Hees PA, Van Elteran PH, Van Lier JH, et al: An index of inflammatory activity in patients with Crohn's disease. *Gut* 1980; 21:279–286.
18. Von Graffenfried B, Krupp T: Adverse effects of cyclosporine in renal recipients and patients with autoimmune diseases. *Transplant Proc* 1986; 18:876–883.

Chapter 30 _____

New Steroids

David B. Sachar

The ideal therapy for patients with IBD would have all the efficacy of steroids, with rapid action, prompt reduction of inflammation, and immediate promotion of well-being without any of the toxicity of steroids. That goal has not yet been achieved, but I shall review efforts that have been made thus far.

At the start is the corticosteroid molecule, of which hydrocortisone is the prototype (Fig 30–1). How does this agent work? Its anti-inflammatory action is conferred by its ability to bind to the glucocorticoid receptor, which in turn depends on these four sites (see Fig 30–1): the double bond at the 4–5 position, the two ketos at the 3 and 20 position, and the 11-hydroxy. These are the four "sacred," absolutely required sites for anti-inflammatory action. Cortisone, when it is first secreted by the adrenal cortex, has a keto instead of a hydroxy at the 11 position, so that it is inactive in terms of glucocorticoid or anti-inflammatory effect until it is metabolized by the liver to an 11-hydroxy to become hydrocortisone. Here, then, is where we begin, with the natural corticosteroids.

In the 1950s efforts were begun to create synthetic corticosteroids that had the same anti-inflammatory activity as hydrocortisone but that did not have so much mineralocorticoid (salt-retaining) effect. That is how prednisolone was developed, simply by creating a second double bond at the 1–2 position (Fig 30–2). That one change in the molecule conferred more anti-inflammatory action with less mineralocorticoid effect. Prednisone, which is used so frequently in this country, has a keto at the 11 position like cortisone, but to become active it has to be metabolized like hydrocortisone to the 11-hydroxy form, prednisolone. This is why topical agents that might include prednisolone compounds,

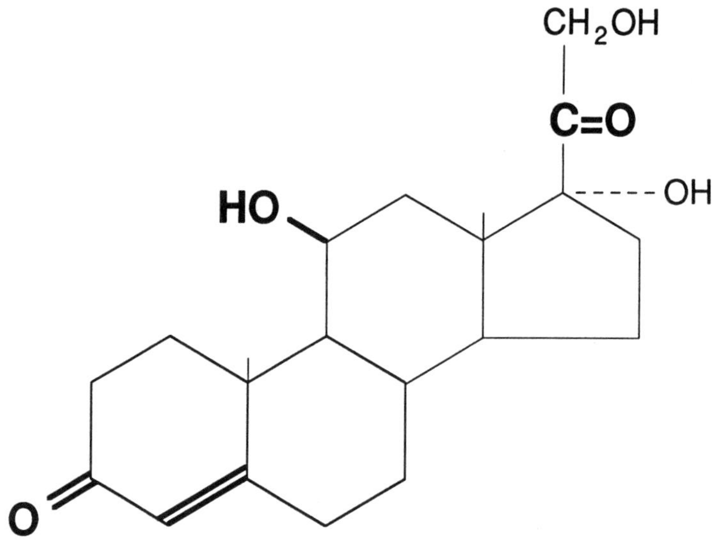

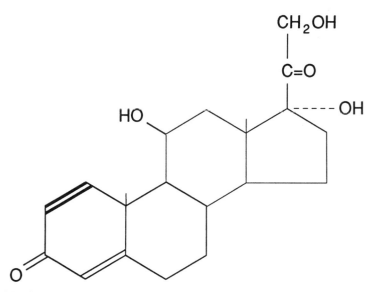

FIG 30–1.
Hydrocortisone. The four sites essential for anti-inflammatory activity are the 3- and 20-ketos, the 4-5 double bond, and the 11-hydroxyl.

FIG 30–2.
Prednisolone. Addition of the 1-2 double bond reduces the mineralocorticoid activity of hydrocortisone.

like the 21-phosphate or the metasulfabenzoate, never contain prednisone because the 11-keto in prednisone has to be systemically metabolized to a hydroxy before the drug can have anti-inflammatory action.

In the 1960s there was an effort to make these agents much more
potent by adding a halogen at the 9 position, usually a fluoride, in order
to block the binding of the corticosteroid to the transcortin receptor
and thereby prevent its clearance. In other words, when their binding
to the transcortin receptor was inhibited by 9-halogenation, these
agents were not so rapidly biotransformed, and their levels stayed up
higher and longer in the systemic circulation. They were thus more systemically potent. Triamcinolone has a fluoride at the 9 position (Fig
30–3); a chloride at the 9 position makes beclomethasone. Although
these agents are much more potent systemically, the halogen at the 9
position blocks their systemic biotransformation, and they are clearly
not going to be any more effective topically.

What happened in the 1970s, therefore, was an effort to get more
topical action from the corticosteroids by means of side chains added
at the 17 and 19 positions. These side chains provided more topical tissue binding and more topical activity, as with triamcinolone acetonide
(Fig 30–4), betamethasone valerate, and beclomethasone dipropionate.

In the 1980s we have seen the continuing development of what we
might call "super topical" agents that depend on further manipulations

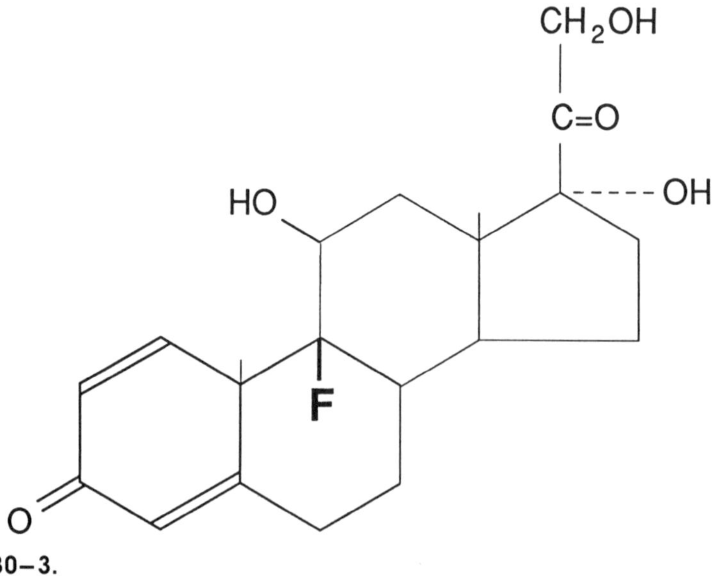

$$CH_2OH$$
$$C=O$$

FIG 30–3.
Triamcinolone. Addition of the 9-fluoride increases systemic potency of prednisolone.

FIG 30−4.
Triamcinolone acetonide. Addition of the side-chain increases topical activity of triamcinolone.

of the side chains. With changes at these side chains it is possible to get more tissue binding and greater affinity for the glucocorticoid receptor, which, as we have said, is what determines the anti-inflammatory action. So agents like budesonide (Fig 30−5) have more than 15 times the potency of prednisolone and about 100 times the potency of hydrocortisone topically. A thiol at the 17 position produces fluticasone propionate, while a different thiol ester at the 21 position yields tixocortol pivalate.

The other desirable feature for agents that we want to act topically but not systemically is very rapid clearance from the systemic circulation. This property is achieved by removing the halogen from the 9 position and thereby unblocking the binding site for the transcortin receptor. The resulting agent thus is not only very active topically because of its side chains, but also, if it gains any access to the systemic circulation, it will be rapidly cleared because the 9 halogen is gone. This is the principle of several of the new steroids currently used in therapy for asthma.

So, in summary, this is what has been happening during the last few decades: starting with hydrocortisone, reducing the mineralocorticoid effect by synthesizing prednisolone, increasing the systemic potency by adding a 9 halogen, making the agent more topically active by adding certain side chains, and then making it "supertopically" active by further manipulating the side chains and removing the 9 halogen. This

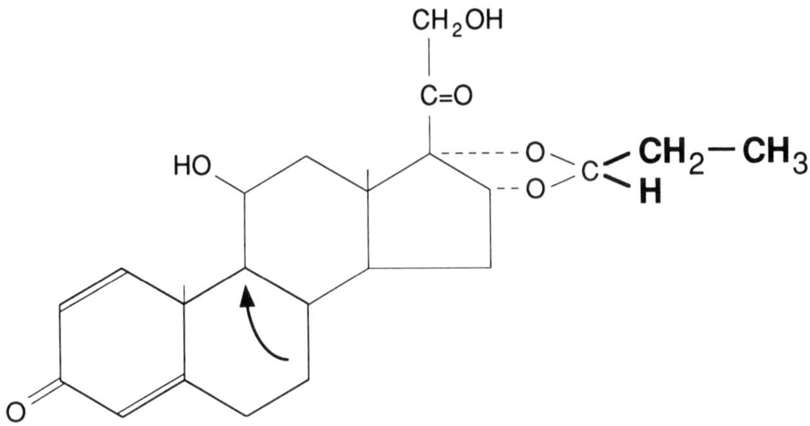

FIG 30–5.
Budesonide. Further alterations of the side-chain and removal of the 9-fluoride confer additional topical potency while reducing systemic effects.

explains the theory, but how are these new steroids doing in practice in patients with IBD?

Principally there are two kinds of potential use for them. First, they could be used for topical therapy as enemas that would be more potent than hydrocortisone or prednisolone enemas but that would have even less systemic corticoid action. Second, they could be used as oral therapy in the hope they would exert a topical action on Crohn's disease of the small bowel or Crohn's disease or ulcerative colitis of the colon. In either event, we would like them to be the magic agents that would give us anti-inflammatory action in the bowel, with all the potency of topical steroids but without any systemic action.

Oral therapy is just beginning to be tested throughout Europe, and the results are not yet complete. Glaxo, Inc. has been making fluticasone propionate, but they are not accomplishing much with oral therapy at this point. Sandoz Pharmaceuticals has been working with tixocortol pivalate orally, but are not yet successful with that either. New work is being done with budesonide, with some early promising data. It is much too early to indicate where these new steroids will fit or which ones, if any, will prove useful. I believe, however, that in the 1990s it is time to think about this approach to therapy, because development of these promising new agents is where a lot of the research will be directed.

Chapter 31 _____

Other New Drugs

Daniel Adler

_____

The vast array of therapeutic maneuvers that have been tried in the patient with inflammatory bowel disease (IBD) is an indicator of the frustration clinicians have in treating a disease of unknown cause and for which there is no recognized cure. A large group of patients refractory to standardized treatment remains. The trials of new agents are, however, also a testament to the quest for improved treatment and represent an amalgamation of clinical and basic science research. A brief review of trials of agents recently introduced to the armamentarium against IBD follows. Most are uncontrolled pilot studies involving small numbers of patients and for short periods of clinical follow-up. Widespread application of these therapeutic possibilities will depend on the results of forthcoming larger, controlled trials.

SUCRALFATE

Sucralfate has been shown effective in healing peptic ulcer and nonsteroidal anti-inflammatory drug–induced ulcers of the upper portion of the gastrointestinal tract. It has been proposed as a possible agent useful in healing mucosal lesions of ulcerative colitis of the distal area of the colon. Two double-blind studies were reported. The first involved 50 patients randomized to be treated with 10 mg sucralfate in 100 mL water, 2 g 5-aminosalicylic acid (5-ASA) in 100 ml water, or placebo (lactose), each by enema for a period of 4 weeks. Utilizing the results of clinical, sigmoidoscopic, and histologic indices, 5-ASA was shown to be statistically superior to both sucralfate and placebo, and sucralfate was not shown to have any advantage over placebo.[2]

In the second study 44 patients with ulcerative colitis were randomized to 4 g sucralfate enemas or 20 mg prednisolone enema. Clinical and sigmoidoscopic improvement was seen in the sucralfate group, but there was no placebo control against which to judge this result. The magnitude of the improvement seen in the sucralfate group was significantly less than that seen in the prednisolone group.[9]

METHOTREXATE

Methotrexate is a folate antagonist with proved anti-inflammatory properties that is used in many "autoimmune diseases." An open trial of this drug for treatment of eight patients with Crohn's disease and eight patients with ulcerative colitis was recently completed. Each of the patients was refractory to conventional therapy, including four in whom treatment with azathioprine was not successful. Nine of twelve (75%) showed significant improvement in clinical activity indices. Six of eight with Crohn's disease had endoscopic and histologic remission, but none in the group with ulcerative colitis experienced complete remission. Steroid sparing was seen in 9 of 12, and was complete in 4. Neither clinical improvement nor complications correlated with serum methotrexate levels.[5] This same investigational group recently reported an update on 26 patients with Crohn's disease and 12 with ulcerative colitis. During an initial induction phase with use of 25 mg intramuscular methotrexate weekly for 12 weeks, 80% of the group with Crohn's disease and 75% of those with ulcerative colitis showed significant clinical improvement and steroid sparing. During the maintenance phase after 12 weeks, 15 mg oral methotrexate was used with taper. Sixteen of 20 patients with Crohn's disease and 7 of 10 with ulcerative colitis were able to maintain remission at 47 and 50 weeks, respectively. Short-term side effects, including nausea, abdominal cramping, hair loss, hypersensitivity, and transaminitis, appear tolerable. Further studies must be performed to define the role of methotrexate in IBD, especially among patients with Crohn's disease.[4]

CHLOROQUINE

Chloroquine, an antimalarial agent, is a drug that accumulates in cellular lysosomes and has been shown to "slow antigen processing" in vitro. It was used by Mayer and Sachar[7] in an uncontrolled pilot study for treatment of 10 patients with ulcerative colitis and four with Crohn's disease, all refractory to conventional therapy. A daily dose of 300 mg for at least 3 weeks was used. Eight of ten (80%) of the patients with ulcerative colitis improved in 3 to 8 weeks, and six achieved complete remission. Based on this pilot study, a prospective double-blind controlled study is in progress at Mount Sinai Hospital.[7] The investigators favored a trial of hydroxychloroquine sulfate (Plaquenil), a related drug, as the therapeutic agent because of an improved side effects profile compared with chloroquine. An oral dose of 400 mg at bedtime is being used in patients with ulcerative colitis. The study is employing a 6-week blinded segment followed by a 6-month open trial. Two patient groups are being used, those steroid dependent and those maintained on sulfasalazine plus other drugs permitted intermittently. Preliminary data indicate an 80% response rate, and a mean time to response of 3 to 4 weeks. Further details are awaited.

ANTIMYCOBACTERIAL THERAPY

The recent isolation of atypical mycobacteria from some Crohn's disease granulomas has rekindled interest in antimycobacterial therapy. Two uncontrolled studies have recently been reported. Thayer et al.[13] reported an uncontrolled trial of six patients treated with 1 g streptomycin 5 days each week for 2 to 4 months, and 300 mg rifabutin daily continued for an indefinite period. In all six patients steroids could be withdrawn, and there was marked improvement in activity indices and healing of fistulas. In a second study, 16 patients with Crohn's disease with early postoperative recurrence in the neoterminal ileum (10 symptomatic) were treated with 5 mg/kg/day rifabutin and 15 mg/kg/day ethambutol for 6 months.[10] Among the five patients who completed the study, none showed endoscopic improvement. In addition, an unusually high prevalence of flulike illness was seen in these patients compared with patients similarly treated who did not have IBD.

NICOTINE

Many epidemiologic studies have documented the association between nonsmoking or discontinued smoking and ulcerative colitis. A recent double-blind placebo-controlled crossover study was presented in which five patients during the treatment arm of the study used up to ten squares (20 mg) of nicotine gum each day for 2 weeks and then crossed over to placebo.[6] This was repeated twice for each patient during the study period. Three of the five (60%) demonstrated improvement in symptom scores and sigmoidoscopic appearance during treatment periods. One patient withdrew because of side effects, and one showed no improvement.

FISH OIL

A major mediator of inflammation in ulcerative colitis has been determined to be leukotrienes of the B class liberated by neutrophils of the inflammatory infiltrate. The major fish oils have been found to compete as a substrate for lipoxygenase enzymes acting on arachidonic acid, decreasing the amount of leukotriene B_4 (LTB$_4$) produced by these neutrophils. A pilot study from Trinity College in Dublin utilized 3 to 4 g of eicosapentaenoic acid daily. A significant improvement in patient symptoms, histology, and neutrophil LTB$_4$ levels compared with control subjects was seen at the end of 12 weeks.[8] Encouraging results have been seen from two other groups in open trial on small numbers of patients for observation periods of up to 4 months.[11, 12]

In contrast, Hawthorn et al.[3] reported the final results of a 1-year double-blind controlled study in which 96 patients were randomized into 4.5 g eicosapentaenoic acid or placebo daily. Patients who were in remission and in relapse were studied.[3] Biochemical analysis revealed a greater than 50% LTB$_4$ suppression in patients treated with the fish oil. Despite this, clinical data did not show any advantage over placebo during the remission or relapse phases.*

LYMPHOCYTE APHERESIS

Lymphocyte apheresis is a technique of removing T lymphocytes by differential centrifugation. A pilot study from Memphis, Tennessee used this technique to remove 80 billion cells in divided treatments during a period of 3 to 4 months in each patient. To date 54 patients with chronically active Crohn's disease have been treated. A statistically valid remission has been achieved, lasting an average of 18 months in 48 out of these patients. Morbidity is minimal, but the technique is expensive and requires complex specialty equipment, at an average cost of greater than $10,000 per patient.[1]

*Editor's Note: A selective 5-lipoxygenase inhibitor (zileuton) being tested by Abbott Laboratories shows promise of efficacy in ulcerative colitis.[2]

REFERENCES

1. Bicks RO: The current status of T-lymphocyte apheresis (TLA) treatment of Crohn's disease (Editorial). *J Clin Gastroenterol* 1988; 11:136–138.
2. Campieri M, Gionchetti P, Belluzi A, et al: 5-Aminosalicylic acid, sucralfate, and placebo enemas in treatment of distal ulcerative colitis (ulcerative colitis). *Gastroenterology* 1988; 94(part 2):A58.
3. Hawthorne AB, Daneshmend TK, Hawkley MZ, et al: Fish oil in ulcerative colitis; final results of a controlled clinical trial. *Gastroenterology* 1990; 98(part 2):A174.
4. Kozarek RA, Patterson DJ, Botoman VA: Methotrexate—the long and short of it. *Gastroenterology* 1990; 98(part 2):A183.
5. Kozarek RA, Patterson DJ, Gelfand MD, et al: Methotrexate induces clinical and histologic remission in patients with refractory inflammatory bowel disease. *Ann Intern Med* 1989; 110:353–356.
6. Lashner BA, Silverstein MD, Kreines MD, et al: Nicotine gum for ulcerative colitis. A series of randomized trials for individual patients. *Gastroenterology* 1988; 94(part 2):A252.
7. Mayer L, Sachar DB: Efficacy of chloroquine in the treatment of inflammatory bowel disease. *Gastroenterology* 1988; 94(part 2):A293.
8. McCall TB, O'Leary D, Bloomfield CA, et al: Therapeutic potential of fish oil in the treatment of ulcerative colitis. *Aliment Pharmacol Therap* 1989; 3:415–424.
9. Riley SA, Gupta I, Mani V: A comparison of sucralfate and prednisolone enemas in the treatment of active distal ulcerative colitis. *Gastroenterology* 1988; 94(part 2):A377.
10. Rutgeerts P, Vantrappen G, Van Izveldt J, et al: Rifabutin therapy in patients with recurrent Crohn's disease after ileocolic resection. *Gastroenterology* 1988; 94(part 2):A391.
11. Salomon P, Kornbluth AA, Janowitz HD: Treatment of ulcerative colitis with fish oil in 3 omega fatty acid: An open trial. *J Clin Gastroenterol* 1990; 12:157–161.
12. Stenson WF, Cort D, Beeken W, et al: A trial of fish oil supplemented diet in ulcerative colitis. *Gastroenterology* 1990; 98(part 2):A475.
13. Thayer WR, Coutu JA, Chiodini RJ, et al: Use of rifabutin and streptomycin in the therapy of Crohn's disease. *Gastroenterology* 1988; 94(part 2):A458.

PART 7 _____

Management of Ulcerative Colitis and Crohn's Disease

Chapter 32 _____

Common Errors in Management of Ulcerative Colitis

David B. Sachar

When we think about ulcerative colitis we should remember that most people with ulcerative colitis in the United States do not have toxic fulminating colitis and are not seeking cyclosporine therapy or surgery. Most patients have distal disease, proctitis, or proctosigmoiditis, and most often the disease is mild. I believe the first mistake made commonly in management of ulcerative colitis is to overtreat mild, limited colitis with potent systemic therapy, high-dose sulfasalazine, or high-dose steroids, when it is perfectly reasonable to think about management with simple, symptomatic treatment.

Part of that same mistake is to forget that many of the symptoms in patients with proctocolitis or ulcerative colitis are symptoms from irritable bowel syndrome, or at least from the neuromotor complications of the colitis but not from the inflammatory, ulcerative, hemorrhagic components of the colitis.

So *Mistake No. 1* is overtreatment with anti-inflammatory therapy instead of relying on simple antidiarrheal symptomatic treatment.

Mistake No. 2 is to refrain from giving patients with ulcerative colitis adequate treatment for their diarrhea, because of fear that if one gives an anticholinergic or narcotic antidiarrheal, toxic megacolon will be precipitated. Certainly when a patient has toxic colitis and impending megacolon, one does not use antidiarrheal therapy, but those patients who are not at imminent risk for the development of megacolon should be adequately treated for their major symptom, diarrhea. As we have learned from Dr. Marvin Kaplan, the use of codeine as a very potent antidiarrheal agent is generally not fraught with the same kind of addictive potential that the narcotics have when used as analgesics (see Chapter 10).

On the other hand, *Mistake No. 3* in treating simple, mild, limited colitis is to overlook the fact that in disease of the distal area the primary bowel symptom is not always diarrhea. It is often constipation, with tiny pelletlike stools, difficulty with evacuation, or tenesmus. We often forget that the condition of such patients can be very much improved with use of bulk formers like Effersyllium or Metamucil or Fiberall. One has to warn the patient not to look at the label and say, "Bulk laxative! I don't need this." Tell the patient not to be frightened by the fact that these products are usually thought of as laxatives, and explain that you are prescribing them to give some bulk and formation to the stool. Also indicate that taking them with large amounts of water, as stated on the label, is not necessary. A daily spoonful of psyllium hydrophilic mucilloid in a small amount of water is often very helpful for the patient with mild colitis of the distal area of the colon.

Besides symptomatic therapy, treatment for colitis of the distal area often includes topical steroids and topical 5-aminosalicylic acid. The indications for these agents are limited to patients with left-sided disease or who have tenesmus or other rectal symptoms as their predominant complaint. *Mistake No. 4* is using topical medication for the wrong indications. When patients have extensive systemically active colitis, unless tenesmus is a very major component of the symptoms, topical medications are simply the wrong treatment.

Mistake No. 5 is to keep treating patients with enemas when they continue to have tenesmus and to overlook the fact that while one has treated the upper area of the rectum, the rectosigmoid, and a little bit of the descending colon, the lower area of the rectum and anus may have been missed. When doing endoscopies on these patients, one often finds that everything looks good except the distal 7 to 10 cm of anorectal area, which may be missed by the liquid enemas and may respond better to 5-aminosalicylic acid or hydrocortisone suppositories.*

We have learned much about sulfasalazine, which is certainly a mainstay of therapy for mild to moderate disease. But *Mistake No. 6* is using this agent for the wrong indication, such as in patients with severe disease who would be better off on a regimen of steroid therapy.

Conversely, *Mistake No. 7* is stopping sulfasalazine too soon once

---

*Editor's Note: In my experience it is still more common to find normal-appearing rectal mucosa on sigmoidoscopic examination after treatment with medication by enema while the disease more proximal remains active. We must allow for the area of concentration of the enema in evaluating response to therapy.

the acute attack has come under control. The relapse rate of ulcerative colitis during a 6-month period on placebo is in the 50% to 60% range, but on 3 g of maintenance sulfasalazine the 6-month relapse rate drops to 14%. On 4 g it drops to 9%, but at that point side effects often become troublesome.

Also with respect to side effects, *Mistake No. 8* is introducing this drug too fast, giving too much too soon, by writing a prescription and saying, "Take two tablets three to four times each day," and not explaining the importance of starting gradually, working up slowly, and taking the medication with food.

Mistake No. 9 is telling patients when they get pregnant that they have to stop taking the drug. Since sulfasalazine is safe in pregnancy and in nursing, and since it is especially important to maintain remission during pregnancy and the puerperium, the drug should not be stopped during pregnancy or breast feeding.

What happens when we get to more active disease, the kind requiring steroids? Mistake No. 1 was overtreating patients with mild disease or distal disease; *Mistake No. 10* is undertreating patients with more active disease when we decide to use steroids. If we start with a little bit of prednisone to take the edge off the symptoms, the patient may get a little better but not well enough, so we increase the dose some more; but the patient is still not doing very well in 7 to 10 days, so we add another 5 to 10 mg. We will never catch up this way. When we decide to use steroids we should start high, induce remission, and not start lowering the dose until that remission is well established.

If Mistake No. 10 is being too timid with steroids, *Mistake No. 11* is using them too long. This is one of the most common errors I encounter. Once a remission has been induced in ulcerative colitis, there is really no role for long-term high-dose steroid maintenance. If the patient still needs a lot of steroids to keep disease in remission, he or she will need either surgery or 6-mercaptopurine, or one of the other new alternative therapies we are currently studying. It is a major and common mistake to keep patients with ulcerative colitis and those with Crohn's disease on a regimen of steroid therapy for too long.

What happens when ulcerative colitis gets severe? At this point patients will need hospitalization and treatment with parenteral steroids. Should the treatment be with adrenocorticotropic hormone (ACTH) or hydrocortisone? At Mount Sinai Hospital Dr. Samuel Meyers and his colleagues answered this question definitively by a randomized prospective study of 66 patients who had been stratified according to whether they had previously received steroid therapy. In these very ill patients, the success rate of intravenous therapy was only about 40%

overall for both ACTH and hydrocortisone. It made a big difference, however, whether the patients had already been receiving steroids at the time of the hospitalization. For patients who had been receiving steroids previously, hydrocortisone was better than ACTH (53% remission vs. 25% remission). For patients who either had new-onset disease or had not been receiving steroids within the previous 30 days, there was a statistically significant difference between response to ACTH (63%) as opposed to hydrocortisone (only 27%).

We concluded from this study that patients with severe ulcerative colitis should be treated with intravenous hydrocortisone if they have been receiving prior corticosteroid therapy, and with intravenous ACTH if they have not.

We have to keep in mind that if a patient receiving intravenous ACTH suddenly develops severe pain in the side or flank, out of proportion to the severity of the colitis, it may not represent a complication of the colitis but is more likely to be adrenal hemorrhage. We have seen four cases in the past 2 years of unilateral spontaneous adrenal hemorrhage in patients receiving intravenous ACTH. It is a simple diagnosis to make, if characteristic symptoms are present. Diagnosis can be made immediately with a sonogram or a computed tomographic scan. After stopping ACTH and using prednisone, there is almost immediate clearing, but one has to be alert to the diagnosis. I do not think this complication is sufficiently common to obviate the conclusion that ACTH is the preferred treatment for severe colitis in nonsteroid patients, but it is something we have to consider.

One of the most prevalent of the common errors is *Mistake No. 12,* giving a nondehydrated patient hydrocortisone or ACTH in a constant infusion with saline solution. The patient blows up like a balloon and is very uncomfortable. At the same time there is occasionally a failure to add the supplementary potassium that is almost invariably needed by patients on high-dose intravenous corticoid therapy. In brief then, Mistake No. 12 is putting too much salt in the intravenous fluids and forgetting the potassium.

Mistake No. 13 is one of the biggest and most pernicious of all. That is what happens if one has a patient with severe ulcerative colitis who is not responding to intravenous steroids or ACTH after a week. While wondering if operation is necessary, one decides to prescribe total parenteral nutrition (TPN), thinking that "bowel rest" will do some good and "buy some time." This reasoning is false and will not work. The role of TPN in the treatment of severe ulcerative colitis has been studied repeatedly, and it never helps. It might even make matters worse. We have been learning recently about the harmful effects of depriving the mucosa of nutrients, such as occurs when these patients are placed on a regimen of nothing by mouth and long periods of TPN. Relying on TPN in this situation is like stepping into quicksand; the more one stalls the deeper one sinks. Having a patient on a regimen of TPN is not magic. With this type of therapy, one is "buying trouble," not "buying time."

This does not mean that if one has a terribly nutritionally depleted patient to prepare for surgery, nutritional repletion should not be used. Nutritional repletion is reasonable, but it is no substitute for decisive therapeutic action. TPN is not going to treat a patient who has ulcerative colitis or provide an extra margin in which prolonging steroid therapy will work. The patient will need surgery or cyclosporine or some other definitive therapy; TPN will not do the job or delay the need for decision.

Another serious error in the treatment of severe colitis, *Mistake No. 14*, is thinking that toxic colitis is synonymous with megacolon. Do not believe that unless you have a dilated colon, more than 6 cm or 9 cm or whatever your magic number is, you do not have to worry. In other words, toxic colitis is occurring when the patient is getting sicker. If the temperature and pulse are going up and the hemoglobin is dropping and the white blood count is going up and the albumin is dropping, the sedimentation rate is rising and the abdomen is getting more quiet and distended and tender, and if the patient is starting to accumulate a little gas over longer than normal segments of colon, it really does not matter how many centimeters in diameter the colon is—this is toxic colitis. Do not wait for toxic colitis to deteriorate to toxic dilatation before starting to treat aggressively.*

What is the management of toxic colitis? The Mount Sinai Hospital regimen often includes passage of a long tube; intravenous hydrocortisone or ACTH is given, as previously discussed. We also administer antibiotics because of the pathologic and clinical evidence that toxic colitis entails dissection of the inflammatory process all the way across the colon wall to the serosa, producing a reactive serositis and a localized paralytic ileus. Blood and crystalloid and electrolyte support are also given as needed.

This brings me to *Mistake No. 15*, which I have committed. It is treating a patient for toxic colitis and forgetting that there is an antidiarrheal order for diphenoxylate hydrochloride (Lomotil) or codeine or

*Editor's Note: Furthermore, a segment of colon outlined by air less than 6 inches in width in the setting of disease activity can herald deterioration without signs of either toxic megacolon or toxic colitis.

tincture of opium or dicyclomine hydrochloride (Bentyl) still on the order books. Watch out for this "forgotten order."

It is Dr. Present who has taught us about the importance of avoiding *Mistake No. 16.* Do not leave the patient lying supine in bed like a turtle on its back. In this position gas accumulates in the anterior portions of the transverse colon. Dr. Present has shown us that rolling or repositioning the patient will transfer the gas to posterior parts of the bowel and mobilize it out the rectum.

Mistake No. 17 is not following patients with toxic colitis closely enough clinically and radiologically. With all the steroids they receive, the classical signs of peritonitis and perforation are very easily missed, so that frequent physical examinations are required not just to look for tenderness but also to make sure that hepatic dullness is intact. X-ray examination needs to be done frequently not only to monitor colonic dilation but also to keep an eye under the diaphragms to make sure there is no perforation. Perforation can be clinically silent in patients receiving high-dose steroids, so follow them closely.

Mistake No. 18 is to fail to appreciate the grave prognostic significance of a hypercoagulable complication, such as venous thromboembolism in a patient with severe colitis. Deep vein thrombophlebitis or pulmonary embolism is a sign of impending perforation and disaster; the patient will need colectomy promptly.

Suppose we do everything right and do not make any of the 18 mistakes—where are we then? What happens to patients with toxic dilation if we do everything right? We can successfully decompress the colon at least half the time. Once those patients are home, they do not all inevitably have colectomy performed within the following year; about half of those who survive toxic dilation have surgery soon thereafter, but half do not! Therefore, *Mistake No. 19* is to jump the gun surgically at the first sign of toxic colitis or at the first moment of colonic dilation. It is a mistake to believe that toxic dilation in colitis automatically means immediate surgery. We are now learning that decompression can be done.

Mistake No. 20 is to drop our guard after decompressing the bowel, thinking the danger has passed. What happens to these patients after decompression? We checked the records of 75 patients with toxic dilation during a 15-year period at Mount Sinai Hospital to see how often death occurred. These days mortality from toxic colitis is low. The few patients who die have perforation. Who has perforation? We see two groups at highest risk. The first group comprises those patients who are sent in from other hospitals after being kept for 6 to 8 weeks on a regimen of steroids or TPN; they finally go into shock and are moribund.

They are sent to the referral hospital, arrive in the emergency room, are taken to the operating room, and die because their arrival was too late.

The second group at risk of dying are those who have had decompression of the colon. Dilation is no longer present, but the underlying colitis has not yet improved. They are still having a lot of toxic manifestations, with tachycardia, some fever and tenderness, some bleeding, some leukocytosis, and hypoalbuminemia. We may be giving them TPN and doing everything supportive, but they are still sick with active colitis. If we continue waiting because the colon is not dilated, thinking everything is okay, that can be a fatal mistake. *The colon does not have to be dilated to perforate!* In fact, by absolute numbers most perforations in ulcerative colitis occur in people whose colon is not dilated. Obviously, as a proportion of cases the dilated colon has a higher probability of perforation, but if one looks at the absolute numbers of all perforations occurring in the hospital during a 10 to 20 year period, most were from patients who did not have colonic dilation. If we are still neglecting decompressed patients with active colitis more than 30 days, that is the group where mortality can still occur.

We have completed a review of 20 common mistakes, some trivial and some important, but all are mistakes nonetheless. Suppose from these 20 we had to pick the one or two worst or most important. My first vote would be Mistake No. 14, thinking that colitis is not toxic or dangerous until it is megacolon. We must recognize toxic colitis early and not wait for dilation. My second vote for the most important mistake would be Mistake No. 20, which is waiting too long when a patient has decompression, the colon is not dilated, but the patient is still sick and not yet "out of the woods." These are the worst two mistakes because these can allow people to die. We have learned a lot during the last 10 years about how to save colons. It may be very important to save colons, but it is more important to save lives.

Discussion

Dr. Sohn: We have just had a very comprehensive review of virtually every important aspect of the clinical care of patients with IBD. We will open the floor to questions. I would like to ask Dr. Korelitz, is it your feeling that 30 days is the high water mark in the management of a severe ulcerative colitis?

Dr. Korelitz: I can imagine circumstances in which we would persist in medical therapy for that long, but it is not the usual picture. In the vast majority a decision has to be made long in advance of 30 days. There might be an occasional case with incomplete improvement and extenuating circumstances to explain it, in which case there is perhaps some justification for pursuing a medical program.

Dr. Sohn: Dr. Cohen, how would you feel about management of severe ulcerative colitis patients surgically?

Dr. Cohen: I agree with Dr. Korelitz. Most of these patients declare themselves when you have them in your own hospital. Most who get into trouble come from other hospitals and their doctors have been "sitting on them." They have been half treated and are on TPN; and these are the ones who get into trouble. We have not taken an active therapeutic intervention with cyclosporine, we have used it on occasion, but we have not used it often. We have operated on this type of patient fairly rapidly. It is amazing how well they get after the colon is removed and they have an ileostomy. We get them eating again fairly quickly, and the young patients improve so rapidly. They looked dreadful, were hanging around the hospital, and suddenly now they begin to improve dramatically. We feel a fairly aggressive approach to that kind of patient is necessary, and surgical intervention on a fairly aggressive basis is warranted. The results are very good.

Dr. Sohn: Dr. Korelitz, your experience does not really coincide with the Sinai experience on ACTH vs. hydrocortisone. Do you know why?

DR. KORELITZ: No, despite the fact that I accumulated experience with intravenous ACTH at Mount Sinai Hospital, so it is difficult to reconcile. You and I both remember patients transferred to Lenox Hill Hospital from other institutions after having failed high-dose intravenous hydrocortisone and surgery had been recommended. On admission I switched them to intravenous ACTH, and not only did they improve but the improvement was dramatic.

Q: To Drs. Sachar and Janowitz about ACTH vs. steroids—I found it puzzling that in the group of patients who failed outpatient oral steroid therapy, and were then brought into the hospital, 53% responded to intravenous hydrocortisone, and that this response was actually better than intravenous ACTH. You had another group of seriously ill patients who had never had prednisone or who had not had it in a month and were not prednisone failures and only 27% of those responded to intravenous hydrocortisone, whereas 60% or so responded to ACTH. And that gave you your statistically significant difference in the B group and therefore the recommendation for ACTH. A 27% response rate is a little low in most studies of even severe colitis, and I wonder why only 4 out of 15 in that group responded. Is that real or some peculiarity in your particular study?.

DR. SACHAR: There are two parts to the question—why is a patient not responding to prednisone on the outside going to do better in the hospital on intravenous hydrocortisone? Maybe they were not absorbing the medication so well and a lot of other things happen when you come into the hospital setting for more intensive therapy.

The harder part is why the so-called "virgin" patients did not respond well to hydrocortisone? One of the peculiarities of the study is that there was only a 40% response rate overall; usually it is a better rate. We limited it to really the very sickest patients.

DR. JANOWITZ: It took Dr. Meyers more than 6 years to get the 30 patients who were not on steroids at the time we saw them so I have a feeling. . .

DR. PEPPERCORN: I naively said in the editorial comment the controversy continues and your letter said how can the controversy continue—you will never do this study another time.

DR. JANOWITZ: Anyway, we were glad to see you were tentatively accepting our conclusion in your most recent analysis.

DR. SACHAR: Dr. Korelitz, about your recommendation for therapeutic abortion in a woman on 6-MP who becomes pregnant or a woman who is impregnated while her spouse is on 6-MP. I do not quite understand it on the basis of the evidence. From the thousands of pregnancies on record of women on Imuran and 6-MP for lupus or transplants or chronic nephritis, there is absolutely no higher incidence of fetal malformation, teratogenicity, or any fetal problems in pregnancy. I cannot help wondering if there is not some medicolegal thinking here. If there is a bad outcome you will be liable for it. If that is part of the anxiety, cannot one just present the data to the patient and say we have this much experience on these many people, we all worry about it, but there has never been any indication of a higher risk to the fetus to people on 6-MP than not. It is not a guarantee, you can have a bad baby, but the chances are no higher than in a group not on 6-MP?

Dr. Korelitz: The answer is probably no. Data and logic go together, but this does not have to do completely with data and logic—it has to do with fear and you have heard it expressed already even with Azulfidine, after many years of evidence that it is safe during pregnancy, there is still so much resistance, not only from patients but from many obstetricians. If that is true of Azulfidine, which has been around since 1940, you can imagine the fear with 6-MP. Maybe part is a malpractice concern, but more is the true concern that "my child" might be the one marred by medication. You really have to deal with that.

Voice: It is actually parents who have to deal with it. I had the same fear, a lot of anxiety and emotions. Fear and anxiety are good reasons for doing a lot of things, but I am not sure they are a good reason for recommending an abortion.

Dr. Korelitz: That is where the partnership concept comes in. You sit with the patient and husband, tell them what we know and do not know about it, they get a vote, and if they turn the ultimate decision back to you on that basis I would arrive at the same conclusion you would.

Q: Same pregnant patient—what about steroids, people who develop colitis and need steroids for the first time during pregnancy or who somehow are on steroids?

A: *I have no problem using steroids in the pregnant patient. I have seen many patients through pregnancy with colitis on steroids, and we have seen colitis develop in pregnancy and steroid treatment used.*

A: *There is no evidence in literature against it—what you can say about sulfasalazine you can say about corticosteroids. In some animal studies there was some increased cleft palate, but it really has not been evi-*

denced in humans. The maxim is to treat pregnant patients in almost identical manner to the nonpregnant short of instrumentation and obvious things like that.

Q: Do any of the experts disagree that there is more than emotion involved in patients' and physicians' fears of some of these agents, including sulfasalazine in pregnancy? If we think biologically if the drug can affect the germ cell as in Azulfidine or if a drug like 6-MP can cause tumors in some patients, why can't that drug biologically do the same thing in other instances?

A: *I do not think any of us approach any of these patients lightly. We fall back on accumulated data. You can argue with sulfasalazine that there has not been really good prospective data taking thousands of people on and off it, but the accumulated retrospective data which come out of 30 to 40 years of experience are overwhelming. I cannot speak about what happens to these people who go off these agents, particularly sulfasalazine. I cannot speak for 6-MP. I would demand that patients do not get pregnant if at all possible when on a regimen of that or metronidazole. The other side of the coin is, if they stop the drug and have a flare-up, as many will, you have a different set of problems. You have to rely on accumulated evidence.*

It is more than retrospective evidence—instead of fear we should have science, but some of that science is pseudoscience. In other words, pseudoscience says sulfonamide can displace bilirubin from albumin and therefore cause kernicterus. But science actually measures the levels and shows they are not quantitatively sufficient to produce the complications you fear. Similarly, pseudoscience says the sulfapyridine in sulfasalazine causes lowering of sperm count, alteration of sperm morphology, lowering of sperm motility, and decrease in sperm-penetrating ability. But science says none of those alterations quantitatively leads to abnormalities of fertilized ovum when fertilization occurs. So we think we are basing some of the fear on science, but maybe not.

DR. SOHN: Would you comment on the effect of a flare-up of IBD on the fetus?

DR. KORELITZ: Data show outcome of pregnancy is statistically not influenced by active ulcerative colitis during pregnancy. There will be an occasional patient where cesarean delivery has to be done, and thereby the fetus is put at risk, but it amounts to nothing statistically.

Q: Isn't it true, Dr. Korelitz, that in Crohn's disease there is a higher incidence of spontaneous abortion in patients who do have active disease, which is one of the reasons for discouraging patients from getting pregnant until the disease is at least under control?

DR. KORELITZ: This is an area where there is a distinct difference between ulcerative colitis and Crohn's disease. The major issue about Crohn's disease in pregnancy is Crohn's disease activity, and if present it should be treated vigorously. That will be a good investment in a favorable outcome of pregnancy.

VOICE: How long do you have to be giving intravenous ACTH before adrenal hemorrhage might be a complication?

DR. SACHAR: That occurs not just in IBD but with ACTH for any purpose. It usually takes a fair amount of time, and it is unusual to see it before 8 to 9 days of therapy; that is why we see so few cases since we give therapy for only 10 days before making a decision to go in another direction.

Q: Dr. Korelitz, is there a place for azathioprine?

DR. KORELITZ: I never quite understood not using 6-MP as opposed to azathioprine because all of the favorable data have been on 6-MP. Theoretically I agree it should not make very much difference except that 6-MP is a metabolic product of azathioprine and therefore a purer entity. Monitoring should be made more accurate with 6-MP.

VOICE: I assume you use prednisolone instead of prednisone, therefore.

VOICE: Can I mention something important for Dr. Korelitz as a practical point for clinicians. Can you comment on 6-MP and allopurinol and give us a warning about that? We have seen near disasters.

A: *You will encounter patients who were put on allopourinol obviously for gout, and if you put them on 6-MP or azathioprine you must use one-fourth to no more than one-half the dose. It is a very potent inhibitor of the breakdown of purines; we have seen some near tragedies in patients, not so much with IBD but with other disorders such as transplants, who are on an otherwise acceptable dose of 6-MP (75 mg) and are put on allopurinol who have the bottom drop out of the bone marrow.*

VOICE: Another point: about one 500 persons has congenital xanthine oxidase deficiency without being on allopurinol. So there is a theoretic 0.2% risk that patients who go on to Imuran or 6-MP might have an inherent defect in its metabolism that might be responsible for the very rare phenomenon of a patient in the first couple of weeks of 6-MP with sudden drop in white count. Rather than try to do red blood cell xanthine oxidase assays on all patients before starting, I wonder if it might be a good idea to do the first white count in a week.

Voice: Dr. Korelitz does that, and we do too, every week for the first month do the white count. That may be aggressive, but while we are on the point—I am very careful about sulfasalazine and neutropenia and agranulocytosis or hemolytic anemia. There was an elderly women who developed hemolytic anemia before our eyes after 2 weeks. I make it a policy to have CBC done in 7 to 10 days to cover the occasional patient who drops quickly. Then another at 2 weeks, a month, or 6 weeks, etc. Relax after 2 to 4 months as the late hematologic effects are pretty rare, and you cannot keep having the patient coming back. I insist they come back for a CBC in a couple of weeks. With 6-MP it is mandatory.

Dr. Korelitz: That reminds me of another point for those in whom you have initiated 6-MP and they are already on Azulfidine and the white count falls, not necessarily dramatically. Sometimes a particularly low white count in that combination is in fact due to the combination, and if eventually you eliminate the Azulfidine it can be corrected. It will not happen often but it has come up.

Question for Dr. Peppercorn: About enteric-coated Azulfidine—do you start with that? Do you use it only if the patient develops toxicity? Is it as effective?

Dr. Peppercorn: Good question. I was going to mention it but I skipped over the toxicity. There are anecdotal uncontrolled data from Europe that enteric-coated forms of sulfasalazine diminish the occurrence of dyspepsia. That is about all we can say. I do not routinely prescribe it as some have suggested, and it is no more efficacious. It is more expensive, but if I have a patient with heartburn and dyspepsia as side effects which are sometimes appreciated with sulfasalazine, I will go to the enteric preparation and I will tell you that anecdotally it is in style. The answer is yes, but I do not routinely use it in the first go around.

Q: Do all the panelists have the same feeling about stopping 6-MP in the male partner in terms of anticipating the possibility of pregnancy?

A: *I do. Largely for possibly irrational reasons, that has been my suggestion as well. I feel that is correct until we know more.*

Q: Any advice on particularly challenging patients such as the woman of childbearing years (late) with insulin-dependent diabetes, colonic Crohn's disease, and joint swelling arthritis? Or possibly the young male who has steroid-dependent ulcerative colitis with psoriasis and psoriatic arthritis?

A: Give the second patient methotrexate, leave the other patient to the rest of the panel.

VOICE: How effective is methotrexate in this situation?

A: *Maybe methotrexate should be elevated on the list of new drugs mentioned, with some of the others. In Dr. Kozarek's latest update, I think he calls it the short and the long of methotrexate, which will be coming out in abstract in the May 1990 issue of Gastroenterology, he has accumulated a reasonable number of patients, all uncontrolled; about three-fourths respond both short term and long term, both in Crohn's disease and ulcerative colitis, the same figures that we hear about 6-MP and 5-ASA. So that is an alternative in the steroid-dependent patient.*

You may not want to put particular patients on 6-MP because of the length of time it takes to take effect. The patient with colitis and psoriasis may do well with a short course of methotrexate, or the acutely sick patient with a short course of cyclosporine. The favorable effect of cyclosporine has been seen in cases of psoriasis as well. You might use it as an alternative treatment.

DR. COHEN: What about surgery for a patient with resistant ulcerative colitis who has not responded to steroids for a period of time. I think we should not forget about its role either. It may help the psoriasis, but in a patient with steroid-dependent ulcerative colitis, that in itself can be an indication for operative intervention.

DR. KORELITZ: However, Dr. Cohen, that might be the only drug the patient has ever been given. What does that mean—steroid dependent? He saw a doctor, was put on steroids which worked, the dose was reduced, symptoms start coming back, and that is the way it was done for years.

We obviously would have to know how he was treated previously. You have a different case scenario when you know the patient was properly managed with combinations of chronic-phase drugs such as sulfasalazine, 5-ASA, and 6-MP. Steroid sparing means different things to different people.

Q: A woman in her thirties, with some pressure in terms of childbearing, who is an insulin-dependent diabetic, fairly uncomplicated with no hospitalizations for coma or diabetic ketoacidosis, who has colonic Crohn's disease and arthritis. She has been on Azulfidine but never on

Flagyl, which she is not keen to take for a prolonged time anyway. Are there any other antibiotics or any other medications?

A: *I think you have to weigh pressure to get pregnant with need to get well from the Crohn's disease. It is not easy, and she should not get pregnant, especially when she is at high risk, until she gets the disease under control. So it is reasonable in this patient, who may not be a surgical candidate, to go through the litany of things. Be sure the sulfasalazine has been adequately tried; if she has distal disease, consider topical therapy. Then you are again left with the same considerations we have been discussing, but doing them after she is under control. Try to wean her off, and then let her get pregnant.*

Chapter 33 _____

Common Errors in Management of Crohn's Disease

Daniel H. Present

_____

I have been fortunate to have been exposed to many patients with inflammatory bowel disease (IBD) at Mount Sinai Hospital. My mentors,
Drs. Henry Janowitz, Richard Marshak, Mansho Khilnani, and Arthur
Aufses, have provided valuable medical, surgical, and radiologic experience with the many complications of IBD. I have also learned much
from colleagues such as Drs. Burton Korelitz and David Sachar, and I
have realized that much of what I read in books and articles regarding
management is incorrect and divergent from my experience with patients. What I will now present is some science and much clinical experience learned from these patients. I predict that some of these conclusions that are at variance with the literature will hold up under the
scrutiny of time. The following are what I believe to be the most common errors in the management of Crohn's disease.

ERROR NO. 1: FAILURE TO MAKE AN EARLY DIAGNOSIS

I have seen many patients whose disease has been misdiagnosed
who had intermittent fever attributed to viral infections. In fact, most
had aphthous ulcerations, which was the clue that the patient has
Crohn's disease, and I look for aphthous ulcers in patients with atypical
irritable bowel syndrome. The simple question, eliciting the history of
nocturnal bowel movements, often suggests Crohn's disease in the differential diagnosis. About 10% to 15% of patients with Crohn's disease
have subtle clubbing of the fingernails. Approximately 90% of patients

with Crohn's disease not diagnosed previously who are explored for appendicitis had bowel symptoms that were present for at least 6 months. The physician too often fails to elicit this history, which would prevent surgical exploration in a patient with suspected appendicitis.

ERROR NO. 2: INCORRECT USE OF SYMPTOMATIC MEDICATIONS

I not infrequently see patients being treated with immunosuppressive drugs, sulfasalazine, metronidazole, and steroids, whereas the major symptom is diarrhea, which has received no symptomatic therapy. If the only symptom is diarrhea, I advise use of antidiarrheal medications rather than the others noted, since there is no controlled evidence that one can alter the long-term natural history by placing the patient on sulfasalazine or steroids. One must also remember, however, that in acute toxicity all antidiarrheal and anticholinergic medications must be stopped to avoid megacolon. Endoscopy is not required for diagnosis of duodenal Crohn's disease, because in most cases it is evident with upper gastrointestinal x-ray examination. Even if one cannot distinguish between ulcer disease and Crohn's disease of the duodenal bulb, it is of little clinical significance to perform an endoscopy since both respond to H_2 blockers, although patients with Crohn's disease require a much higher dose.

Hospitalized patients with IBD who are receiving steroid therapy are often given antacids to prevent ulcers, and this results in diarrhea with the mistaken impression that the patient is not improving. Likewise, iron compounds are difficult to tolerate in patients with IBD, often causing significant symptoms, and patients should be observed closely for worsening after these agents have been added to the regimen.

ERROR NO. 3: INCORRECT USE OF DIAGNOSTIC MODALITIES

In ulcerative colitis colonoscopy is the diagnostic modality of choice; however, this is not true in Crohn's disease. Barium enema is much more accurate than colonoscopy, especially regarding fistulization. One can also obtain good detail of the more proximal area of the colon when strictures are present. The single-contrast barium enema is preferred to a double-contrast study, especially regarding the discomfort factor, and refluxing the terminal area of the ileum is easier with a single-contrast enema.

Modigliani et al.,[11] in a recent study, have shown that there is absolutely no correlation of clinical activity with endoscopic findings in Crohn's disease, and there is, therefore, no indication for periodic colonoscopy in clinical management. On the other hand, a flexible sigmoidoscopy provides diagnostic certainty that the rectum is spared and can subsequently be anastomosed if surgery is required. Colonoscopy is usually not needed for differential diagnosis, because this can be ascertained clinically. Biopsies are usually nonspecific, and granulomas are found in only 5% to 10% of patients with Crohn's disease of the colon.

ERROR NO. 4: FAILURE TO HEAR THE PATIENT'S COMPLAINTS

To preface this point, I have an interesting story of a patient with Crohn's disease and obstruction of the small bowel. The managing gastroenterologist advised surgery, and at consultation I agreed. However, the patient asked if there was any medication that she had not received that might be effective. She had not been treated with antibiotics; however, I advised her that at this stage in obstruction that antibiotics are usually ineffective. Nonetheless, she wanted to be treated, and I placed her on a regimen of ampicillin (500 mg four times a day) and wrote a consultation letter indicating that I agreed with the referring physician's opinion but had prescribed ampicillin on the patient's request. She called back a month later asking to have the prescription renewed, and on questioning of her status she reported feeling perfectly fine, with no gastrointestinal symptoms. I asked her to have her local physician renew the prescription, but she said, "He did not believe in antibiotics." I sheepishly wrote him another note stating that I was surprised that the patient had improved and that she will probably have obstruction again in the near future, but that we should persist with antibiotics. She called a month later for another prescription because the gastroenterologist still did not believe in antibiotics. The patient was transferred to another local physician and did well for 3 years until she finally had obstruction and underwent elective surgery. This case history indicates that one must "listen" to patients even if their responses disagree with current opinion and knowledge.

In a similar vein, we must distinguish between clinical symptoms and radiologic appearance of Crohn's disease. I saw an x-ray film of a small intestine with tremendous dilatation and an ileosigmoidal fistula that had been present for years. In the last 6 years since this x-ray examination was done, the patient still has the same symptoms, namely, diarrhea that is easily controlled with sulfasalazine and antibiotics. He has few obstructive symptoms, and we should learn from this that we do not treat x-ray films, but, rather, symptoms.

ERROR NO. 5: THE FALLACY OF STEROID EFFICACY

I am amused when I am asked what informed consent I obtain when starting immunosuppressive drugs. I retort by asking physicians what informed consent they obtain before initiating steroids, since the latter are more toxic than 6-mercaptopurine (6-MP). I would first like to review the uncontrolled data in the literature on steroids in Crohn's disease by illustrating three series that show short-term efficacy. Jones and Lennard-Jones[6] showed 22 of 30 patients whose condition improved. Sparberg and Kirsner[20] had improvement in greater than 50% and in Cook and Fielding's series,[3] two of three responded. Steroids do work on a short-term basis, but Crohn's disease is a disease of a lifetime. Long-term data from the same groups showed that of the 22 patients of Jones and Lennard-Jones[6] whose condition improved, 4 subsequently died, 8 had surgery, and 7 were unable to stop steroids. Sparberg and Kirsner[20] reported that although 50% showed improvement, the disease progressed while they were on a regimen of steroid therapy, and there was no prevention when steroids were used for treatment after resection. Cooke and Fielding[3] noted that not only did steroids not work long term, but that these patients had both an increased need for surgery and an increased serious complication rate. Therefore, the uncontrolled data fail to show that steroids are effective on a long-term basis. What of the controlled data as to steroid efficacy in Crohn's disease? The National Cooperative Crohn's Disease Study showed short-term efficacy for 17 weeks.[22] There was one surprising and likely incorrect conclusion that steroids were not effective in Crohn's colitis. The European Cooperative Study showed efficacy for 6 weeks in all sites in the bowel.[9]

What are the long-term data? There are four controlled trials in the literature regarding prevention. In Bergman and Krause's[1] 97 patients there was no difference in recurrence rates when the patients were treated with placebo or steroids. In Smith et al.'s[19] trial of 64 patients followed up for 3 years, there was no improvement in relapse rate, and there was no effect on recurrence or extension of disease in both arms of the trial. When we now return to the National Cooperative Crohn's

Disease Study, this showed no benefit of steroids compared with placebo in preventing flare-ups, and therefore no indication for long-term maintenance. The European Cooperative Study had one subgroup of patients suggesting efficacy for maintenance that was not statistically significant. Therefore, none of the four controlled trials showed any benefit of steroids in maintenance of Crohn's disease.

One trial in which intravenous steroids were administered also showed no long-term efficacy regarding the rate of relapse. It appears that one cannot alter the natural history of Crohn's disease with steroids. Even more disturbing are the data from the National Cooperative Crohn's Disease Study revealing that if one places a patient on a regimen of steroid therapy, only one-third can discontinue the drug and stay well. Therefore, when initiating steroid therapy 60% of one's patients may be committed to long-term usage. The only deaths reported in the literature occurred in the European study in patients who had a mass and abscess that were hidden by steroid administration.*

If one then restates the question, "Are steroids indicated in Crohn's disease?" my conclusion is, *hardly at all*. Certainly, there is no long-term indication for steroids in Crohn's disease.† When steroids are used, errors are often made in improper administration. As Dr. Sachar pointed out, in ulcerative colitis, do not initiate steroids at low levels and work up to higher doses, but, rather, start at higher levels and gradually taper. There is no convincing evidence in the literature regarding alternate-day vs. single-dose vs. divided-dose administration. In the experience I have gleaned from patients with active disease, it appears to me that a single dose does not work as well as when the dose is spread through the day. When the patient is improved one can then retreat to a single dose or alternate-day dose, but, once again, in my experience if one is administering alternate-day doses, the patient is probably well enough that steroids are not needed.

As to dosage, we do not have this information in studies of Crohn's disease so we have to look at the ulcerative colitis data. In one trial 40 mg and 60 mg were more effective than 20 mg daily; however, the 60 mg dose had more side effects. We conclude that the initial dose should be 40 to 60 mg daily. We have discussed the data with use of adrenocorti-

---

*Editor's Note: I question whether steroid therapy per se was responsible for the deaths.

†Editor's Note: I emphasize that steroids are not maintenance drugs. One area in which I disagree with Dr. Present, however, concerns steroids for the therapy of acute or severe Crohn's disease. Under these circumstances we will often use them to bring the patient into or toward remission to "buy time" for a chronic-phase drug like oral 5-aminosalicylic acid (5-ASA) or 6-MP to get established (see Chapter 27, "Use of Steroids and 6-Mercaptopurine in Inflammatory Bowel Disease."

cotropic hormone (ACTH) therapy in ulcerative colitis, and, although there is nothing in the literature to support the contention, my experience is that ACTH works equally as well for treatment of patients with Crohn's disease.

ERROR NO. 6: FAILURE TO USE ANTIBIOTICS IN THE MANAGEMENT OF CROHN'S DISEASE

What is the evidence for efficacy of antibiotics? There is the underground use by experienced clinicians. Dr. Theodore Bayless often uses tetracycline in children who have IBD. Dr. Joseph Kirsner likewise uses sulfamethoxazole with trimethoprim (Septra), and Dr. John Carbone uses ampicillin. Drs. Brandt and Bernstein use metronidazole, and I use all of these antibiotics, often rotating them and sometimes administering double antibiotic therapy. The double-blind controlled trials are limited and poor regarding antibiotics except for metronidazole. Metronidazole in Ursing et al.'s[23] study was shown equal to sulfasalazine, and after crossover the patients on a regimen of metronidazole fared better. A multicenter trial that has been reported only in abstract, comparing metronidazole at 10 mg/kg/day vs. 20 mg/kg/day vs. placebo, found metronidazole at both doses to be statistically superior to placebo in treatment of Crohn's disease.

The indications for metronidazole are mild to moderate bowel activity, and I prefer using this agent before initiating steroids. Metronidazole works best with colonic involvement and fistulous disease. If a patient has been receiving steroids for a long time, I often add metronidazole before attempting to taper the dosage. I try not to use this drug for long-term maintenance, and prefer to rotate to less potentially toxic antibiotics. In my personal practice 5% or less of patients with Crohn's disease of the small bowel are treated with steroids, but instead sulfasalazine or antibiotics (or both) are effective management. Regarding toxicity, this has been reviewed, but I would like to reemphasize that paresthesias are common and may not disappear for long periods of time after stopping metronidazole.[2]

ERROR NO. 7: FAILURE TO USE IMMUNOSUPPRESSIVE DRUGS IN CROHN'S DISEASE

I will not go into detail since this topic has been covered, except to emphasize a few points. The first is that the literature regarding efficacy in uncontrolled trials showed it to be 70%.[15] The literature on controlled trials is clear if the reports are carefully analyzed. Willoughby's controlled trial showed positive findings for maintenance of remission. Rhodes showed no efficacy in a 2-month trial that was not long enough to demonstrate efficacy. Watson's 6-month trial showed no maintenance of remission. In Klein's group azathioprine showed no statistical significance, but no patient who took azathioprine underwent surgery, whereas some of the patients receiving placebo did require surgery. Rosenberg's trial showed statistical significance and ability to reduce steroids. O'Donohue, in a maintenance trial, showed statistically significant prevention of flare-ups. As was noted, the National Cooperative Crohn's Disease Study showed efficacy, but this was not statistically significant.

We performed the longest controlled trial in Crohn's disease with patients receiving either placebo or 6-MP for 1 year, with subsequent crossover to the opposite arm for a second year.[16] Of 29 responders, 26 were receiving 6-MP compared with 3 taking placebo. 6-MP, in addition to having a 67% response rate, was steroid sparing as well as effective in closing fistulas. This is presented in representative x-ray films in two patients showing healing of gastrocolic and colovesical fistulas. Healing occurred in both patients within 6 months, and has been maintained for 7 years and 12 years, respectively.

Data from Dr. Korelitz and me indicate that if we maintain the patients on a regimen of therapy with 6-MP after response, 90% to 95% will maintain remission. We believe that 6-MP often alters the natural history of chronic Crohn's disease.

Our complication rate is very low. In 400 patients treated for a mean of almost 6 years mortality was less than 1%.[18] Morbidity occurs in less than 10%, much of which is quickly reversible when the drug therapy is stopped. With our current knowledge we believe that total colectomy is not indicated before a trial with 6-MP in Crohn's colitis.

ERROR NO. 8: FAILURE TO TREAT TOXIC MEGACOLON IN CROHN'S DISEASE MEDICALLY

Although the literature is vague in separating toxic megacolon in patients with ulcerative colitis from those with Crohn's colitis, in our series of 19 patients 13 had ulcerative colitis and 6 had Crohn's colitis.[17] The regimen includes the passage of a long tube, parenteral antibiotics, and steroids. It must be noted that if a patient lies supine in bed on a pillow, the most anterior portion of the bowel is the transverse colon, and air tends to accumulate at this site. As we have described in our rolling technique, if one places the bed flat, rolling the patient prone for 15 minutes every 2 hours, the air redistributes and is passed more easily out of the colon. The combination of the long tube and rolling prevents massive dilatation of the transverse colon. This decompression of the colon allows the physician time to treat the active inflammation with steroids and antibiotics. We decompressed 19 of 19 patients in our series, with some taking 7 to 8 days. What specifically happened to our patients with Crohn's disease? After decompression, our long-term follow-up indicates that each one has retained the colon. Two of the four required immunosuppressive drugs to quiet the colonic inflammation. I conclude that toxic megacolon in Crohn's disease should be treated medically and that colectomy should be deferred.

ERROR NO. 9: FAILURE TO SEPARATE PERIANAL DISEASE FROM BOWEL ACTIVITY

Many patients have perianal disease alone as a presenting symptom, without bowel symptoms. Physicians will use steroids to treat perianal disease, but I have never seen a study in the literature stating that steroids are effective for any type of perianal disease. If the presenting symptom is fistulization or fissure, the patient should be treated with broad-spectrum antibiotics. For the more complicated fistulas patients should be treated with metronidazole or 6-MP. Regarding the surgical approach, I have had great success with the Park's procedures for rapid relief of symptoms, with subsequent maintenance on a therapy regimen of 6-MP or metronidazole.

ERROR NO. 10: FAILURE TO USE NUTRITIONAL SUPPORT PROPERLY

Physicians often put excessive dietary restrictions on patients with Crohn's disease, and severe limitation of food items is really not appropriate. There is no correlation in the literature of activity with specific types of food. Although milk is often restricted, very few patients are truly lactose intolerant. When the bowel disease is quiescent, many patients can tolerate lactose, whereas during activity dairy products increase symptoms.

What is the role of oral nutritional therapy long term and what is the role of total parenteral nutrition (TPN)? Regarding bowel rest and

TPN, I think the number one error at every medical center for management of patients with IBD is treating patients with ulcerative colitis with TPN and non per os (NPO). Controlled trials show no efficacy with this modality.[10] On the other hand, TPN works well for Crohn's disease, and if one looks at a review of 254 patients with Crohn's disease, their remission rate is 65%. TPN is not to be used alone, however, and in the patient who has been chronically ill, it is best to initiate 6-MP as TPN is started, and by the time the patient might show relapse after having received a course of TPN alone, the 6-MP has begun to take effect.

There is no advantage in controlled trials of oral nutritional therapy compared with steroid administration in Crohn's disease.[12] I believe these data are true, but I do not believe there is any role for utilizing nutritional therapy alone in Crohn's disease. Adult patients will not maintain this modality for long periods of time, and when one stops oral nutritional therapy the relapse rate is high. From a practical point of view, patients will prefer medications.

Is bowel rest required when nutritional therapy is initiated? From a study by Greenberg et al.[5] comparing patients who were NPO with TPN vs. partial oral nutrition plus TPN vs. a defined formula diet, at the end of 1 year all groups showed equal response. One therefore does not have to prohibit food. My philosophy about this correlates with Levenstein's et al.'s[8] study, which randomized one group of patients to a restricted diet and in another allowed a liberalized normal Italian diet. After 1 year there was no difference in the two groups regarding outcome, symptoms, hospitalizations, surgery, or new complications. Lifting dietary restrictions does not appear to cause deterioration in Crohn's disease.

ERROR NO. 11: IMPROPER USE OF MEDICATION DURING PREGNANCY

This is a major error made by obstetricians who are afraid of medications such as sulfasalazine and steroids, despite evidence to show efficacy and lack of toxicity at all stages of pregnancy. In fact, there are no data to support the toxicity to either mother or fetus of 6-MP during pregnancy. If the patient has active disease, these medications should be maintained.

ERROR NO. 12: FAILURE TO RECOGNIZE CORRECT INDICATIONS FOR SURGERY

Although I am a strong advocate of varied combinations of medications in the treatment of Crohn's disease, this all changes with a short segment of disease, especially in a patient who is on a long-term regimen of steroid therapy. It is preferable to refer this type of patient to the surgeon. In 4 to 6 weeks they are restored to excellent health, with an improved quality of life. Short segments of disease with clinical and radiologic obstruction or patients with fistulization and an inflammatory mass are best treated surgically.[14] This philosophy would not apply in patients who have already had prior multiple resections.

Although surgery for some patients is rewarding, it should not be performed for the wrong reasons. Internal fistulas per se (such as an ileosigmoid fistula with minimal symptoms) are not an indication for surgery. Hydronephrosis per se also does not warrant surgery, since chronic renal infections and renal failure do not occur with long-term observations. As was noted in a previous section, total colectomy without an adequate trial of 6-MP is incorrect. Korelitz has reported a large series of patients with bladder fistulas, many of whom responded to medical therapy.[9a]

ERROR NO. 13: FAILURE TO EDUCATE PATIENTS PROPERLY

When one has many patients with IBD, it is impossible to answer all questions, and therefore the patient has to become more involved in management of his or her disease and put "in charge" of the illness. Physicians cannot be dogmatic about the illness and say do this and do that, but must give patients some control of the disease. I am perfectly willing to learn from my patients; if they want to stop or to change medications we discuss the pros and cons, and I allow the patient great leeway in the final decision. Patients need to learn to cope with a chronic illness. They can receive help from mutual support groups sponsored by the Crohn's and Colitis Foundation of America (formerly the National Foundation for Ileitis and Colitis).[21] This Foundation also raises money for research that is so badly needed.

I have presented 13 major errors, but there are several others that we should note, e.g., failure to use sulfasalazine properly. Peppercorn[13] notes that there is no controlled evidence that sulfasalazine works in Crohn's disease of the small bowel; however, we have all seen subsets of patients who do respond. Do 5-ASA drugs prevent flare-ups? There are

now two studies showing that 5-ASA agents may be preventive in terms
of maintenance for patients with Crohn's disease, and I predict that the
disease in a large subset of patients will be maintained with prophylactic 5-ASA agents, as is done in ulcerative colitis.

Failure to recognize cancer risk may be an error in that epidemiologic studies indicate a 4- to 20-fold increase of cancer in patients with
Crohn's disease.[4] The cancers we see are occurring in patients younger
than normally expected. Two of three cancers occur in involved areas,
and we are also familiar with cancers in bypassed small bowel segments. Dysplasia may also precede cancer in Crohn's disease, as Hamilton showed in a retrospective review. Korelitz et al.'s[7] data also showed
a number of patients with Crohn's disease and dysplasia in whom cancer developed later. I think surveillance may also prove to be an important modality in preventing cancer in patients with Crohn's disease.

A major error of academicians is the failure to design appropriate
trials. The errors made include great variation in patient selection, e.g.,
the inclusion of acutely ill patients with chronically ill patients in the
same trial. Another error is the failure to differentiate between patients
with and without internal fistulization in the same trial. If one is studying chronically ill patients, the investigator should have made certain
personally that all the modalities had failed to help the patient. This
will avoid a high placebo response. In the 6-MP study by Korelitz and
me, we had an 8% placebo response compared with a 30% placebo response in most series. Durations of studies are also important since
Crohn's disease is a chronic process, and one must be severely critical
of efficacy studies of short duration.

In summary, management of Crohn's disease can be greatly improved by careful attention to the medical literature and by the personal experience obtained by listening to and observing patients.

REFERENCES

1. Bergman L, Krause U: Postoperative therapy with corticosteroids and sala-
zosulphapyridine after radical resection for Crohn's disease. *Scand J Gastroenterol* 1976; 11:651.
2. Brandt LJ, Bernstein LH, Boley SJ, et al: Metronidazole therapy for perianal
Crohn's disease. *Gastroenterology* 1982; 83:383–387.
3. Cooke WT, Fielding JF: Corticosteroid or corticotrophin therapy in Crohn's
disease (regional enteritis). *Gut* 1970; 11:921–927.
4. Ekbom A, Helmick C, Zack M, et al: Increased risk of large bowel cancer in
Crohn's disease with colonic involvement. *Lancet* 1990; 336:357–359.
5. Greenberg GR, Fleming CR, Jeejeebhoy KN: Controlled trial of bowel rest

and nutritional support in the management of Crohn's disease. *Gut* 1988; 29:1309–1315.

6. Jones JH, Lennard-Jones JE: Corticosteroids and corticotrophin in the treatment of Crohn's disease. *Gut* 1966; 7:181–187.

7. Korelitz BI, Lauwers GY, Sommers SC: Rectal mucosal dysplasia in Crohn's disease. *Gut* 1990; 31:1382–1386.

8. Levenstein S, Prantera C, Luzi C: Low residue or normal diet in Crohn's disease. A prospective controlled study in Italian patients. *Gut* 1985; 26:989–993.

9. Malchow H, Ewe K, Brandes JW, et al: European Cooperative Crohn's Disease Study (ECCDS). Results of drug treatment. *Gastroenterology* 1984; 86:249–266.

9a. Margolin ML, Korelitz BI: Management of bladder fistulas in Crohn's disease. *J Clin Gastroenterol* 1989; 11:399–402.

10. McIntyre PB, Powell-Tuck J, Wood SR, et al. Controlled trial of bowel rest in the treatment of severe acute colitis. *Gut* 1986; 27:481–485.

11. Modigliani R, Mary JY, Simon JF, et al: Clinical, biological and endoscopic picture of attacks of Crohn's disease. *Gastroenterology* 1990; 98:811–818.

12. O'Morain C, Segak AW, Levi AJ: Elemental diet as primary treatment of acute Crohn's disease. A controlled trial. *Br Med J* 1984; 288:1859–1862.

13. Peppercorn MA: Advances in drug therapy for IBD. *Ann Intern Med* 1990; 112:50–60.

14. Present DH: Surgical management of IBD: Traditional and innovative. Crohn's disease part 2. *Pract Gastroenterol* 1988; 12:12–22.

15. Present DH: 6-Mercaptopurine and other immunosuppressive agents in the treatment of Crohn's disease and ulcerative colitis. *Gastroenterol Clin North Am* 1989; 18:57–71.

16. Present DH, Korelitz BI, Wisch N, et al: Treatment of Crohn's disease with 6-MP—a long term randomized double blind study. *N Engl J Med* 1980; 302:981–987.

17. Present DH, Wolfson D, Gelernt IM, et al: Medical decompression of toxic megacolon by "rolling." *J Clin Gastroenterol* 1988; 10:485–490.

18. Present DH, Meltzer SJ, Krumholz MP, et al.: 6-Mercaptopurine in the management of IBD. Short and long term toxicity. *Ann Intern Med* 1989; 111:641–649.

19. Smith RC, Rhodes J, Heatley RV, et al.: Low dose steroids and clinical relapse in Crohn's disease: A controlled trial. *Gut* 1978; 19:606–610.

20. Sparberg M, Kirsner JB: Long term corticosteroid therapy for regional enteritis. *Am J Digest Dis* 1966; 11:865–880.

21. Steiner P, Banks PA, Present DH: *People Not Patients—A Source Book for Living With IBD*. New York, National Foundation for Ileitis and Colitis, 1985.

22. Summers RW, Switz DM, Sessions JT, et al: National Cooperative Crohn's disease study: Results of drug treatment. *Gastroenterology* 1979; 77:847–869.

23. Ursing B, Alm T, Barany F, et al.: A comparative study of metronidazole and sulfasalazine for active Crohn's disease. *Gastroenterology* 1982; 83:550–562.

Final Discussion

Dr. Korelitz: Dr. Peppercorn, you saw Dr. Faber's data on Asacol. What has been your final conviction so far on the role of oral 5-ASA in Crohn's disease?

Dr. Peppercorn: We use oral Pentasa, which is the ethylcellulose microsphere slow-release form, and we were part of that study. Our experience is both with that study in a control trial, and a fair amount, not as many as you have here, in an open trial, and it is about as good as sulfasalazine overall in Crohn's disease. I do have some notable patients who did not respond to sulfasalazine with ileal Crohn's disease, nonobstructing, who did seem to get better when put on oral 5-ASA. I think the jury is still out as to whether it will be a great advance; obviously in the sulfa-allergic patient it will be. Dr. Faber and I were talking about this—it looks more like oral 5-ASA products have their own share of toxicity, including pericarditis, pancreatitis, maybe bone marrow reaction, and neurologic symptoms. I think the major advance is that you do not have sulfa moiety, and patients truly allergic will tolerate them. I do not see it as a tremendous advance over what was tried with sulfasalazine.

Dr. Korelitz: I think what you and we are picking up is that oral 5-ASA does work better in small bowel disease with narrowing and strictures than if the advantage was only elimination of the side actions. The favorable results might have something to do with the stricture. The drug stays longer just proximal to this stricture and in that sense has an opportunity for the coating to be dissolved, the drug to be released on that level, and to work longer and do something more than we had anticipated.

A Physician: The Pentasa study, which will be reported at the 1990 AGA meeting, at least in abstract, did not separate ileal disease vs. colon vs. ileocolitis, and that is a question that remains. That will be nice if it really is an advance, but it is too early.

334

Dr. Korelitz: Dr. Present, when we have a sick patient with Crohn's disease, how will we make the decision whether to use steroids or intravenous cyclosporine?

Dr. Present: Steroids are standard for an acutely ill patient at this time unless there is an inflammatory mass. If the patient has an inflammatory mass I treat acute Crohn's disease with triple antibiotics, neither steroids nor cyclosporine, until I can see that the process is under control with CT scan, making sure there is no abscess. If there is none, it has been my experience that triple antibiotics quiet the process, and then I can make a more rational decision later. Overall, I always try to avoid steroids and even to avoid cyclosporine until I am sure of the infectious component. Triple antibiotics with TPN is my treatment of choice. Then I decide later on.

Dr. Korelitz: Dr. Present did not answer the question, which gives me the opportunity to note that this is one of the very few areas where he and I disagree. If I have a sick patient with Crohn's disease I use intravenous steroids, despite the presence of a mass, even if I know the mass is an abscess. I cover any possible sepsis by using antibiotics at the same time, but the abscess, according to my reasoning, is based on the primary bowel disease, and treatment for this still must be emphasized. Our data show that this approach to therapy has been very effective and without risk. I still would like to pursue the question about treatment in Crohn's disease, let us say without an abdominal mass, as to how we will choose between intravenous cyclosporine and intravenous steroids.

Dr. Sachar: I have to go along with Dr. Present that there is more experience with steroids, and I think cyclosporine should be confined to centers where it is studied meticulously in terms of everyday clinical use. If the choice comes down to intravenous cyclosporine or steroids, I would use the steroids if there are no contraindications.

Dr. Korelitz: Do you agree, Dr. Peppercorn?

Dr. Peppercorn: Yes, I think we have to be careful. Dr. Present's data are very impressive. The problem is lack of controls, and maybe Dr. Present can address this—we certainly have had patients on the intravenous steroids who were 2 to 3 days away from colectomy. For some reason we or they held off, and a number of them in the second and third week do not require surgery. You may say those 15 without a question were 24 hours away from operation. The data are impressive, but I would be cautious about this. I am concerned about the long-term effects that are really not addressed. It looks very safe—but we need more data even short term.

DR. PRESENT: We are doing a double-blind control trial at three centers, UCLA, University of Chicago, and Mount Sinai (the ulcerative colitis part around January 1991). The Crohn's disease trial is to start 1 year later. In my experience it is very rare not to be able to quiet down acute Crohn's disease in the hospital with TPN, NPO, and antibiotics. It is very rare, and is the chronic issue one must talk about, since I rarely have a patient with Crohn's disease who needs surgery "acutely."

VOICE: I take that position also. We talked about Crohn's disease before—the patient who comes in with a complication (fever and mass are usually a complication of the disease), true, due to the underlying disease, but we all have our experience, and I have rarely seen a patient who has not quieted down on bowel rest and broad-spectrum antibiotics. Then you can institute the primary therapy. We have seen the study that shows mortality with a mass was there only when there was a mass and fever. We have seen a couple of disasters—people who seem to have their sepsis masked and felt well until they suddenly deteriorated. I am wary, and I do not see the advantage of steroids in the first few weeks.

DR. PRESENT: The sick patient coming in with an acute mass and tenderness and fever either does not need steroids or will straighten out with antibiotics and bowel rest, and the patient who comes in acutely sick with obstruction does not need anything at all—only time and intravenous fluids. I think that obstruction will open, and I never use steroids in that situation, although most people do. They give the patient a dose of steroids to take down swelling and open up obstruction. It opens in 3 days and it is great—but bring the patient in and do not give steroids and the obstruction opens up in 3 days as well.

DR. KORELITZ: Patients I know do not like to hang around in the hospital. Dr. Sohn, I remember in the old days we were taught that perirectal abscesses were never touched because if you did you cause a lot of trouble. Is there any justification now for not draining a perirectal abscess?

DR. SOHN: Dr. Present made the point in the most recent talk that the perianal disease does not follow the bowel disease. The patients with Crohn's disease tend to get perirectal abscesses for reasons that have never been defined, but once they are established they follow the rules of a perirectal abscess, in general, like those that occur in the absence of Crohn's disease. There is no one who would treat a perirectal abscess without instituting adequate drainage. Antibiotics are adjunctive; I guess cyclosporine is too.

Dr. Korelitz: Dr. Present, if we should get a patient with pancreatitis developing after 6-MP, do you think we should try Imuran?

Dr. Present: The experience has been that the incidence is the same whether you use Imuran or 6-MP, and the question has been asked whether to use Imuran or 6-MP. I do not know why anyone would want to use Imuran, as Dr. Korelitz has said; just because the company makes more money on it and the drug is still under patent is no reason to use it. There was no therapeutic advance in production of Imuran. It was just that the hematologists learned how to use the 6-MP better; they said Imuran was less toxic, but it was just a question of learning how to use the drug, since Imuran was broken down to 6-MP. If you do have hepatic abnormalities, it may break down to some inactive groups. There is only one control trial using both, and they were equally as effective, but there is no reason not to use both. If you have true pancreatitis or true allergy to one you are allergic to the other.

A Physician: How high do you push the dose?

Dr. Present: When we did the initial study not every patient in the trial had to be pushed to leukopenia. We found that was not essential in terms of most patients responding. But if I have a patient who has failed 4 to 6 months, I will try to push that patient to leukopenia empirically. I have seen a couple where it seemed to work, but I was not sure because in some people even in our control trial it took 8 months. But at about 6 months is when I give a trial for at least 1 to 2 months to leukopenic doses.

Dr. Korelitz: And what usually is that dose? What is the largest dose you have given?

Dr. Present: The largest I have used is 200 mg, but that is very rare. The highest usually that I use now is 125 mg of 6-MP.

Dr. Korelitz: Dr. Sachar, in the different approaches to the management of dysplasia in ulcerative colitis, Dr. Waye has often said that if you find low-grade dysplasia and there is some ulcerative colitis activity in the bowel, treat it and get rid of it and then do another surveillance colonoscopy with biopsies. What do you think about that? Do we have any justification?

Dr. Sachar: It depends entirely on the definition of dysplasia. If it is unequivocal dysplasia representing a neoplastic change in the tissue, there is no need to repeat anything or do anything. Dysplasia is dysplasia. If on the other hand, as is often the case, there is difficulty in distinguishing between "true dysplasia" and reactive atypia or regenerating epithelium under inflammatory attack, those cases are generally reported out as indefinite, probably "negative." In that situation by all means you should treat to reduce the inflammatory component and repeat. The issue is not to see whether dysplasia goes away. The issue is to see if it is or is not actually dysplasia.

Dr. KORELITZ: I must say I have never seen the course of steroids resolve the issue. All the considerations you say are true, but I do not recall a single case where treatment resolved it.

Dr. PRESENT: I make further distinction between high-grade and low-grade dysplasia. I am a firm believer that high-grade dysplasia indicates carcinoma now or within the next 1, 2, or 3 years. The question is still in doubt with low-grade dysplasia read by a good pathologist; e.g., the St. Mark's series where the patients with low-grade dysplasia (about 20% to 25%) went on to high-grade dysplasia and 75% to 80% never showed dysplasia again, never went on to high-grade dysplasia, and never went on to carcinoma. My own data in my office—we had nine low-grade dysplasias of which two went on to high grade, and we removed the colons—seven have not recurred and have not been found again. So I am still not convinced about low-grade dysplasia being an absolute indication for the disease. I really strongly warn the patients that they have to help make that decision with me, but I do not feel the sequence of low grade to high grade has been definitely followed.

Dr. KORELITZ: Let me ask you, Dr. Present, if you feel the same about the following three situations:

1. Low-grade dysplasia associated with a mass lesion
2. Low-grade dysplasia found in multiple sites in the colon on one examination
3. Low-grade dysplasia repeatedly demonstrated on subsequent examinations

Dr. PRESENT: In all of those I think a mass indicates carcinoma, probably there and then. I think multiple sites indicate fertile soil which will develop cancer. Repeat dysplasia to me says this patient really has something wrong.

Dr. KORELITZ: I think that is unanimous. Dr. Sohn, someone asked about a 41-year-old woman with Crohn's disease who had an ileostomy 5 years ago presumably for fistula disease. She developed pyoderma a couple of years after the surgery. Two years later she was steroid dependent with side effects, maintenance cyclosporine, 150 mg two times per day, analgesic dependent (Percocet) and four to five stools per day. Suggestions?

DR. SOHN: Does she have an ileostomy?

DR. KORELITZ: Questioner, was there extensive resection with the ileostomy?

Q: I believe the patient had a total colectomy. I have not seen the complete record, but from the information we had it looks like there was major resection.

DR. KORELITZ: In addition to the fact that she is steroid dependent and on cyclosporine, what is the evidence for primary bowel disease? What is the status now?

Q: The bowel disease appears stable. My concern now is long-term implications of what this patient is on. I should have indicated that she presented with a small dose of 20 mg prednisone, but there is evidence of bone effects and other effects.

DR. KORELITZ: Why can't we get the patient off steroids? If she is in remission why do we continue steroids?

Q: Mainly symptomatic.

DR. KORELITZ: I can summarize. This is one of the errors Dr. Present listed. An accurate diagnosis is necessary in order to treat properly. My conviction is that you must get the patient off steroids.

DR. SACHAR: I am not making a diagnosis here, but I would like to raise consciousness to an issue in a patient who comes with a story of having had a colectomy, no records, no reports, complaining of all kinds of symptoms, on steroids, cyclosporine with no documentation of any bowel disease present, it was a lesion which was diagnosed as pyoderma—beware of factitious disease and beware of Münchausen syndrome.

DR. KORELITZ: That is a very good point—one which we all see once in a while.

DR. SOHN: Dr. Present, there seemed to be another discrepancy between you and Dr. Korelitz. You mentioned in your talk that a resection permits proximal extension of Crohn's disease and Dr. Present recommended resection for limited Crohn's disease. Do you believe the hypothesis Dr. Korelitz presents that a resection permits proximal extension of the disease?

Dr. Present: I think that has been traditional in the disease. If you operate it comes back. It always comes back; the question is how much time you get to resume a normal life before it returns. Distal recurrence and progression are much more unusual, so it is the proximal recurrence we deal with all the time.

A Physician: Dr. Korelitz, while on this topic could you address the role of 6-MP prophylactically postoperatively in preventing the inevitable recurrences with anastomoses?

Dr. Korelitz: Dr. Present and I hope to do this study, namely, prophylactic 6-MP following resection. We agree that we would set up the study following two resections. We have not yet decided if we would do it even after one resection. 6-MP and azathioprine are the only drugs demonstrated to have prophylactic value in preventing recurrence of Crohn's disease. I am sure some patients would not accept it after one resection; others would demand it.

Dr. Present: I agree with Dr. Korelitz.

Dr. Sachar: When you talk about "after first or second resection" there are still different populations of patients to be considered. We talk about a patient who comes to first resection after 12 years of disease, a slow stenosis; that patient is not in the high-risk group for rapid symptomatic recurrence and would not be a good model of the population on which to do such a test. Either do your study on people who had two or three resections or on the person who comes in with rapidly progressive disease, short onset of fistulization complications, and has undergone surgery. We know from the studies in Belgium that by following endoscopically (not clinical but research), that might be a way to select the patient population on whom to do such a study—as soon as you see the early appearance of the confluent lesion or the large lesion or the large linear ulcer, that is the hallmark of a bad rapid postoperative course with a bad prognosis.

Dr. Korelitz: Dr. Present, how do you reconcile that with leaving the patient alone if they have no symptoms?

Dr. Present: As Dr. Sachar said, that is the perfect area to study. We plan at Mount Sinai a postoperative prevention—starting the patient on Pentasa immediately postoperatively and watching for colonoscopic findings, clinical and radiographic findings. That study remains to be done with a number of agents, and I would like to see both—with the new oral 5-ASA and with 6-MP—perhaps the new ASAs for the first resection and 6-MP for the second resection.

Dr. Korelitz: Let's do it!

Dr. Sohn: That is only if the 5-ASA does not work.

A Physician: What are the panelists' thoughts on management of a patient we have seen over the last 4 to 6 months, an 18-year-old female who seems to have a short segment of ileitis. She has bleeding as the only manifestation of the short segment of ileitis. She has had maroon blood per rectum three to four times over the last 4 to 6 months, once hemodynamically compromising, and has required 6 to 7 units of blood. She had a Meckel scan, upper endoscopy, and colonoscopy. We were not able to get into the ileum, but the small bowel series shows a clear segment of cobblestoning, which is fairly classical in the terminal ileum.

Dr. Sachar: I do not know if the panel will agree with me on this, but we have studied such cases at Mount Sinai Hospital, looking at all the patients with Crohn's disease in terms of principal manifestations of major hemorrhage that caused hemodynamic compromise, and retrospectively we came to the conclusion they should have resection because, medically managed, they end up with the worst long-term prognosis. You are describing short-segment ileitis with multiple repeated major bleeding. I do not see why not to do a resection, but I am not sure the panel will agree.

Dr. Sohn: I would also worry about the possibility of a lymphoma. Is that a consideration?

Voice: We have done a CT scan as well, looking for significant lymphadenopathy or signs of something other than Crohn's disease—we do not have a tissue diagnosis because we have not been able to reach the ileum endoscopically.

Dr. Korelitz: My own experience is that massive bleeding from ileitis is an early phenomenon, not late. Therefore, knowing this, if the patient could be treated vigorously with steroids, if they are seen through that period, I do not think resection will ever be necessary. They will then fall into the common pool with the other cases of ileitis.

Questioner: We tried her initially on Flagyl, but she bled through that. On prednisone, she became cushingoid and very unhappy. Then she bled through that. We added Azulfidine, and she had a very severe allergy to it. She is still reluctant to undergo limited ileal resection, which is what we recommended when she became cushingoid on steroids.

Dr. Korelitz: I think that, given the total history, I would go along.

A Physician: What about trying immunosuppressives?

Dr. Korelitz: No! After hearing the additional follow-up and duration of therapy—I would operate.

A Physician: With absolutely no other manifestations like diarrhea? No pain, sedimentation rate about 30?

A Physician: Diagnostically, you might send her to Dr. Waye's office. He is likely to get into the terminal ileum, and if he does not they can use a long scope through the small bowel and get a look at this, as you might be dealing with another entity such as tuberculosis, lymphoma, etc. It is atypical, although I have seen such patients. You might think about it before surgery.

A Physician: We had a couple of such patients, and they really do quite well if you resect that segment. For some reason those ulcers are sitting on a vessel, and if you get that segment out, even if the ulcers recur, they do not necessarily bleed again.

A Physician: Question for Dr. Peppercorn—I disagree with Dr. Present about steroids. I have worked with Dr. Franz Goldstein, who uses alternate-day long-term prednisone and seems to have successes. If they fail, then one treats with Imuran. What is your feeling?

Dr. Peppercorn: There is nothing like success to build confidence in your approach. I think the key in IBD is careful care of the patient. There are a lot of different ways to carve up the pie. Dr. Present has tremendous success as he is very diligent and treats this and that and gets away without using steroids, and therefore does not get into trouble with them. I am a little more liberal with the use of steroids, but I agree that there are the obvious potential effects.

Where I disagree somewhat is that I feel there is a role in a limited number of patients, and the European study touches on this, who do very well on 5 or 7.5 mg/day or alternate day (10 mg every other day). When you try to taper the dosage for too long, and this may be the issue you are bringing up, you can never wean the patients off. If you do get them off for too long, they have a flare-up. When you get them back on they do beautifully. After going through three or four courses of tapering and weaning, you settle on a so-called maintenance dose.

I do not believe these people are ever in complete remission, and therefore it does not quite go against the idea that steroids do not maintain remission. I feel the bottom line is that we all have patients like this—Dr. Bayless told me he has 200 patients on low-dose alternate-day steroids who are not all coming in with osteonecrosis, diabetes, and hypertension. I suppose the aseptic necrosis long term is the main thing to fear. We just don't see diabetes and hypertension. There are some cataracts on low doses. Some of these people are reluctant to go on immunosuppressives. The usual litany of things. I think this is a rule in a very small group of people with Crohn's disease who just seem to do OK on those low doses of steroids, I am not convinced that the low doses are any more toxic or dangerous long term because I have seen people go 20 to 25 years on these drugs until they die of heart disease or something else.

Dr. Korelitz: But the complications of the steroid, depending on which complication it is, can come all of a sudden. You do not always know when. It can be 22 years and one day.

Dr. Peppercorn: I accept that with every therapy. There may be patients who go 25 years on 6-MP and who start to develop lymphoma. We just don't know—we experiment as it is evolving. All one can say, as with sulfasalazine in pregnancy, if we look at the accumulated experience there are enough of us who have seen these patients (I have not been in practice for 25 years, but I follow patients who have been on low-dose steroids) and there is not a great incidence, but I think there is a role. It may be you should never have started them on it because you cannot wean them off. Once they are on they do OK.

A Physician: To Dr. Korelitz—about a woman in her mid thirties who had indeterminate colitis, with no small bowel involvement. The disease started about 8 years ago as rectal disease and then extended. The rectum is relatively spared ever since. I am not clear what she has. She was significantly allergic to Asacol, with significant fevers complicating its use. About 1½ years ago she had a very severe exacerbation during which time she was taken care of by Dr. Korelitz, who suggested 6-MP, which the patient refused. She had been surprisingly relatively well on Asacol, at a fairly high dose. She now seems to have intermittent low-grade fevers, which I suspect may be from the Asacol. My question—I agree she needs 6-MP and thus far I have not been able to convince her, but I will try harder—over what time course or how exactly would you reduce the drug that she seems to be having allergic problems to and how would you institute a drug that takes a long time to work?

Dr. Korelitz: If you really concluded she has an allergic reaction to Asacol, I would stop it now regardless of what I would do next.

A Physician: This lady almost lost her colon last time, and my point is I am afraid to leave her with nothing while I am waiting for 6-MP to work.

Dr. KORELITZ: Steroids could be used briefly should an exacerbation occur, and most likely this would work. It would "buy time" for 6-MP to get launched.

A PHYSICIAN: What is the pattern of the fever? Are you sure it is a drug reaction? Most drug fever does not occur one to two times per week.

Q: This lady does not live in New York City and does not come in as often as she should. She has fevers to 101° F, last a few days, and are unassociated with any other symptoms, no bowel symptoms, no respiratory symptoms. It is my suspicion it is allergy to the drug.

A PHYSICIAN: You may be correct, but it is an unusual manifestation of drug fever. Usually once it comes it stays, and it would be unusual to have intermittent fever. I would wonder if there is occult disease, a pocket or abscess, and I would go that route before thinking about switching. I have seen, just parenthetically, patients who are not doing quite so well on sulfasalazine who wanted to switch to something else and our protocol permitted them to do so. We stopped the drug and they deteriorated very quickly. I would be hesitant unless you will support them with something else like steroids, which I would be afraid of in the sense of the setting of intermittent fever which is unexplained. I would be careful about just stopping the first drug cold.

Dr. KORELITZ: If the fever is due to the underlying disease, presumably it favors Crohn's disease rather than ulcerative colitis. This reminds me of another question—occasionally I get a patient with ulcerative colitis who runs fever. What do you think of that? Dr. Present, do patients with ulcerative colitis, short of any complication, have fever?

Dr. PRESENT: They usually don't unless they are systemic, unless they are clinically very active—those are patients usually sick enough to be in the hospital, if they run fever in ulcerative colitis, unless there is another reason for the fever.

Dr. KORELITZ: Can the fever be related to the primary bowel activity?

Dr. PRESENT: It can when they are very sick. We admit such patients. Truelove's original criteria included fever in an acutely ill patient, but if they have fever with ulcerative colitis they are sick or fever is due to something else.

A PHYSICIAN: Is there a place for stricturoplasty?

Dr. SOHN: Sometimes we can do that; sometimes the short strictures are longer than you think and you cannot do stricturoplasty, but if it is a short stricture that lends itself to a stricturoplasty, we will do it.

A PHYSICIAN: For a single short one?

DR. SOHN: No, only for multiple strictures, unless we are concerned about a short bowel.

DR. KORELITZ: It is important to trust your surgeon in this respect after discussing the case with him beforehand.

A PHYSICIAN: I read the literature and I had trouble with ileoanals and a lot of trouble with the stricturoplasty story because they are reported from very good surgeons like at the Cleveland Clinic with 120 stricturoplasties. I have a huge practice and I do not see those patients who are amenable to stricturoplasty. Most of mine have a segmental resection — take it out and that is the end. Most of these patients on whom they do stricturoplasties do not have significant strictures.

DR. SOHN: That has been our finding also, and we rarely have patients who need stricturoplasty. Once, in a patient who had about seven strictures, we resected six in a short segment. There was one about 2 feet away that we did a stricturoplasty on. I agree they may be doing them in cases where we would not be operating.

DR. SACHAR: I know of a few dozen such cases at Mount Sinai Hospital where the indication has been diffuse jejunoileitis since childhood, the whole bowel with multiple links and chains of sausages, where invariably a combination of some resection for some active areas and multiple stricturoplasty have been indicated with some very good short-term results.

DR. SOHN: I would suggest that this requires a controlled trial because I have a great number of patients who had a single section removed without stricturoplasty who did well for 10 to 15 years. So I would consider leaving the rest of the disease behind.

DR. KORELITZ: Dr. Faber, do you treat asymptomatic Crohn's disease when you have positive x-ray findings?

DR. FABER: I would not treat for active disease if there is none, but rather my orientation would be to give a prophylactic medication to prevent recurrent activity. Which drug, whether sulfasalazine, 5-ASA, metronidazole, or 6-MP, would be influenced by the nature of the x-ray findings, the location, duration of disease, and response to medications in the past.

A PHYSICIAN: Dr. Mendelsohn suggested NSAIDs are contraindicated in IBD. For the patient with IBD and oligoarthropathy, does the panel share that viewpoint?

A: *Contraindicated is too strong. I do try to discourage them as Dr. Korelitz or Dr. Present do, but in the real world of taking care of these patients sometimes the ankylosing spondylitis or the inflamed knee takes precedence and you have to go with it. Just be aware that they may make the disease worse. There are many people on NSAIDs who have IBD whose disease does not get worse. You have to recognize there are some whose disease clearly will get worse.*

DR. KORELITZ: Another area in which we all agree.

A PHYSICIAN: What is a short segment?

DR. SOHN: If you have to remove less than a foot of bowel, I consider that a short segment.

A PHYSICIAN: What operation do you perform for toxic colitis?

DR. SOHN: I think the optimal operation is total abdominal colectomy with an ileostomy and a sigmoid mucous fistula. One other option is a Hartmann procedure where you oversew the end of the rectum. I think Dr. Cohen just published a paper comparing that with the mucous fistula. There are fewer complications with the mucous fistula. Having hemorrhage from the rectum, you might have to remove the rectum at that time. But by doing the total abdominal colectomy or what can be termed a subtotal colectomy, you are leaving the rectum in for the patient to decide what option he would want to have—abdominoperineal or sphincter-saving procedure.

A PHYSICIAN: Do we have any data on withdrawal of the oral 5-ASA agents in terms of relapse rate, severity of relapse, etc?

A: *I am not aware of any. There may be. It seems my own experience and that around the country have been relapse with the topical agents, so I cannot answer and don't know if it is a real phenomenon in the sense of being any more common than if you withdrew topical hydrocortisone or sulfasalazine. Our impression is that it may be. We are seeing patients with a kind of refractory who you bring under control, whose set of T lymphocytes are lurking; then when you release them, they go wild. I just don't know—it is a concern to me. The simple answer is that I don't have any data on the oral, but I wanted it to come up because it is something we should be aware of. On the other hand, how can you take someone with new-onset mild distal colitis, give them a course of 5-ASA enemas, put them into remission, and then commit them to long-term prophylactic therapy when they may not ever have another problem or may have a problem 5 years from now. I have trouble with that even though I am concerned about this kind of severe relapse.*

Dr. Present: I will take the other turn because if you look at the data on localized proctitis with proctosigmoiditis, the extension rate in that group is somewhere around 10% to 12%. Of those who extend, 80% lose the colon. So you are talking about a group of people who, when they initially present—if they are in the bad risk group that extends, are likely to lose the colon. I therefore take all new patients who present with proctitis and proctosigmoiditis in their first time out and treat them with sulfasalazine preventively for 2 years; I have not had a single patient extend in the last 5 years. That is empirical thinking going from one to the other. Trials remain to be done, but I can't justify patients taking rectal medication, because they will not do it anyway. I think oral medication should be used at the onset of proctitis; I am overtreating a number of people, and I recognize that—but I think it is worth it.

A Physician: What do to you do at 2 years?

Dr. Present: I stop it at 2 years because the data show 90% of those who extend do it in the first 2 years.

Dr. Korelitz: I agree completely with this with one exception—at 2 years I would only reduce it.

A Physician: Do you operate on a patient who had ileitis for years, has had obstruction, and whose x-ray shows stricturing?

Dr. Korelitz: You mean symptomatic or not? You can't go by duration. You have to go by symptoms, which also means to what extent is it fibrosis and to what extent is it active inflammation? I think that is the crux of the issue.

A Physician: Dr. Sachar, what is the prognosis in cancer arising in ulcerative colitis?

Dr. Sachar: 1. I think it is something of a myth that the cancer associated with ulcerative colitis is any more aggressive in behavior or prognosis than cancer arising in the general population. There are a lot of data on this showing that the long-term survival rate is exactly the same. 2. Prophylactic colectomy really is not a practical consideration, and there is no one in the United States recommending it. The answer to your question is, yes. The cancers associated with Crohn's disease are identical in all clinical and pathologic features with the cancers seen in ulcerative colitis. The same multiplicity, distribution, Dukes classifications, association with dysplasia, age incidence, hazard rate, and risk, given the same duration and extent of disease. The Crohn's disease risk is exactly the same as the ulcerative colitis risk. I think we are all starting to recognize that.

I think they will do worse not because of that but because they are very difficult to diagnose. Most present as obstruction, and you cannot tell if it is the Crohn's disease or superimposed carcinoma, especially since we see stricture in Crohn's colitis all the time—so it is hard to diagnose. You wait long and I guess the outlook is worse. Dr. Present, your comment about the bypassed loop—when you showed increased risk in the bypassed loop—I would like to suggest the modification because I do not believe there is any increased risk in the cancer in the bypassed loop given the same total duration of disease. It is a duration phenomenon. There is, of course, a much greater risk of the cancer being undetected once it develops in a bypassed loop. The actual biological risk I do not feel is any different.

Finally, before closing, Dr. Korelitz, I can't believe there is anyone who could fail to be impressed by the enormous concentration of talent and intelligence and experience represented by 15 faculty members from Lenox Hill Hospital, an extraordinary concentration of both clinical material in terms of patients and clinical talent in terms of the faculty. I think it is in large measure a tribute to Dr. Korelitz personally that by his experience and by his example as a clinician and scholar he has attracted around him as a magnet such an extraordinary concentration of talent.

Index

risk of, following ileoanal
anastomosis with proximal
pouch for ulcerative colitis,
178, 181, 182–183
surveillance for, biopsy in, 124
in ulcerative colitis, 204
prognosis in, 347
Candidiasis complicating
corticosteroids, 276–277
Carcinoembryonic antigen (CEA) as
tissue marker in cancer,
217–218, 234
Carcinoma (*see* Cancer)
Carcinoma-associated antigens
(CA-199 and CA-50) as tissue
markers in cancer, 218
Cataracts complicating
corticosteroids, 275
Causative agent, putative,
characteristics of, 16–17
Cell counts in differential diagnosis of
inflammatory bowel disease,
122–123
Chloroquine, 300–301
Cholangiocarcinoma in inflammatory
bowel disease, management
of, 223–224
Cholangitis, sclerosing
in inflammatory bowel disease,
management of, 223–224
primary
antineutrophil cytoplasmic
autoantibodies in, 9
in inflammatory bowel disease,
32–33
Coagulation abnormalities of
corticosteroids, 281–282
Cobalamin deficiency in inflammatory
bowel disease, 72–73
Cobblestoning in Crohn's disease,
radiologic or endoscopic
evaluation/follow-up of,
108–109
Codeine for diarrhea, dependence on,
98
Colectomy, prophylactic, in ulcerative
colitis, 219
Colitis
collagenous, 53–54 (*see also*
Collagenous colitis)

granulomatous (*see* Crohn's disease)
indeterminate, 120–121
microscopic, 54 (*see also*
Microscopic colitis)
NSAID-induced, 49, 63
self-limited, inflammatory bowel
disease differentiated from,
119–120
toxic, surgery for, 346
ulcerative (*see* Ulcerative colitis)
Collagenous colitis
antineutrophil cytoplasmic
autoantibodies in, 8
diagnosis of, 56–57
differential diagnosis of, 58–59
pathogenesis of, 55
prognosis of, 59–60
sprue and, 53–54
treatment of, 59
Collagenous sprue, collagenous colitis
and, 53–54
Colon
disease of
cause of, 49
nonsteroidal anti-inflammatory
drugs and, 48
role of prostaglandins in, 47–48
Colonoscopy, 100
barium enema following, 110
in evaluation and follow-up of
colonic inflammatory bowel
disease, 105–114
in initial evaluation and follow-up
of colonic inflammatory
bowel disease, 105–114,
126–130
in surveillance of ulcerative colitis,
199–200, 206–207
Computed tomography (CT), 102–103
Continent ileostomy for ulcerative
colitis, advantages/
disadvantages of, 159,
160–161
Contraception, inflammatory bowel
disease and, 36, 63–64
Copper deficiency in inflammatory
bowel disease, 72
Corticosteroids
for inflammatory bowel disease,
262–264

x-ray or endoscopic
evaluation/follow-up of,
106–107
Ultrasound, 101

V

Vasodilation complicating
corticosteroids, 279
Vitamin A deficiency in inflammatory
bowel disease, 75
Vitamin B_{12} deficiency in
inflammatory bowel disease,
72–73
Vitamin C deficiency in inflammatory
bowel disease, 73–74
Vitamin D deficiency in inflammatory
bowel disease, 74–75

Vitamin deficiencies in inflammatory
bowel disease, 72–76
Vitamin E deficiency in inflammatory
bowel disease, 75–76
Vitamin K deficiency in inflammatory
bowel disease, 75

X

X-ray for initial evaluation and
follow-up of colonic
inflammatory bowel disease,
105–114, 126–130

Z

Zinc deficiency in inflammatory
bowel disease, 71–72